The Management of Malignant Disease Series

General Editor: Professor M. J. Peckham

The Management of Testicular Tumours

Edited by Michael Peckham

Professor of Radiotherapy (University of London)
Institute of Cancer Research, London and Surrey
Civilian Consultant in Radiotherapy to the Royal Navy

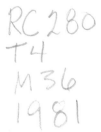

Edward Arnold

© Edward Arnold (Publishers) Ltd 1981

First published
by Edward Arnold (Publishers) Ltd
41 Bedford Square, London WC1B 3DQ

British Library Cataloguing in Publication Data
The Management of testicular tumours. – (The
   Management of malignant disease
   ISSN 0144-8692; 3)
   1. Testicle – Cancer
   I. Peckham, Michael
   616.99′4′63   RC280.T4

   ISBN 0-7131-4326-6

Filmset in 10/11pt Baskerville and printed in Great Britain by
Butler and Tanner Ltd, Frome and London

Contributors

Barrett, A. MB, BS, FRCR
Senior Lecturer and Honorary Consultant Radiotherapist, Institute of
Cancer Research and Royal Marsden Hospital, London and Surrey.

Cameron, K. M. BSc, MB, ChB, FRCPath
Senior Lecturer in Pathology, Institute of Urology, London.

Hendry, W. F. ChM, FRCS
Consultant Urologist, Royal Marsden Hospital, London.

Heyderman, Eadie MB, BS, BDS, LDSRCS, MRCPath
Senior Lecturer and Honorary Consultant, Department of Histopathology,
St Thomas' Hospital Medical School, London.

Husband, Janet E. MRCP, FRCR
Consultant Radiologist and Honorary Senior Lecturer, Royal Marsden
Hospital and Institute of Cancer Research, London and Surrey.

Juttner, C. A. MB, FRACP
Consultant Clinical Haematologist, Institute of Medical and Veterinary
Science and The Royal Adelaide Hospital, Adelaide, Australia.

Kohn, Joachim Med. Dip. (Lw'ow), FRCPath, DCP
Consultant Clinical Pathologist, Royal Marsden Hospital; Visiting Clinical
Scientist, Ludwig Institute for Cancer Research, Sutton, Surrey and
Research Fellow, Department of Clinical Chemistry, University of Surrey.

Macdonald, J. S. FRCP(E), FRCR
Consultant Radiologist and Honorary Senior Lecturer, Royal Marsden
Hospital and Institute of Cancer Research, London and Surrey.

McElwain, T. J. MB, FRCP
Head, Division of Medicine, Institute of Cancer Research and Royal
Marsden Hospital, London and Surrey.

Neville, A. Munro PhD, MD, ChB, MRCPath
Director of the Ludwig Institute for Cancer Research (London Branch),
Sutton, Surrey.

Peckham, M. J. MD, MRCP, FRCP(G), FRCR
Professor of Radiotherapy, Institute of Cancer Research and Royal Marsden
Hospital, London and Surrey.

Raghavan, Derek MB, BS, FRACP
Medical Oncologist, Royal Prince Alfred Hospital, Camperdown, Australia.

Selby, Peter J. MRCP, MD
Medical Registrar, University College Hospital, London.

Preface

Since malignant tumours of the testis predominantly afflict young men, it is particularly gratifying that one of the most important advances in oncology to have occurred during the past few years should have been in the management of these hitherto lethal tumours. Until relatively recently the outlook for men with metastatic non-seminomatous germ-cell tumours was bleak and to those who experienced the frustration and feelings of helplessness when confronted by uncontrollable, rapidly progressive malignancy, the fact that many of these patients are now curable is indeed a remarkable and exciting achievement.

The success of modern therapy is tempered by its intricacy and toxicity so that delivery of optimal treatment demands the skills of a team as well as attention to detail. Progress has been good but important problems remain. A minority of patients still die of tumour and treatment may be associated with considerable toxicity.

This book is based to a great extent upon experience at the Royal Marsden Hospital and, although primarily a description of investigation and treatment methods, makes reference to some of the biological aspects of relevance and interest in germ-cell malignancy.

Special thanks are due to Elizabeth Austin for her dedicated assistance in data documentation and to Marion Anderson for her invaluable help in preparing the manuscript for publication.

MJP

Contents

1

General introduction: biological diversity and predisposing factors

M. J. Peckham

Testicular tumours are uncommon but important since they predominantly afflict young men in their most productive years, often at a time of major family responsibility. During the past few years there have been major advances in clinical management, particularly the introduction of effective chemotherapy. This, together with developments in clinical staging procedures, the use of tumour markers and a better understanding of major factors influencing patient prognosis have led to striking improvements in treatment results.

Tumours of the testis are diverse with respect to histopathology, clinical evolution, age at presentation and therapeutic sensitivity. The majority of testicular tumours fall into the general category of germ-cell tumours which are divided into two broad subgroups—seminoma and malignant teratoma. To avoid terminological confusion (see Chapter 2) the latter are referred to sometimes as non-seminomatous germ-cell tumours of the testis. Seminoma and malignant teratoma may occur alone, or together in the same testis as a combined tumour. The histogenesis of seminoma and teratoma and the possible relationship between the histologically distinct components of combined tumours in terms of cellular origin, remain unsolved but fascinating problems.

Seminomas tend to present at an early stage and the cure rate with orchidectomy and radiotherapy exceeds 90 per cent (Chapter 10). Malignant teratomas can be divided into the two broad categories of early-stage and advanced-stage disease. Approximately 80 per cent of the first category can be cured by orchidectomy and radiotherapy or orchidectomy and retroperitoneal node dissection, whereas hitherto, the prognosis for patients with metastatic malignant teratoma has been poor. As described in Chapters 11 to 15, chemotherapy used alone or in conjunction with radiation and/or surgery has resulted in a major improvement in survival rates for patients with advanced disease, and the major challenge for the future is the development of treatments appropriate to each clinical situation, with particular stress on the minimization of toxicity and the preservation of normal tissue function, including potency and, where possible, fertility.

The purpose of this book is to describe current approaches to patient management, but it would be an omission not to review briefly several aspects of the biology of testicular tumours, since this provides a useful background to the better understanding of these unusual neoplasms.

The biological diversity of testicular tumours

Histology (see Chapter 2)

Figure 1.1 shows the distribution of testicular tumours by histopathological subtype, drawn from the large experience of the British Testicular Tumour Panel (Pugh and Cameron, 1976). The most common tumour type is seminoma and some 14 per cent of patients show histological evidence of both seminoma and teratoma components within the same tumour.

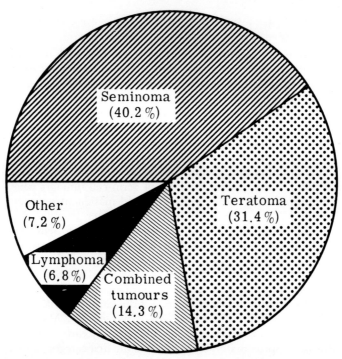

Fig. 1.1 Distribution of testicular tumours by histological subtype. (Data from Pugh and Cameron, 1976.)

Figure 1.2 (a–f) shows the differing age distributions of the major histopathological subtypes. The peak incidence of the whole group lies between the ages of 25 and 35 years (Fig. 1.2a). The initial part of the age distribution curve comprises the rare testicular tumours of childhood, including paratesticular embryonal sarcomas and the alphafetoprotein-producing yolk-sac tumour (Fig. 1.2f). Malignant lymphomas are predominantly tumours of old age (Fig. 1.2b). Seminoma (Fig. 1.2d) and teratoma (Fig. 1.2c) show peak incidences approximately one decade apart at 35 to 39 years and 25 to 29 years respectively. Combined tumours, where both seminoma and teratoma elements are identified, present within this general age range, but tend to show a peak incidence between seminoma and teratoma at 30 to 34 years (Fig. 1.2e).

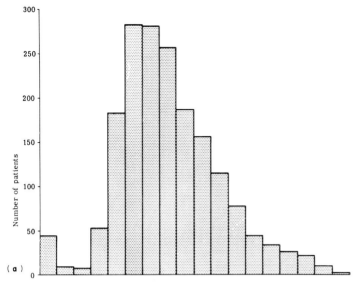

Fig. 1.2 Distribution of testicular tumour by age. **(a)** Whole group.

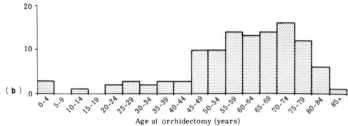

Fig. 1.2 Distribution of testicular tumour by age. **(b)** Malignant lymphoma.

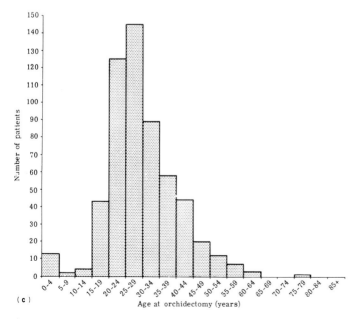

Fig. 1.2 Distribution of testicular tumour by age. **(c)** Malignant teratoma. (Data from Pugh and Cameron, 1976.)

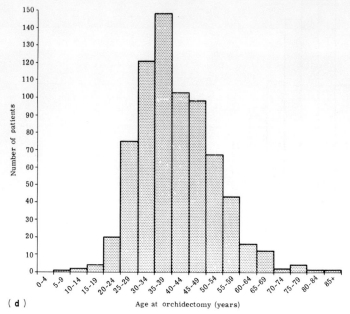

Fig. 1.2 Distribution of testicular tumour by age. **(d)** Seminoma.

(d)

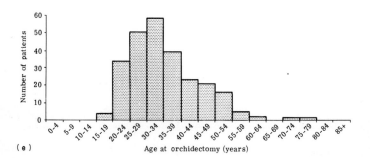

Fig 1.2 Distribution testicular tumour age. **(e)** Combi tumours.

(e)

The heterogeneous nature of testicular teratomas is emphasized by the range of histological appearances which may be seen in different metastases from the individual patient. However, data bearing on this important point are limited.

Information from two sources is summarized in Table 1.1. In the series from Ray *et al.* (1974), in 37 of 108 (34 per cent) of patients with embryonal carcinoma (malignant teratoma undifferentiated) primary tumours, the metastases in the abdominal nodes showed other associated histological elements. Of 32 patients with combined teratoma and seminoma primary tumours, 2 had pure seminoma metastases without an identifiable teratoma component.

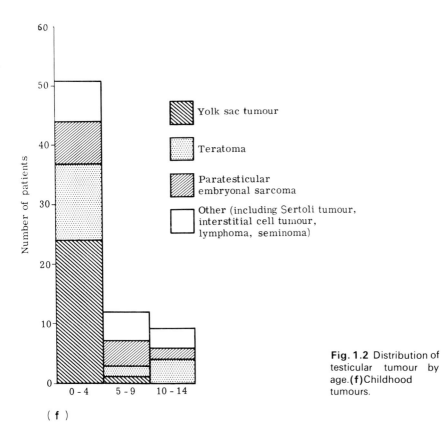

Fig. 1.2 Distribution of testicular tumour by age. **(f)** Childhood tumours.

Table 1.1 Histology of metastases in relation to histology of primary testicular tumour

References	Histology of primary tumour	Total patients	Histology of metastases				
			TD	MTI	MTU	MTT	Sem
Pugh and Cameron	MTI + Sem	15	1	2	9	1	2
(1976)	MTU + Sem	17			15	2	
	MTT + Sem	2				2	
Ray *et al.* (1974)	Sem	2					2
	EC	34			34 (5)*		
	TC	1			1 (1)		
	Chorio	1			1 (1)		
	YS	1			1		
	EC + Sem	32			30 (5)		2
	EC + TC ± Sem	32		1	30 (20)		
	EC + TC + Chorio ± Sem	13		2	11 (5)		

* Figures in parentheses indicate metastases containing elements other than MTU. EC, embryonal carcinoma (taken as synonymous with MTU); TC, teratocarcinoma (taken as synonymous with MTI); Chorio, choriocarcinoma; YS, yolk-sac tumour; TD, teratoma differentiated; MTI, malignant teratoma intermediate; MTU, malignant teratoma undifferentiated; MTT, malignant teratoma trophoblastic; Sem, seminoma.

Functional pathology

In approximately two-thirds of men with testicular tumours, elevated serum levels of alphafetoprotein (AFP) or human chorionic gonadotrophin (HCG), or both, are present and provide a useful means of monitoring the course of the disease and the effectiveness of treatment (see Chapter 4). The identification of these tumour products, using immunocytochemical techniques on tissue sections, has provided a further indication of the complexity and heterogeneity of malignant teratomas and seminomas. This aspect is discussed in Chapter 3. Recently, it has been possible to grow human testicular teratoma tissue as xenografts in immune-suppressed mice. Production of AFP and HCG has been demonstrated by the identification of both markers in mouse serum and in fluid from the cystic centre of the xenografted tumour. The combined use of immunocytochemistry and in-vitro tumour cell cloning methods should provide the means whereby the functional elements of the tumour can be dissected apart and studied separately (see Chapter 5).

Tumour growth rate

Testicular teratomas are rapidly growing tumours, whereas most, but not all, seminomas tend to follow a more indolent course. Tumour growth rates are calculated readily in teratomas by measuring the dimensions of pulmonary metastases on sequential chest radiographs. When this is done a volume doubling time can be calculated and this tends to be short— 10–30 days (Fig. 1.3).

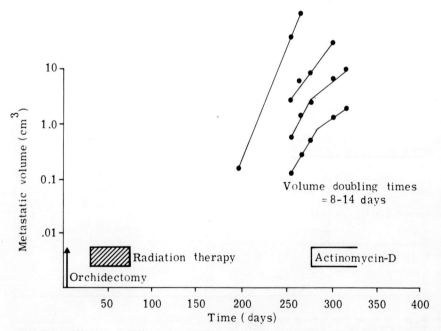

Fig. 1.3 Testicular teratoma: growth rate of pulmonary metastases detected seven months after orchidectomy and in association with failure to eradicate bulky para-aortic lymph node metastases.

Considerable variation is observed between individual patients. This is illustrated in Fig. 1.4, where the modal doubling time is approximately 20 to 25 days. However, there is a wide range of growth rates from rapidly growing tumours to indolent tumours doubling in two to three months. The rapid growth rate of malignant teratoma has important implications for clinical

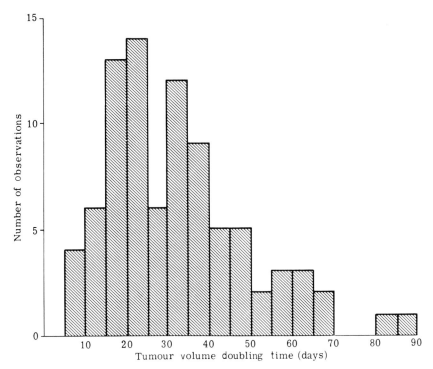

Fig. 1.4 Distribution of tumour volume doubling times in testicular teratomas. (Pooled data from Garreta *et al.* (1970) and the Royal Marsden Hospital series.)

management since, as described in Chapter 13, if relapse occurs after primary treatment, it tends to present within the first year. Similarly, uncontrolled tumour tends to lead to rapid demise of the patient. In addition to the growth rate variation seen between individual patients, sometimes different growth rates are observed between different metastases in the same patient (Fig. 1.5). Where differences in the growth rate of individual metastases are observed, this may be a reflection of differences in histology between the various deposits. Indeed, in some instances, spontaneous cessation of growth or even tumour regression may occur (*vide infra*).

Cellular origin and differentiation

Testicular teratomas are postulated to arise from gametocytes early in spermatogenesis, the pluripotency of the cell of origin being reflected in the diversity

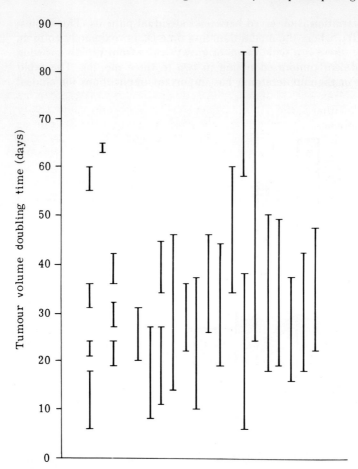

Fig. 1.5 Range of tumour volume doubling times in testicular teratoma. Each line represents the range of doubling times of different metastases within an individual patient. The figure illustrates the variation in growth rate between individual patients and between different metastases in some patients. (Data from Garreta *et al.*, 1970.)

of histological appearances of the established tumour. The rare primary teratomas and seminomas of extragonadal sites, pineal, mediastinal, retroperitoneal and sacrococcygeal (see Chapter 17), are envisaged to arise from primordial germ cells normally colonizing the gonadal ridges in embryonic life and which have failed to migrate from the primitive mesoderm (yolk sac) to the gonads during fetal development.

Teratomas and seminomas arise at an unidentified stage in the rapidly proliferating system where spermatids arising by meiotic division from spermatogonia replicate to produce spermatozoa.

Studies in a spontaneous mouse teratoma have shown that the tumour cells arise within the seminiferous tubules, at first lying within the intact basement membranes of the tubules (Stevens, 1964). Electron microscopy studies of human seminoma demonstrate cells of varying degrees of differentiation exhibiting the features of spermatocytes and spermatogonia as well as undifferentiated cells (Pierce, 1966), on this basis seminoma may be regarded as a tumour of seminiferous epithelium arising from stem cells already committed to differentiate into the spermatocytic series.

The cellular origin of male malignant teratomas is unknown. Linder *et al.* (1975), using chromosome banding techniques to study ovarian teratoma tissue, concluded that since teratomas were uniformly homozygous for 17 chromosome polymorphism they had arisen by parthenogenesis from single germ cells after the first meiotic division. Early in-situ teratomas arising from germinal epithelium and confined to the lumina of the tubules have been documented in man (Waxman, 1976). The combination of both seminoma and teratoma elements within the same tumour mass suggests a common origin and chromosome studies have failed to demonstrate populations of cells with different karyotypes in combined tumours (Martineau, 1969). Large abnormal aneuploid cells are present in a proportion of men presenting with infertility, testicular atrophy or maldescent. Approximately 50 per cent of patients with these in-situ changes show progression to invasive germ-cell tumours which may be seminomas or teratomas (Skakkebaek and Berthelsen, 1978), suggesting that these tumours may arise from a common malignant stem cell.

That human teratomas can differentiate is shown by the presence in some tumours of easily identifiable adult somatic tissues such as muscle, nervous tissue, cartilage and gastro-intestinal epithelium (see Chapter 2). The spontaneous mouse teratoma referred to above has been studied extensively to provide some understanding of the spontaneous maturation process. In this tumour, which arises in the seminiferous tubules in early gestation (Stevens, 1964), the development of differentiated teratoma can be traced from undifferentiated tumour. In some strains of mice, germ-cell tumours can be produced by grafting embryonic genital ridges into adult testes. The resultant tumour cells, when grown in an ascitic form, produce embryoid bodies resembling normal five- to six-day embryos (Pierce *et al.*, 1960).

Artzt *et al.* (1973) have reported that syngeneic antisera raised against primitive cells of a rat teratoma react specifically against male germ cells and also appear to possess cell-surface antigens in common with normal cleavage stage embryos. Diwan and Stevens (1976) have reported subsequently that the primary ectoderm and endoderm of six-day mouse embryos grafted into the testes of adult mice give rise to teratocarcinoma composed of undifferentiated embryonal cells and mature derivatives of the germ layers, including respiratory and alimentary epithelia. The multipotentiality of teratoma stem cells has been investigated extensively by Kleinsmith and Pierce (1964). In cloning experiments, transplantation of single tumour cells results in tumour formation in 11 per cent of mice, the tumours showing a wide range of somatic tissues. Differentiation in the mouse teratoma system has been shown to be influenced by environmental factors. Restitution by the tumour cells of haemopoiesis and immune function in irradiated recipients has been investigated by Auerbach (1971) and, in a series of elegant transplantation experiments in which the nuclei of teratoma cells were transferred to the ova of female recipients of a different strain, Mintz and Illmensee (1975) have shown that normal offspring can be produced, bearing some of the genetic characteristics of the mouse strain from which the teratoma was derived.

So far as the clinical significance of these experimental observations is concerned, it indicates that tumour cell evolution may be influenced both by cellular control mechanisms and extracellular factors. There are parallels between the murine model and testicular tumours in man. Although human teratomas are classified for convenience into the broad categories of malignant teratoma undifferentiated (MTU), intermediate (MTI and trophoblastic (MTT), a considerable diversity of cell types is evident within individual tumours and in MTI a wide range of adult mature tissues may be juxtaposed to undifferentiated malignant components. In some cases the tumour may be composed exclusively of fully mature tissues (teratoma differentiated), yet metastases may occur which themselves show histological evidence of differentiation. 'Maturation' in metastases generally occurs as a result of therapy and may, of course, reflect the elimination of the malignant component leaving a residue of mature tissue. The possibility of spontaneous or therapy-induced differentiation, however, needs to be considered. In patients undergoing intensive chemotherapy, the presence of well-differentiated teratoma in residual tumour tissue is not uncommon. However, differentiation after minimal therapy is also well documented (Smithers, 1969). An example is shown in Fig. 1.6 in a patient with an undifferentiated primary malignant teratoma receiving minimal chemotherapy for bilateral lung metastases more than eight years ago. One large metastasis, appearing after treatment, has disappeared

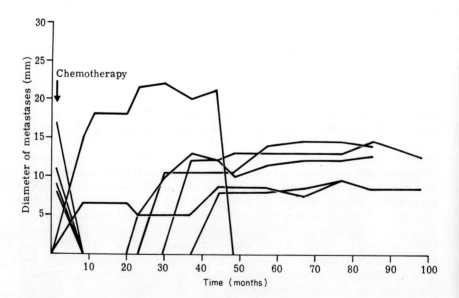

Fig. 1.6 Patient with Stage IV malignant teratoma undifferentiated (MTU) receiving one course of single-agent chemotherapy and showing simultaneous regression and progression of metastatic disease with subsequent long-term stabilization in the absence of further therapy.

spontaneously and several other lesions, after an initially rapid phase of growth, have remained unchanged for five years. The histology of the residual opacities might well show a completely differentiated structure composed of mature somatic tissues.

An unexplained and rare phenomenon of considerable interest is the apparent spontaneous regression of primary tumours in some patients. Azzopardi *et al* (1961) described a series of patients dying of widespread tumour dissemination in whom no primary tumour could be identified in the testes. In these patients the testes showed characteristic lesions composed of well-defined fibrous scars, often with ghosted remnants of seminiferous tubules. In some cases there were small foci of differentiated teratoma or microfoci of seminoma cells. The unusual appearance of these scars suggests the spontaneous resolution of the primary malignancy in the face of florid progression of metastatic disease elsewhere in the body.

Epidemiology and predisposing factors

Testicular cancer is rare in Africa and Asia and varies considerably from one European country to another (Table 1.2). The highest age-adjusted rates are encountered in Northern Europe and, interestingly, in Maoris in New Zealand. In Nordic countries there is considerable variation from 1.1 per 100 000 males in Finland to 4.9 in Denmark.

Within countries there may be marked variation in incidence between different ethnic groups. Thus, as shown in Table 1.3, the incidence rate in Negroes in the United States is approximately one-third of that of Whites. However, the incidence in Negro populations outside the United States may be considerably lower. In the African Negro, for example, it is approximately one-twentieth of the incidence observed in White populations. These observations suggest that both racial and environmental factors may be relevant in aetiology and that the observed difference between Negroes in Africa and the United States may result from exposure in the latter group to environmental agents. However, the situation may be more complex, since testicular tumours appear to be more common in the professional classes. Thus, racial differences may be explained, at least in part, by socio-economic and environmental factors.

In addition to variation between countries and between races, cancer registries in several countries have reported increasing incidence rates. Figure 1.7 summarizes data for Denmark collected by Clemmenson (1974) and shows a rise from 3.4 per 100 000 males in 1943–1947, to 5.4 in 1963–1967. Similar, and as yet unexplained, increases have been reported in this country and in the United States (Table 1.3). The increase in incidence of testicular tumours has been reported in both high and low incidence areas. Thus, age-adjusted rates rose from 3.2 to 6.7 in Copenhagen over twenty years. In Japan, a low incidence country, the rate rose from 0.15 to 0.38 during a similar period (Lee *et al.*, 1973).

The increase appears not to have changed the distribution of histological subtypes, although variability of diagnostic criteria makes intercomparison of dubious value. It is of interest that orchioblastoma (yolk-sac carcinoma) is reported to be relatively more common in Africans (Templeton, 1972). There

Table 1.2 Incidence rates for testicular cancer by country. (Data from Muir and Nectoux, 1979)

	Country/race	Rate (Average annual rate, age adjusted to world population and expressed per 100 000)
Europe	Denmark	4.9
	Norway	4.3, 4.6*
	Switzerland	4.4
	Fed. Rep. Germany	3.0, 4.7
	UK	2.4–3.0
	Sweden	2.5
	Iceland	2.1
	Hungary	1.0, 1.8
	Poland	0.6–2.3
	Yugoslavia	1.9
	Finland	1.1
United States	White	2.8–4.5
	Black	0.5–1.0
Africa	African	0.0, 0.1
	Israel Jews	1.6
	non-Jews	0.2
Asia	India	0.7
	Japan	0.7–1.2
	Singapore	0.3–0.9
Oceania	Hawaii	
	Chinese/ Hawaian/ Caucasian	2.3–3.0
	Filipino/ Japanese	0.3
	New Zealand	
	Maori	4.3
	non-Maori	3.7

* More than one rate indicates several studies from the same country.

Table 1.3 Testis tumour incidence per 100 000 males in two surveys carried out in the United States (Devesa and Silverman, 1978)

	White males	Non-white males
Second National Cancer Survey 1947–1948	2.6	1.5
Third National Cancer Survey 1969–1971	3.6	0.8

is evidence of an urban excess in some countries but not in others. Clemmenson (1974) found a twofold preponderance in Copenhagen compared with rural Denmark.

The factors underlying increasing incidence and geographical and racial differences in tumour incidence have not been identified. Sexual activity, trauma, mumps orchitis and temperature variation (particularly elevated

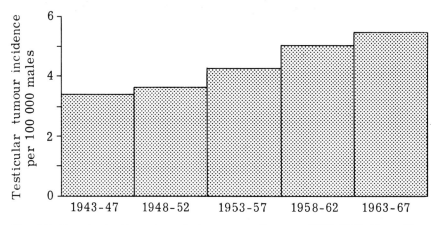

Fig. 1.7 Changing incidence in testicular tumours, Denmark, 1943–1967. (From Clemmenson, 1974.)

testicular temperature related to tight-clothing fashions) have all been postulated as possible aetiological factors, but supportive evidence is lacking and they remain purely speculative.

Testicular maldescent (see below) is a known risk factor and Morrison (1976) has reported in a case-control study that testicular tumours are 2.9 times as common in men with a history of inguinal hernia. In England and Wales, cancer registration data show an excess of cancer of the testis among chemists (Muir and Nectoux, 1979).

Testicular maldescent and tumorigenesis

Testicular maldescent is well recognized as being associated with an increased risk of tumour formation. In the eighth month of intra-uterine life the testis migrates through the inguinal canal into the scrotum, during normal development. Descent may be arrested at any point along the normal course of migration and generally three main forms of maldescent are recognized—the intra-abdominal testis, the inguinal testis and the high scrotal testis.

Estimates of the incidence of true cryptorchidism (as opposed to the retractile testis) have varied widely, but the figure is probably less than 1 per cent of the total male population. In the majority of cases, maldescent is unilateral and there is some evidence to suggest that the normally developed testis develops compensatory hypertrophy before puberty (Laron and Zilka, 1969).

Histological abnormalities can be identified in the testes of patients with maldescent. In the first six months of life there are no apparent differences between maldescended and normal testes. Between 3 and 8 years of age the maldescended testis shows smaller tubules, and spermatogonia are sparse with no evidence of mitoses. In older boys spermatogenesis is absent.

A total of 75 boys with undescended testes were studied by Sudmann (1971). True cryptorchidism was present in 64 patients, was more common on the right and was bilateral in one-quarter of cases. The most common location of the testis was near the superficial inguinal ring. In 20 boys, aged 6 to 14 years, pre-operative biopsies were performed; 4 showed no spermatogonia and 16 showed considerable diminution of germinal epithelium. In all cases the tubule diameter was considered subnormal. Chorionic gonadotrophin brought 31 per cent of palpable testes into the scrotal sac. Abnormalities of the germinal epithelium have been reported also in previous studies (Salle *et al.*, 1968). It is of interest that abnormalities have been noted in the normally descended testis in patients with unilateral cryptorchidism (Canlorbe *et al.*, 1966).

Bramble *et al.* (1974) have reported on 23 men treated surgically for bilateral maldescent. Orchidopexy was carried out between the ages of 7 and 14 years. The overall fertility rate was 47.6 per cent, as judged by sperm count, and apparently fertility was not influenced by the age of orchidopexy. The major effect of maldescent is on spermatogenesis and tubular damage results in an increase in serum follicle-stimulating hormone (FSH) levels. Woodhead *et al.* (1973) studied 47 men, aged between 18 and 21 years, with unilateral maldescent. Of this group, 36 per cent were found to be oligospermic.

In-situ tumours in cryptorchid testes have been identified by fine-needle biopsy. Waxman (1976) described a 19-year-old male with maldescent and an apparently normal testis which was placed in the scrotal sac. Needle biopsy at the time of orchidopexy showed atrophic seminiferous tubules and absent spermatogenesis. Abnormal germ cells were observed, the majority of which showed obvious evidence of malignancy. At orchidectomy, the testis was of normal size and consistency. Histologically, most of the tubules were atrophic and there was no spermatogenesis. Malignant germ cells were seen lining the tubules and within the lumen, but could not be identified outside the tubule walls. This observation is similar to a report from Skakkebaek (1972) describing apparently identical cells in biopsies from two infertile men. A recent report adds to this experience of apparent carcinoma in situ in patients being investigated for infertility (Skakkebaek and Berthelsen, 1978). In-situ changes were observed in 18 men, aged between 26 and 36 years, who were being investigated for infertility and in whom there was no suspicion of tumour. Subsequently, 9 of the 18 developed malignancies, the interval varying from one month to six years. In an electron microscopy study of these abnormal testes, Nielsen *et al.* (1974) have concluded that the cells identified as malignant germ cells originated probably from an early developmental stage (A-spermatogonis or gonocytes or prespermatogonia). The nuclear DNA contents were high, in the tetraploid range, and mitotic activity was pronounced.

It is well established that the risk of malignant change is higher in the patient with a history of maldescent than in normal males of the same age in the general population (Whittaker, 1970). In most series of testicular tumour patients, however, only a minority (5 per cent to 10 per cent) will have a history of maldescent. Gilbert and Hamilton (1940), in a survey of more than 7000 case records of testicular tumour patients, found a history of ectopy in 840 men (16 per cent). These authors, on the basis of a calculated incidence of maldescent in the total male population of 0.23 per cent, estimated the risk of malignant change in the patient with a history of maldescent to be increased by a factor of forty-eight times.

There is no clear evidence that the risk of tumour in the maldescent patient is reduced substantially by orchidopexy. Furthermore, it is of interest that 20 per cent of tumours developing in subjects with a history of maldescent appear in the normally descended testis. In the Testicular Tumour Panel series of 1812 patients, 123 men (6.8 per cent) had a history of maldescent. Of the 123 tumours, 22 (17.9 per cent) arose in an intra-abdominal testis. It has been suggested that the risk of tumour formation in an intra-abdominal testis may be as high as 1 in 20.

Several examples of intersex states associated with germ-cell tumours are reported in the literature. Szokol *et al.* (1977) reported a 24-year-old patient who considered herself to be female, but who had both male and female body features with absent vagina and hypospadiatic urethral orifice on the clitoris. A testis was found in a congenital hernial sac. Subsequently, an intra-abdominal testis and ovary were identified. The testis contained a combined germ-cell tumour predominantly seminoma. This true hermaphrodite was 46 XY karyotype. It is thought that the Y chromosome is necessary for tumour development in a dysgenetic gonad and, if this is present, the risk of tumour formation is about 25 per cent (Schellhas, 1974). Doll *et al.* (1978) have reported a seminoma in a 12-year-old boy with 46 XY/45 XO mosaicism. The tumour developed in an undescended testis in the groin.

Bilateral incidence of testicular tumours

One other factor is recognized which predisposes to testicular tumour formation, and that is a history of malignancy in the contralateral testis. Thus, the man who has one testicular tumour is at increased risk of developing a second. The risk is small and is shown in Table 1.4. It is well recognized also that the risk is highest for malignant lymphoma (see Chapter 18).

The incidence of bilateral tumours, as might be expected, is considerably higher in patients with a history of maldescent. As shown in Table 1.5, almost half the patients developing bilateral tumours have a history of maldescent.

Table 1.4 Incidence of bilateral testicular tumours

	Seminomas and teratomas	Malignant lymphomas
Testicular Tumour Panel Series (Pugh and Cameron, 1976)	29/1688 (1.71%)	28/124 (22.5%)
Royal Marsden Hospital (Sokal *et al.*, 1980)	21/760 (2.76%)	2/24 (8.3%)

Table 1.5 Bilaterial testicular tumours and history of maldescent

	Total patients with bilateral testicular tumours	Number with history of maldescent
Royal Marsden Hospital	15	7 (46%)
Testicular Tumour Panel Series	57	26 (45.6%)

Both tumours may appear synchronously or there may be an interval, which in our experience has varied from four months to fifteen years (Fig. 1.8). Furthermore, bilateral cryptorchidism strongly predisposes the patient to the development of bilateral testicular malignancy. Thus, Gilbert and Hamilton (1940) reported that 24.6 per cent of 69 men with bilateral maldescent developed two tumours, compared with an incidence of 0.7 per cent in patients

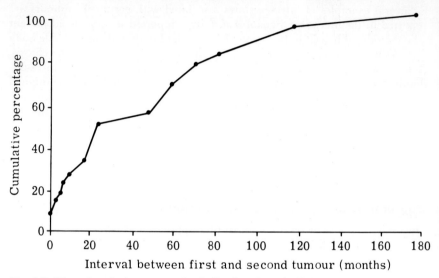

Fig. 1.8 Bilateral testicular tumours (excluding lymphoma). (Sokal *et al.*, 1980.)

developing one testicular tumour and in whom there was no history of maldescent. We have studied a total of 760 men who were referred with testicular tumours between 1952 and 1976 (Sokal *et al.*, 1980). Of this group, 21 patients (2.8 per cent) developed bilateral tumours. In 9 of these 21 patients (43 per cent) the second tumour was diagnosed within two years of the first. The range, however, was wide (4–180 months). Of 15 patients in whom a history of maldescent was sought, 7 (47 per cent) had a history of unilateral or bilateral maldescent.

The incidence observed in the Testicular Tumour Panel series was 25/1557 (1.6 per cent). These figures exclude malignant lymphoma where the incidence of bilateral involvement is known to be higher (8 per cent in our series; see Chapter 18).

It is of interest that chromosome studies of one patient with bilateral seminomas showed different modal chromosome numbers and marker chromosomes in each tumour, suggesting separate origins (Martineau, 1969).

Recently, Berthelsen *et al.* (1979) have studied biopsy specimens of the contralateral testis in 50 patients with testicular malignancy and reported that 3/21 patients with seminoma and 1/29 with non-seminomatous germ-cell tumours had carcinoma in situ without clinical signs. One patient developed clinical evidence of invasive malignancy forty-six months later.

Mumps orchitis and testicular tumour

It has been suggested that mumps orchitis may be an aetiological factor in the development of testicular malignancy. However, Ehrenget and Schwartan (1977), reporting data collected on 494 testicular tumour patients in Germany, found only 2 cases of unilateral mumps orchitis with subsequent tumour development. There was a history of epididymitis on the site of the tumour in 4.9 per cent of patients (median interval 8.6 years). It is of interest that 61 (12.3 per cent) of patients had simultaneous atrophy of the tumour-bearing testis. This report indicates that a history of mumps orchitis is uncommon in testicular tumour patients and unlikely to be an aetiological factor. As an extension to the study, 87 patients with mumps orchitis were followed up and none had developed tumours seven to seventeen years later.

References

Artzt, K., Dubois, P., Bennett, D., Coudamine, H., Babinet, C. and Jacob, F. (1973). *Proceedings of the National Academy of Sciences* **70**, 2988.

Auerbach, R. (1971). In *Cell Interactions and Receptor Antibodies in Immune Responses*, p. 393. Ed. by O. Mâkelâ, A. Cross and T. U. Kosunen. Academic Press, London and New York.

Azzopardi, J. G., Mostofi, F. K. and Theiss, E. A. (1961). *American Journal of Pathology* **38**, 207.

Berthelsen, J. G., Skakkebaek, N. E., Mogensen, P. and Sørensen, B. L. (1979). *British Medical Journal* **ii**, 363.

Bramble, F. J., Houghton, A. L., Eccles, S., O'Shea, A. and Jacobs, H. J. (1974). *Lancet* **ii**, 311.

Canlorbe, P., Gotlié, S., Guillon, G. and Lange, J.-C. (1966). *Annals of Pediatrics* **13**, 270.

Clemmenson, J. (1974). Statistical studies in the aetiology of malignant neoplasms. *Acta Pathologica et Microbiologica Scandinavica*, Suppl. 247. Munksgaard, Copenhagen.

Devesa, S. S. and Silverman, D. T. (1978). *Journal of the National Cancer Institute* **60**, 545.

Diwan, S. B. and Stevens, L. C. (1976). *Journal of the National Cancer Institute* **57**, 937.

Doll, D. C., Kandzari, S., Jenkins, J. J., Amato, S. and Jones, B. (1978). *Cancer* **42**, 1823.

Ehrenget, W. and Schwartan, M. (1977). *British Medical Journal* **ii**, 191.

Garreta, L., Debonniere, C., Bergiron, R., Cioppani, F., Josipouici, J. J. and Thomas, J. P. (1970). *Bulletin du Societé Medico-Chirurgical des Hôpitaux et Fomations Sanitaires des Armées* **2**, 93.

Gilbert, J. B. and Hamilton, J. B. (1940) *Surgery, Gynaecology and Obstetrics* **71**, 731.

Kleinsmith, L. J. and Pierce, G. B. (1964). *Cancer Research* **24**, 1544.

Laron, Z. and Zilka, E. (1969). *Journal of Clinical Endocrinology and Metabolism* **29**, 1409.

Lee, J. A., Hitosugi, M. and Petersen, G. R. (1973). *Journal of the National Cancer Institute* **51**, 1485.

Linder, D., McCaw, B. K. and Hecht, F. (1975). *New England Journal of Medicine* **292**, 63.

Martineau, M. (1969). *Journal of Pathology* **99**, 271.

Mintz, B. and Illmensee, K. (1975). *Proceedings of the National Academy of Sciences* **72**, 3585.

Morrison, A. S. (1976). *Journal of the National Cancer Institute* **56**, 731.

Muir, C. S. and Nectoux, J. (1979). *National Cancer Institute Monographs* **53**, 157.

Nielsen, H., Nielsen, M. and Skakkebaek, N. E. (1974). *Acta Pathologica et Microbiologica Scandinavica, A* **80**, 235.

Pierce, G. B. (1966). *Cancer* **19**, 1963.

Pierce, G. B., Dixon, F. J. and Verney, E. L. (1960). *Laboratory Investigation* **9**, 583.

Pugh, R. C. B. and Cameron, K. M. (1976). In *Pathology of the Testis*, p. 199. Ed. by R. C. B. Pugh. Blackwell, Oxford.

Ray, B., Hajdu, S. I. and Whitmore, W. F. (1974). *Cancer* **33**, 340.

Salle, B., Hedinger, C. and Nicole, R. (1968). *Acta Endocrinologica* **58**, 67.
Schellhas, H. F. (1974). *Obstetrics and Gynaecology* **44**, 298.
Skakkebaek, N. E. (1972). *Acta Pathologica et Microbiologica Scandinavica, A* **80**, 374.
Skakkebaek, N. E. and Berthelsen, J. G. (1978). *Lancet* **i**, 204.
Smithers, D. W. (1969). *Lancet* **ii**, 949.
Sokal, M., Peckham, M. J. and Hendry, W. F. (1980). *British Journal of Urology* **52**, 158.
Stevens, L. C. (1964). *Proceedings of the National Academy of Sciences (Washington)* **53**, 654.
Sudmann, E. (1971). *Acta Chirurgica Scandinavica* **137**, 815.
Szokol, M., Kondrai, G. and Papp, Z. (1977). *Obstetrics and Gynecology* **49**, 358.
Templeton, A. C. (1972). *African Journal of Medicine and Medical Sciences* **3**, 157.
Waxman, M. (1976). *Cancer* **38**, 1452.
Whittaker, R. H. (1970). *British Journal of Hospital Medicine* **25**, 37.
Woodhead, D. M., Pohl, D. R. and Johnson, D. E. (1973). *Journal of Urology* **109**, 66.

2

The pathology of testicular tumours

K. M. Cameron

Before discussing the pathology of the neoplastic testis, a short account of the structure of the gonad is appropriate.

The normal testis is an ovoid body which, in the adult, measures approximately 4.5 × 3.0 × 2.5 cm. Its surface is covered by the visceral layer of the tunica vaginalis, except posteriorly in the region of the epididymis. Beneath the serosa is a dense fibrous coat, the tunica albuginea, the posterior part of which is thickened to form the mediastinum from which vertical septa extend into the organ and subdivide it into 200 to 300 lobules, each containing one to four convoluted seminiferous tubules. These drain into a series of ducts—the tubuli recti—which emerge from the lobules and enter the mediastinum to form a network of epithelial lined channels—the rete testis. Efferent ducts pass from the rete into the head of the comma-shaped epididymis which lies along the lateral aspect of the posterior part of the gonad and overlaps its summit. Two vestigial remnants, the appendix testis and appendix epididymis, are present in relation to the head of the epididymis while from its lower end, or tail, the vas deferens arises and traverses the inguinal canal together with the vessels and nerves constituting the spermatic cord.

Within the seminiferous tubules are two populations of cells—sustentacular or Sertoli cells and germ cells which, by the process of spermatogenesis, give rise to spermatozoa. The stem cell, or spermatogonium, divides by mitosis to form more stem cells and also primary spermatocytes. By a process of meiotic or reduction division, secondary spermatocytes and spermatids, with half the normal complement of chromosomes, are formed. The process of differentiation of spermatid to spermatozoon is called spermiogenesis. The supporting Sertoli cells lie between the spermatic cells which are enmeshed in their cytoplasm.

Separating the seminiferous tubules is the interstitium of the testis, composed of loose, fibrous tissue containing blood vessels, a few macrophages and mast cells and, in the fetal and adult organ, clusters of Leydig (interstitial) cells. The latter constitute an endocrine organ producing androgenic hormones.

Neoplasms may arise from any of these structures and cell types. The germ cell has long been accepted as the progenitor of the seminoma. The origin of the teratoma, on the other hand, has been much disputed but, due to the experimental work of Stevens (1967) and of Pierce and his associates (Pierce and Beals, 1964), this tumour also is now generally acknowledged to arise from germ cells, occasionally with some reservations (Pugh and Cameron, 1976). Teilum's suggestion (1959) that the endodermal sinus tumour (adenocarcinoma of the infant testis) is also a germ-cell tumour, in which differentiation has occurred to extra-embryonic tissues resembling the yolk sac, has clarified the situation further and the present concept of germ cell neoplasia is expressed in Fig. 2.1.

Leydig and Sertoli cells occasionally give rise to tumours which may be associated with hormonal changes. Neoplasms of the appendages also occur.

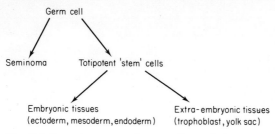

Fig. 2.1 Present concept of germ cell neoplasia.

Classification (Table 2.1)

The rational treatment of testicular, as of other, tumours depends on a sound classification, the basis of which has in the past been most commonly histogenetic. The identification of tumour markers and their increasing use in both

Table 2.1 Histological classification

Tumours of testis
Seminoma(s)
  classical
  spermatocytic
Teratoma
  teratoma differentiated (TD)
  malignant teratoma intermediate (MTI)
  malignant teratoma undifferentiated (MTU)
  malignant teratoma trophoblastic (MTT)
Combined tumour
  seminoma and teratoma in the same testis (CT)
Yolk-sac tumour (YST)
Interstitial (Leydig) cell tumour (ICT)
Sertoli cell/mesenchyme tumour (SMT)
Malignant lymphoma
Miscellaneous
  carcinoid
  carcinoma of the rete testis
Metastases

Paratesticular tumours
Adenomatoid tumour
Cystadenoma of epididymis
Tumours of connective tissue and muscle
  benign—fibroma, leiomyoma etc.
  malignant—embryonal sarcoma, fibrosarcoma
Mesothelioma
Metastases

diagnosis and management have raised the possibility of a more biological approach to the subject. Nevertheless, the situation is not yet clarified sufficiently to justify revision of the current classifications (Parkinson and Beilby, 1980) which are complemented, however, by the biochemical and histochemical findings.

The nomenclature used in this chapter will be that published by the British Testicular Tumour Panel (TTP) in 1976. The equivalent American terminology is shown in Table 2.2.

Table 2.2 Tumour nomenclature

British TTP (Pugh, 1976)	Friedman and Moore (1946)	Mostofi and Price (1973)	World Health Organization (1977)
Seminoma	Seminoma	Seminoma	Seminoma
Teratoma differentiated (TD)	Teratoma	Teratoma mature immature	Teratoma mature immature
Malignant teratoma intermediate (MTI)	Teratocarcinoma	Embryonal carcinoma with teratoma	Teratoma with malignant transformation, embryonal carcinoma and teratoma
Malignant teratoma undifferentiated (MTU)	Embryonal carcinoma	Embryonal carcinoma—adult polyembryoma	Embryonal carcinoma polyembryoma
Malignant teratoma trophoblastic (MTT)	Chorioepithelioma	Choriocarcinoma with or without embryonal carcinoma and/or teratoma	Choriocarcinoma with or without embryonal carcinoma and/or teratoma
Yolk-sac tumour	—	Infantile embryonal carcinoma	Yolk-sac tumour

Tumours of the testis

Seminoma

This is the most common testicular tumour, accounting for 39.5 per cent of the 2739 tumours collected by the TTP from 1958 to 1973, and believed to arise from the seminiferous epithelium of the mature or maturing testis, though rare cases are recorded in younger children. The peak incidence is in the fourth decade.

Two types of seminoma are recognized generally—the classical and the spermatocytic. A variant of the classical seminoma, anaplastic seminoma, has been proposed by Mostofi and Price (1973).

The classical variety is by far the more common and approximately 96 per cent of seminomas are of this type (Thackray and Crane, 1976). The testis is usually symmetrically enlarged with congested veins running over the external surface and converging on the mediastinum (Fig. 2.2)—a feature common to most tumour-bearing testes. The tumour itself is usually well demarcated (Fig. 2.3), uniform in appearance, though often lobulated, and whitish in colour with occasional yellow areas of necrosis. Microscopically, the lesion is composed of fairly uniform cells which are arranged in sheets (Fig. 2.4) or clusters and are round or polygonal with clear or finely granular cytoplasm—the clarity being associated with their content of glycogen and lipid. Multinucleated

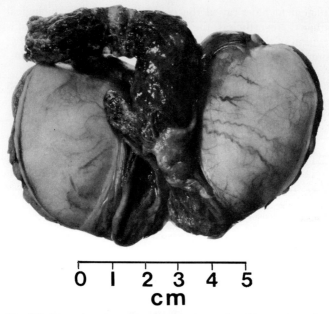

Fig. 2.2 External surface of tumour-bearing testis with tortuous veins on the outer surface.

tumour giant cells, some of which resemble syncytiotrophoblast, are sometimes present and were recorded in 6 per cent of the TTP series.

These giant cells may, in some cases, be shown by immunoperoxidase staining methods to contain human chorionic gonadotrophin (see Chapter 3). Friedman and Pearlman (1970) found that the presence of the giant cells worsened prognosis and suggested the name 'seminoma with trophocarcinoma' for such lesions. However, as they do not have the high malignant potential of trophoblastic teratomas, this name is not considered to be justified.

A variable amount of stroma, which may be granulomatous, is present and lymphocytic infiltration is a common feature (Fig. 2.4). Areas of testicular scarring, thought to result from tumour retrogression (Azzopardi and Hoffbrand, 1965), are seen sometimes in relation to seminomas and may occasionally be the only finding in the testes of patients with metastatic disease.

Mostofi and Price (1973) have described a subgroup, anaplastic seminoma, accounting for about 10 per cent of the seminomas in their series and recognized by increased cellular pleomorphism and the presence of three or more mitotic figures per high-power field. These tumours are reported by some workers to be clinically more aggressive (Maier and Sulak, 1973), a point which will be discussed in Chapter 10, but others deny that this is true when staging is taken into consideration (Percapio *et al.*, 1979).

Local spread to involve the rete testis, usually in the interstitial tissue, is very common; sometimes the spread occurs along the tubular basement membrane, elevating the rate epithelium to give a very distinctive histological picture (Fig. 2.5). In the TTP series, 57 per cent of the seminomas which were suitable for staging were confined to the testicular body and rete (pathological stage P1), 23 per cent were invading the epididymis and/or the lower part of the cord

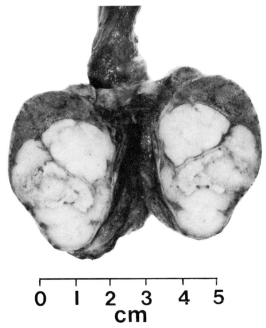

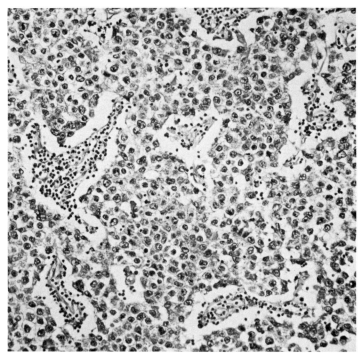

Fig. 2.3 Cut surface of seminoma showing lobulation and an irregular central area of necrosis.

Fig. 2.4 Seminoma consisting of sheets of polygonal cells and stroma infiltrated with lymphocytes. H. & E. ×40. Enlargement ×4.

(P2) and 20 per cent had extended to the upper cord (P3) (Thackray and Crane, 1976).

Between 10 and 12 per cent of patients with seminoma have detectable metastases when first seen (Mostofi and Price, 1973; Thackray and Crane, 1976). Rarely, metastatic tumours in patients with testicular seminoma contain teratomatous components, suggesting that the primary tumour was in reality a combined seminoma and teratoma in which the teratomatous component had been overlooked.

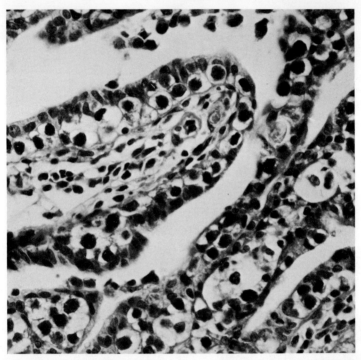

Fig. 2.5 Invasion of the rete testis by vacuolated seminoma cells which are spreading between the tubular basement membrane and the lining epithelium. H. & E. × 100. Enlargement × 4.

Patients presenting with retroperitoneal seminoma form an interesting group. In some, one or both testes are missing from the scrotum and the tumour is considered to have arisen from an undescended gonad. In the remaining patients with apparently normal scrotal testes, several possibilities have to be considered: the tumour may be a metastasis from an occult or retrogressed testicular primary; it may have arisen in a supernumerary undescended testis or be one of the rare primary extragonadal seminomas which are found occasionally in the retroperitoneum, thymus, pineal gland or hypothalamus (see Chapter 17).

Undescended testes
Patients with a history of cryptorchidism have a higher incidence of testicular tumours than the remainder of the population and such a history was given by

6.3 per cent of men in the TTP series. Seminoma was again the most common tumour to be found in this group. It is interesting to note that in approximately 25 per cent of cases of unilateral maldescent the tumour arose in the scrotal testis.

The *spermatocytic seminoma* (originally described by Masson, 1946) occurs in an older age group than the classical variety and most seminomas in patients over the age of 70 appear to be of this type. Grossly, these tumours tend to be softer than the classical variety, often mucoid and sometimes cystic. They are composed of sheets of cells which show marked variation in size and whose cytoplasm is denser than that of the classical tumour and contains no glycogen (Fig. 2.6). Their nuclei are rounded; the larger cells have finely granular nuclear chromatin, but in the smaller cells it is condensed. Giant cells with only three or four very large nuclei are commonly present. Mitoses are usually numerous and may be atypical. In contrast to the classical seminoma, lymphocytic infiltration is not seen and there is no granulomatous reaction. Growth within seminiferous tubules, which may be present in either type of seminoma, is particularly prominent in the spermatocytic variety.

Prognosis
Due to their marked radiosensitivity, the outlook for patients with seminoma is extremely good and the spermatocytic variety in particular behaves in a benign fashion. In the classical case the presence or absence of metastases at

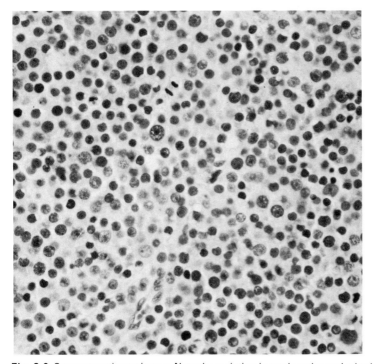

Fig. 2.6 Spermatocytic seminoma. Note the variation in nuclear size and mitotic activity. H. & E. ×100. Englargment ×4.

orchidectomy is the most important factor in determining the outcome, while a high lymphocytic content in the tumour is reported to be an advantageous histological feature (Thackray and Crane, 1976). The most common sites of metastases were the lymph nodes, lungs, liver, bone, kidney and adrenal gland.

Teratomas

As already stated, this group of tumours is now widely accepted to be of germ-cell origin and is sometimes designated 'non-seminomatous germ-cell tumours'. In the mouse, their most primitive cells have been shown to be stem cells which can both reproduce themselves and differentiate towards embryonic and extra-embryonic tissues (Pierce, 1962, Pierce *et al.*, 1962; see Fig. 2.1). Pure tumours, composed of 'stem' cells, embryonic tissues, trophoblast or yolk-sac tissue, do occur but the majority contain a mixture of these elements leading to a very wide variety of appearances.

Nomenclature

In the American classifications, the most primitive form, composed of highly malignant multipotential cells that may, however, show very early somatic differentiation, is called 'embryonal carcinoma'. To tumours consisting of recognizable fetal or adult type tissues, the term 'teratoma' is applied and it is accepted that degrees of somatic differentiation are transitional steps from embryonal carcinoma to teratoma (Dixon and Moore, 1952). The name 'choriocarcinoma' is used for tumours composed of cyto- and syncytiotrophoblast in villus-like arrangement. The American system of classification is to identify and list each component present, e.g. teratoma plus embryonal carcinoma, though for this particular combination the term 'teratocarcinoma' has sometimes been coined (Friedman and Moore, 1946).

In contrast, the British TTP has elected to unify the group by calling all its members teratomas and classifying them, with the exception of the trophoblastic variety, according to their most highly differentiated areas. (While this is contrary to the usual practice in oncology, it accords well with clinical behaviour.) The most primitive, malignant teratoma undifferentiated (MTU), is equivalent to embryonal carcinoma; malignant teratoma intermediate (MTI) equates with teratocarcinoma, and teratoma differentiated (TD) is synonymous with teratoma. Malignant teratoma trophoblastic (MTT) is equivalent to choriocarcinoma either in its rare pure form or when associated with embryonal carcinoma and/or teratoma. The combination of teratoma and seminoma is referred to by the British as a combined tumour.

Table 2.2 summarizes the terminology of four classifications. The British and early American ones are easily interchangeable and have been proved useful in predicting clinical behaviour, both in early stage disease (see Chapter 13) and in advanced stage patients treated with chemotherapy (see Chapter 14). The later American and WHO classifications are rather more complex and aim to provide the clinician with more detailed information by listing each tumour component present. How clinically useful this approach has been is not known.

The TTP nomenclature will be adhered to in the following descriptive pathology.

Approximately one-third of all testicular tumours are teratomas. They are most common in the third decade and the number of cases falls off rapidly after the age of 50 years. The majority of teratomatous testes are enlarged (Fig. 2.7) and the better-differentiated tumours are usually cystic, while the poorly or undifferentiated ones are largely solid in type.

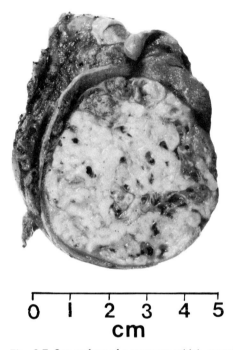

Fig. 2.7 Cut surface of a teratoma which contained much cartilage.

Teratoma differentiated (TD)
This is the most highly differentiated of the group, accounting for 4.9 per cent of 569 teratomas in the TTP series. It contains no histologically malignant areas though, especially in children, some of the tissues may be immature. This tumour occurs most commonly in young children, in whom it often shows a microscopic resemblance to the better-differentiated ovarian teratomas—consisting of differentiated tissues representing all three germ layers and frequently arranged in organoid fashion to form structures resembling, for example, alimentary or respiratory tubules (Fig. 2.8). In children with the diagnosis, the outlook is excellent and in no child of 10 years or under in this series of the TTP did the tumour behave in a malignant fashion. In contrast, some of the adults in whom this diagnosis has been made have died of metastatic disease. Therefore, the TD cannot be considered as a benign tumour.

Malignant teratoma undifferentiated (MTU)
This subtype, at the other end of the teratoma scale, contains no differentiated tissues and consists largely of carcinoma-like cells arranged either in sheets or broken up by slits and acini to give an adenocarcinomatous appearance (Fig.

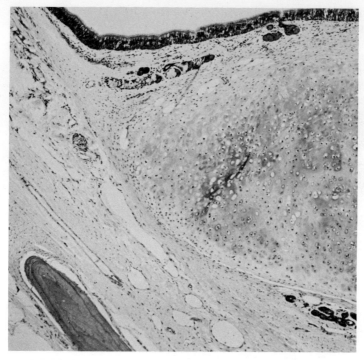

Fig. 2.8 TD showing organoid arrangement of ciliated epithelium, glands and cartilage. A spicule of bone is also present. H. & E. ×40. Enlargement ×4.

2.9). The cells have pleomorphic, often overlapping nuclei with large nucleoli and mitotic figures are numerous. Tumour stroma may sometimes be present. In the TTP series, 36.6 per cent of teratoma were of this type.

Malignant teratoma intermediate (MTI)

This contains both differentiated areas (similar to TD) and undoubtedly malignant areas—as seen in MTU—(Fig. 2.10). It therefore holds an intermediate position histologically, and this is evident also from a prognostic veiwpoint. The MTI formed the largest subgroup in the TTP series, accounting for 54.8 per cent of all teratomas.

Malignant teratoma trophoblastic (MTT)

This variant is diagnosed when three histological criteria are satisfied in some part of a teratoma. Cyto- and syncytiotrophoblast must both be present and the two must be arranged in a papillary pattern with the syncytial tissue forming a surface layer over the cytotrophoblast (Fig. 2.11). Only rarely is the entire tumour composed of trophoblastic tissue (the pure choriocarcinoma of the American classifications); areas having a similar structure to the other subdivisions of teratoma are usually present. The tumour is uncommon and only 3.7 per cent of the TTP series satisfied the rigid criteria of this teratoma subgroup. The prognosis is extremely poor, the great majority of patients dying of disseminated disease within one year of orchidectomy. It should be noted

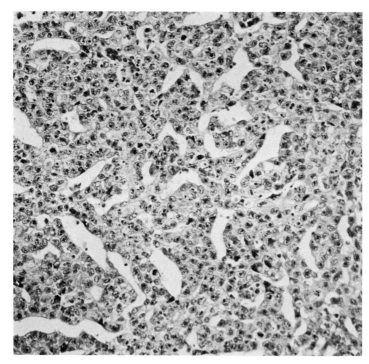

Fig. 2.9 MTU. Sheets of carcinoma-like cells divided up by slits to give an adenocarcinomatous appearance. H. & E. ×40. Enlargement ×4.

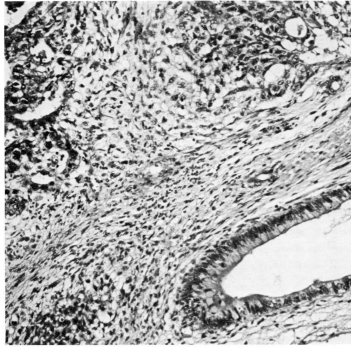

Fig. 2.10 MTI. A differentiated area is present at the lower right-hand side, with undifferentiated areas above. H. & E. ×40.

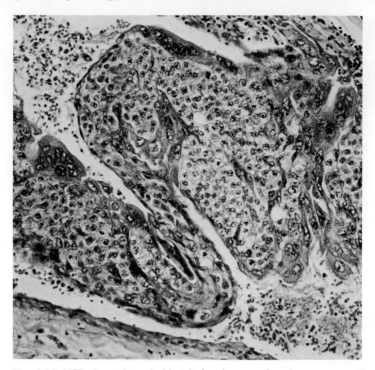

Fig. 2.11 MTT. Syncytiotrophoblast is forming a surface layer over papillary masses of cytotrophoblast. H. & E. ×40. Enlargement ×4.

that irregular syncytial masses may be found in intermediate and undifferentiated malignant teratomas and, in the experience of the TTP, do not have an adverse effect on prognosis.

It is of interest, however, that recent work (see Chapter 3) has shown the presence of HCG within such syncytial masses and the suggestion has been made (Neville *et al.*, 1978) that their presence in MTI tumours does worsen the outlook.

The relationship between pathological staging and the teratoma subgroups is shown in Table 2.3. All the TDs and the majority of MTIs are in stage P1 (i.e. confined to the testis and rete) while in the undifferentiated group, approximately two-thirds of the tumours have spread outside the testis.

Table 2.3 Pathological staging: 233 teratomas (from Table 6.5 in Pugh, 1976)

Stage	TD	MTI	MTU
P1	8	82	33
P2	–	22	34
P3	–	19	35
	8	123	102

Prognosis

The TTP series reflects the outcome of treatment before the advent of effective chemotherapy. All the patients were treated by orchidectomy, followed by radiotherapy unless contra-indicated as, for example, in young children with differentiated teratomas. Retroperitoneal lymph node dissection was performed only rarely and chemotherapy used infrequently and usually as a last resort.

The three-year corrected survival rate (CSR) is 47 per cent overall and 92 per cent for TD, 52 per cent for MTI and 38 per cent for MTU. If the CSR for stage 1 tumours in each group is compared, however, the difference in survival between MTI and MTU is reduced considerably, the relevant figures being 65 per cent for MTI and 61 per cent for MTU. The most common sites for metastases were lung, abdominal and mediastinal lymph nodes, liver, brain, kidney and bone.

In general, secondary deposits of teratoma appear to be less well differentiated than the primary tumour. In an occasional case differentiation is better in the metastasis, a finding which has led to the suggestion that tumour maturation may occur (Smithers, 1969). Rarely, disseminated MTT may be found in a patient whose primary tumour was a TD, MTI or MTU.

Combined tumour

This term describes a neoplasm in which both teratomatous and seminomatous components can be identified. The seminoma is always of the classical type and is usually smaller than the teratoma. The combined tumours are not uncommon and formed the third largest group (13.5 per cent) of the TTP series. The prognosis is essentially that of the teratomatous component, although in the MTI+S group it is very slightly better than for MTI alone (Pugh and Cameron, 1976).

In-situ neoplasia

It is not uncommon to find neoplastic cells within surviving seminiferous tubules in both seminoma- and teratoma-bearing testes. In recent years, collections of atypical germ cells have been described within tubules in testicular biopsies from infertile men who have later developed invasive germ-cell tumours (Skakkebaek, 1978). These cells, which are considerably larger than the normal spermatogonia and show pleomorphism and mitotic activity, are usually the only germ cells in the tubule—in contrast to the random distribution of the occasional abnormal germ cells found in fertile men.

Yolk-sac tumour

This is a rare, rapidly growing tumour which, in the pure form, occurs almost exclusively in the testes of infants and young children. Its many synonyms— adenocarcinoma of the infant testis (Magner and Bryant, 1951), orchioblastoma (Teoh *et al.*, 1960), endodermal sinus tumour (Teilum, 1959) and infantile (juvenile) embryonal carcinoma (Mostofi and Price, 1973)—are an indication of the uncertainty that has long persisted concerning its histogenesis. As

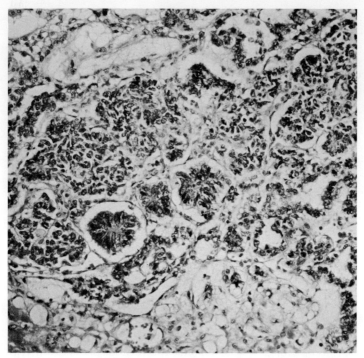

Fig. 2.12 Yolk-sac tumour showing papillary adenocarcinomatous and reticulated areas. H. & E. ×40. Enlargement ×4.

these tumours are regarded now as being of germ-cell origin with differentiation towards extra-embryonic yolk-sac structures, the name yolk-sac tumour seems appropriate. It is the most common testicular tumour of childhood, occurs most frequently under the age of 3 years and may even be present at birth. In the 53 cases in the TTP series (1.9 per cent of all testicular tumours) the mean age at presentation was 17 months (Brown, 1976).

Grossly, the tumour forms a whitish or yellow mass which tends to be haemorrhagic and mucinous and is sometimes cystic. It generally replaces most of the testis and may invade the epididymis or cord.

The microscopic appearance is fairly uniform throughout. The tumour is essentially an adenocarcinoma (Fig. 2.12) with tubular and papillary areas in which the cells are cubical, columnar or flattened and show varying degrees of vacuolation and sometimes mucus secretion. Also present are reticulated microcystic areas composed of rather delicate-looking vacuolated cells and clusters of more compact, deeply staining cells. Perivascular cell formations (the so-called Schiller–Duval bodies) are very characteristic but may be difficult to find in the testicular yolk-sac tumour. Stroma is often scanty and sometimes myxomatous looking and may contain pools of mucin.

Mitotic activity is usually quite marked but is not a good guide to prognosis. Better indicators are the age of the patient and duration of symptoms, the outlook being considerably improved under the age of 2 years and with clinical histories of less than three months (Table 2.4).

Table 2.4 Yolk-sac tumours—TTP 1958-1967 (three-year corrected survival rates (%))

Overall	Age (years) 0-2	over 2	Duration of symptoms (weeks) <11	>11
64	76	58	83	43

In some malignant teratomas in adults, areas resembling yolk-sac tumours are to be seen, though the exact histological criteria for their diagnosis are not agreed universally. Talerman (1975) recorded such areas in 38 per cent of 68 cases and found their presence to be prognostically unfavourable. This aspect of teratomas has aroused much interest since the finding of raised levels of alphafetoprotein (AFP) in the serum of certain patients with germ-cell tumours. Theories postulating AFP synthesis by vitelline cells of yolk-sac origin are convincing and recent studies give support to this view (see Chapter 3). A similar tumour occurs in the ovary and in extragonadal sites.

Interstitial (Leydig) cell tumour

Leydig cells, which produce androgenic hormones, are dispersed widely in the interstitial tissues of the testis. Tumours arising from these cells or their fibroblast-like precursors are uncommon and only sometimes show endocrine activity. Their reported frequency ranges from 1.6 per cent (Symington and

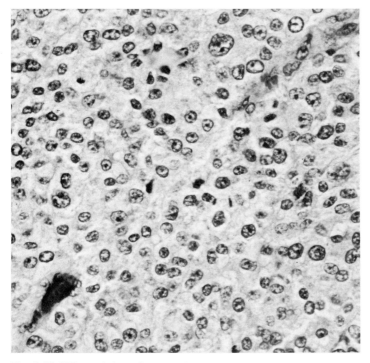

Fig. 2.13 ICT consisting of sheets of pleomorphic granular cells with prominent nuclear membranes and nucleoli. H. & E. ×100. Enlargement ×4.

Cameron, 1976) to 3 per cent (Mostofi, 1973) of all testicular tumours. The majority occur in the third to sixth decades, though they also may arise in, children and the elderly and generally present as testicular swellings which, on palpatation, are unusually hard and well circumscribed. Endocrine symptoms are not uncommon, taking the form of precocious virilization in the young child and of gynaecomastia in the adult.

Grossly, the tumour is rounded and well circumscribed with a characteristic yellow-brown colour and the majority are under 6 cm in diameter (Symington and Cameron, 1976). Areas of necrosis or haemorrhage and cyst formation are unusual.

Histologically, there are compact masses of cells which are polygonal or fusiform in shape and brightly eosinophilic. Their cytoplasm, which is usually granular but sometimes vacuolated, may contain lipofuschin granules, but usually crystalloids of Reinke are not demonstrable. The nuclei of the neoplastic cells have distinct membranes, reticulated chromatin and prominent nucleoli (Fig. 2.13). Pleomorphism is sometimes quite marked and mitotic figures may be numerous, but neither of these features necessarily indicates a poor prognosis.

In contrast to the findings in interstitial-cell hyperplasia, seminiferous tubules are characteristically absent from these lesions. There may be a collagenous or a more cellular stroma in which sometimes focal calcification or even ossification is seen.

Prognosis

Regardless of the histological appearances, the clinical behaviour of most interstitial-cell tumours is benign. In the TTP series, 9 per cent were malignant—a figure which agrees with that quoted by others. In this, as in other endocrine tumours, the only conclusive criterion of malignancy is the presence of histologically proved metastases. Nevertheless, the tumours which do metastasize tend to be large and poorly circumscribed with areas of necrosis and histologically they show evidence of local spread and vascular invasion.

The sites of metastases are retroperitoneal and mediastinal lymph nodes, bone and lung.

Sertoli cell/mesenchyme tumours

These rare tumours, composed of varying amounts of Sertoli-like cells and/or stromal elements, accounted for only 1.2 per cent of the TTP series. They have been called 'androblastomas' by Teilum (1949, 1958), who considers that they epitomise the development of the male gonad. Occurring at all ages, they are most common in the first four decades and usually present as painless, testicular swellings. A minority of the patients have gynaecomastia.

Grossly, the tumours are firm, whitish to cream-coloured and well demarcated and the larger examples are commonly cystic.

The histological appearance varies widely both from case to case and in the individual lesion—with the rare pure Sertoli-cell tumours at one end of the range and lesions resembling fibromas or thecomas at the other; the great majority, however, contain varying proportions of epithelial-like and stromal tissue. In the epithelial areas the neoplastic cells have round or oval nuclei,

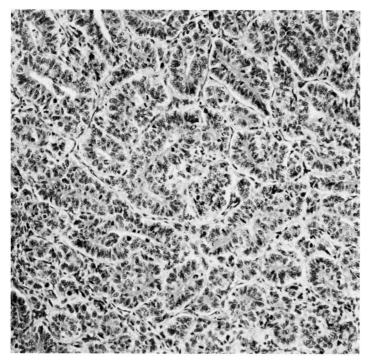

Fig. 2.14 Sertoli-cell tumour showing tubules lined by radially arranged cells. H. & E. ×40. Enlargement ×4.

with a fine chromatin network and small nucleolus and a variable amount of cytoplasm which is sometimes vacuolated. The cells may be arranged in sheets, but a common pattern is of 'tubules', with or without a lumen, lined usually by a single layer, though sometimes by multiple ones, of radially arranged cells resembling Sertoli cells of variable maturity (Fig. 2.14). An alternative pattern is of broad trabeculae of cells outlined by an ill-defined basement membrane.

In tumours which are predominantly stromal, the epithelial element commonly takes the form of irregular islands of polygonal cells with scanty cytoplasm and deeply staining nuclei. Microfollicles and Call–Exner-like bodies may be seen within these cell masses and also there may be cysts bearing some resemblance to Graafian follicles. Leydig cells are present occasionally.

The majority of these tumours behave in a benign fashion, approximately 10 per cent being malignant (Mostofi, 1973). In the TTP series, the malignant growths all showed invasion of lymphatics and/or blood vessels and, commonly, local spread to the rete, epididymis or lower cord. The sites of metastases were the retroperitoneal and mediastinal lymph nodes, liver, lung, brain and bone.

Tumours of dysgenetic gonads (gonadoblastomas)

These are very rare lesions, occurring most commonly in intersex patients and composed of germ cells, other sex-cord derivatives and stromal elements. As they appear to recapitulate gonadal development, Scully (1953) called them gonadoblastomas and divided his cases into three clinical types—phenotypic females (80 per cent), who may be either non-virilized or virilized, and phenotypic males with cryptorchidism, hypospadias and female internal genitalia. The karyotype of these patients is usually 46XY, as in the normal male.

The lesions may be bilateral and sometimes completely replace the gonads, thus obscuring the nature of these organs. They are usually firm in consistency, irregular and greyish-brown in colour and focal calcification is sometimes present.

Microscopically, the appearances are distinctive. Fibrous septa separate masses of cells of two distinct types and sizes. The larger cells have the appearance of germ cells, while the smaller resemble Sertoli cells and form a single layer around the edge of the cell masses and also around Call–Exner-like bodies (Fig. 2.15). The latter, which have been shown by electron microscopy

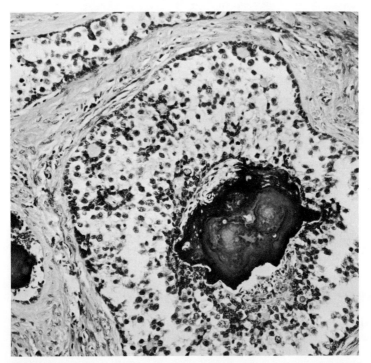

Fig. 2.15 Tumour of dysgenetic testis. Note the two cell types, Call–Exner-like bodies and central calcified mass. H. & E. ×40. Enlargement ×4.

to consist of basement membrane material (Mackay *et al.*, 1974), enlarge, calcify and coalesce, eventually replacing the tumour masses to become embedded in fibrous tissue. In the majority of cases, mature Leydig cells can be seen in the interstitial tissues.

Approximately 50 per cent of the tumours contain seminomatous areas, which vary in size from microscopic foci to large masses and sometimes metastasise. Rare cases of non-seminomatous germ-cell tumours in association with gonadoblastomas have been reported also (Hart and Burkons, 1979).

Malignant lymphoma

Malignant lymphoma not infrequently involves the testis. In most instances this is an early manifestation of already disseminated disease (Woolley *et al.*, 1976), but the finding of a few cases of long survival after orchidectomy shows that primary malignant lymphoma of the testis does exist (Gowing, 1976; Paladugu *et al.*, 1980).

Here the concern is with patients in whom testicular enlargement was a prominent clinical manifestation and led to orchidectomy. Lymphomas were the fourth largest group of tumours in the TTP series, of which they formed 6.7 per cent.

The tumour may develop at any age, but essentially affects the older male with a peak incidence in the seventh and eighth decades. Figure 2.16 shows the striking difference in age distribution between lymphomas and germ-cell tumours in the TTP series, in which the ages ranged from $1\frac{1}{2}$ to 93 years, with 78 per cent of the patients over the age of 50.

Grossly, the testis is enlarged and hard and the tumour usually cream or buff-coloured and poorly demarcated with a homogeneous, though sometimes lobulated, cut surface. Involvement of the epididymis and spermatic cord is common. Microscopically, there is diffuse infiltration of the interstitial tissues with neoplastic cells (Fig. 2.17), which tend to be poorly differentiated and either of the lymphocytic series or of larger 'stem cell' type. The cytological pattern is frequently very pleomorphic and 'poorly differentiated malignant lymphoma' appears to be an adequate description (Gowing, 1976). Plasma-cytic differentiation is seen occasionally. There was no case of Hodgkin's disease in the TTP series.

The remains of widely separated seminiferous tubules can still be distinguished in the lymphomatous testis (Fig. 2.17) and silver impregnation shows a characteristic network of concentric peritubular reticulin fibres caused by penetration of neoplastic cells between the connective tissue fibres surrounding the tubules. Venous invasion is common, with penetration of the neoplastic cells between the muscle fibres and elevation of the endothelium.

Bilateral tumours

The malignant lymphoma is the most common tumour to involve both testes—either synchronously or successively. In the TTP series approximately 3 per cent of all tumours were bilateral and half of these were lymphomas.

Prognosis

This is extremely poor, the majority of the patients dying of disseminated disease within two years of orchidectomy. In the TTP series, the three-year CSR was only 32 per cent and the five-year figure was 24 per cent.

Miscellaneous tumours

Carcinoid

Carcinoid tumours occur rarely in the testis—either as a constituent of a teratoma or, more commonly, in the pure form. In the latter case, the tumour may be a metastasis from an intestinal carcinoid, of which it is sometimes the presenting feature, or a primary neoplasm. Whether this represents

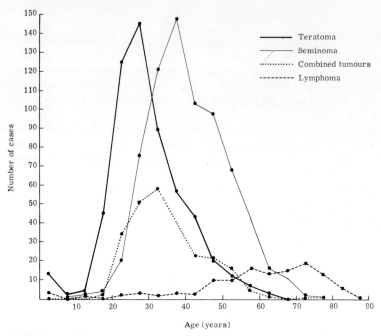

Fig. 2.16 Age distribution at time of orchidectomy for teratomas, seminomas, combined tumours and malignant lymphomas. (Figures taken from Table 4.7 of Pugh, 1976.)

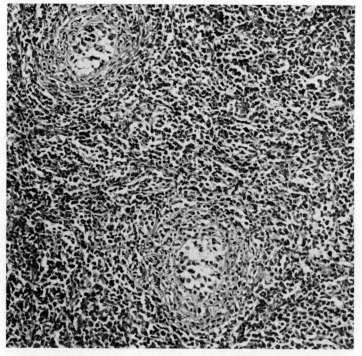

Fig. 2.17 Malignant lymphoma showing two seminiferous tubules surrounded and widely separated by sheets of small cells. H. & E. ×40. Enlargement ×4.

one-sided development of a teratoma or an origin from locally occurring argentaffin cells, not yet identified, is impossible to say.

There were six men with apparently primary carcinoids of testis in the TTP series. Their mean age was 48 years and in none was there evidence of hormonal effects. During follow-up periods of two to twenty-five years there were no recurrences. Although metastases from an apparent testicular primary have been recorded rarely (Berdjis and Mostofi, 1977), the prognosis in the vast majority of reported cases has been excellent (Talerman *et al.*, 1978).

Carcinoma of the rete testis

This very rare tumour, with the structure of a tubular or papillary adenocarcinoma, usually spreads from the mediastinum to involve the vaginal sac and may be difficult to differentiate from a mesothelioma. It metastasizes early and consequently the prognosis is poor.

Secondary tumours

Metastases from primary neoplasms of other organs are found occasionally within the testis, enlargement of which may be the presenting symptom of the disease. The most common tumours to metastasize to the gonad are, in order of frequency, prostatic, bronchogenic and intestinal carcinomas.

Paratesticular tumours

Adenomatoid tumour (adenoma of Müllerian vestiges)

This benign neoplasm of the male and female genital tract is, in the male, most commonly situated in the epididymis. It has been reported also in the testicular tunica, spermatic cord and testis close to the tunica albuginea (de Klerk and Nime, 1975).

The lesion consists of clefts and spaces lined by flattened or cuboidal cells within a stroma of fibrous tissue and smooth muscle; focal lymphocytic infiltration is not uncommon.

Cystadenoma of the epididymis

The cystadenoma is an uncommon, benign tumour, sometimes occurring bilaterally in men with Lindau's disease. As its name implies, it is cystic and contains colloid and papillary outgrowths lined by tall columnar cells with vacuolated cytoplasm.

Embryonal sarcoma (rhabdomyosarcoma)

Occurring most commonly under the age of 20 years, this paratesticular sarcoma, thought to arise from embryonic mesenchyme, may or may not show rhabdomyoblastic differentiation. The age distribution shows two distinct peaks—one in early childhood and the other after puberty.

Grossly, the tumour is usually continuous with the spermatic cord and often very large, causing compression and occasionally invasion of the testis. The cut surface is whitish and whorled, or sometimes brown, and may contain patches of necrosis and haemorrhage.

The histological structure varies from case to case and within a single neoplasm. Myxomatous tissue with stellate and fusiform cells, areas of undifferentiated small dark cells and rounded or strap-like cells with brightly eosinophilic cytoplasm and sometimes cross striations may all be present.

These tumours tend to metastasize widely and, in the past, the prognosis has been extremely poor with death occurring usually within two years of diagnosis. Of the 22 patients in the TTP series, 12 (55 per cent) died of their tumours. However, Olney and his colleagues (1979) state that with the proper use of surgery, radiotherapy and combination chemotherapy an overall two-year survival rate of over 73 per cent should now be obtainable.

Other sarcomas

Paratesticular leiomyosarcomas and fibrosarcomas occur in the older male and are histologically similar to those occurring at other sites in the body. In the TTP series, 5 of the 15 men with leiomyosarcomas and 7 out of 10 with fibrosarcomas died of disseminated disease within three years of operation. Their ages ranged from 41 to 83 years.

Mesothelioma

This is an uncommon tumour arising from the mesothelium lining the vaginal sac. It may be benign or malignant. In making this diagnosis, care must be taken to exclude the cases of mesothelial proliferation and sequestration not uncommonly seen in the walls of hydroceles.

Grossly, there is usually an associated hydrocele. The mesothelium may be locally or diffusely involved and the tumour is papillary, solid or a mixture of both.

Microscopically, the pattern is commonly papillary and tubular and the cell type cubical, columnar or sometimes flattened, but solid sheets of cells, which are occasionally spindle shaped, also occur. As the tumour may be mimicked by metastatic adenocarcinoma, it is essential that continuity between neoplastic cells and mesothelium should be established. The fact that the cells do not produce epithelial mucin may also help in the differential diagnosis. The pure papillary tumours are nearly always benign in behaviour, while those with a more complex pattern may recur (Mostofi and Price, 1973).

(The statistics of the British Testicular Tumour Panel have been used in this chapter with the kind permission of the Chairman.)

References

Azzopardi, J. G. and Hoffbrand, A. V. (1965) *Journal of Clinical Pathology* **18**, 135.
Berdjis, C. C. and Mostofi, F. K. (1977) *Journal of Urology* **118**, 777.
Brown, N. (1976). In *Pathology of the Testis*, Chapter 12. Ed. by R. C. B. Pugh. Blackwell, Oxford.
Dixon, F. J. and Moore, R. A. (1952). *Tumor of the Male Sex Organs: Atlas of Tumor Pathology*, Section VIII Fascicles 31b and 32. AFIP, Washington, DC.
Friedman, M. and Pearlman, A. W. (1970). *Cancer* **26**, 46.
Friedman, N. B. and Moore, R. A. (1946). *Military Surgeon* **99**, 573.
Gowing, N. F. C. (1976). In *Pathology of the Testis*, Chapter 11. Ed. by R. C. B. Pugh. Blackwell, Oxford.

Hart, W. R. and Burkons, D. M. (1979). *Cancer* **43**, 669.

de Klerk, D. P. and Nime, F. (1975). *Urology* **6**, 635.

Mackay, A. M., Pettigrew, N., Symington, T. and Neville, A. M. (1974). *Cancer* **34**, 1108.

Magner, D. and Bryant, A. J. S. (1951). *American Medical Association Archives of Pathology* **51**, 82.

Maier, J. G. and Sulak, M. H. (1973). *Cancer* **32**, 1217.

Masson, P. (1946). *Revue Canadienne de Biologie* **5**, 361.

Mostofi, F. K. (1973). *Cancer* **32**, 1186.

Mostofi, F. K. and Price, E. B. Jr. (1973). *Tumors of the Male Genital System: Atlas of Tumor Pathology*, Second Series, Fascicle 8: AFIP, Washington, D.C.

Neville, A. M., Grigor, K. M. and Heyderman, E. (1978). In *Recent Advances in Histopathology*, Chapter 2. Ed. by P. P. Anthony and N. Woolf. Churchill Livingstone, Edinburgh, London, New York.

Olney, L. E., Narayana, A., Loening, S. and Culp, D. A. (1979). *Urology* **14**, 113.

Paladugu, R. R., Bearman, R. M. and Rappaport, H. (1980). *Cancer* **45**, 561.

Parkinson, C. and Beilby, J. O. W. (1980). *Investigative Cell Pathology* **3**, 135.

Percapio, B., Clements, J. C., McLeod, D. G., Sorgen, S. D. and Cardinale, F. S. (1979). *Cancer* **43**, 2510.

Pierce, G. B. (1962). *Journal of Urology* **88**, 573.

Pierce, G. B. and Beals, T. F. (1964). *Cancer Research* **24**, 1553.

Pierce, G. B., Midgley, A. R., Ram, J. S. and Feldman, J. D. (1962). *American Journal of Pathology* **41**, 549.

Pugh, R. C. B. (1976) *Pathology of the Testis*, Ed. by Pugh, R. C. B. Blackwell, Oxford.

Pugh, R. C. B. and Cameron, K. M. (1976) In *Pathology of the Testis*, Chapter 6. Ed. by R. C. B. Pugh. Blackwell, Oxford.

Scully, R. E. (1953). *Cancer* **6**, 455.

Skakkebaek, N. E. (1978). *Histopathology* **2**, 157.

Smithers, D. W. (1969). *Lancet* **ii**, 949.

Stevens, L. C. (1967). *Journal of National Cancer Institute* **18**, 549.

Symington, T. and Cameron, K. M. (1976). In *Pathology of the Testis*, Chapter 8. Ed. by R. C. B. Pugh. Blackwell, Oxford.

Talerman, A. (1975). *Cancer* **36**, 211.

Talerman, A., Gratama, S., Miranda, S. and Okagaki, T. (1978). *Cancer* **42**, 2696.

Teilum, G. (1949). *Journal of Clinical Endocrinology* **9**, 301.

Teilum, G. (1958). *Cancer* **11**, 769.

Teilum, G. (1959). *Cancer* **12**, 1092.

Teoh, T. B., Steward, J. K. and Willis, R. A. (1960). *Journal of Pathology and Bacteriology* **80**, 147.

Thackray, A. C. and Crane, W. A. J. (1976). In *Pathology of the Testis*, Chapter 5. Ed. by R. C. B. Pugh. Blackwell, Oxford.

Woolley, P. V., Osborne, C. K., Levi, J. A., Wiernik, P. H. and Canellos, G. P. (1976). *Cancer* **38**, 1026.

3

The functional pathology of testicular tumours

Eadie Heyderman, Derek Raghavan and A. Munro Neville

At the present time, conventional histological classification together with careful clinical staging form the basis of prognosis and treatment. The recent recognition of the functional properties of certain germ-cell tumours and the introduction of immunocytochemical procedures have provided a new approach to the understanding and classification of such lesions.

The localization of marker substances produced by testicular tumours has been mainly in those tumours with extra-embryonic elements. These tumours may be of trophoblastic or of yolk-sac type, producing respectively the most useful eutopic markers of disease progression—human chorionic gonadotrophin (HCG) and alphafetoprotein (AFP). Although HCG-like activity has been demonstrated by radio-immunoassay in the normal testis (Braunstein *et al.*, 1975), no reports of the histological localization of either HCG or AFP in the normal testis have yet appeared.

The purpose of this chapter is to examine some of these functional aspects and to indicate their potential relevance in classification and patient management.

There are three main problems related to classification and marker production which may be elucidated using immunocytochemical techniques.

1. Patients whose tumours are classified histologically in the same group and whose clinical staging is identical may have very different clinical behaviour.

2. Patients whose tumours lack conventional trophoblastic differentiation may have raised levels of circulating placental proteins (Braunstein, McIntire and Waldmann, 1973; Muggia *et al.*, 1975).

3. In patients who have elevation of more than one serum marker there may be a differential response of these markers to therapy (Braunstein, McIntire and Waldmann, 1973; Raghavan, Gibbs, Nogueira Costa *et al.*, 1980).

Methodology

Many of the earlier studies of the functional aspects of testicular germ-cell tumours were carried out using immunofluorescent methods (Engelhardt et al., 1971). More recently, the immunoperoxidase technique (Fig. 3.1) has been introduced (de Lellis *et al.*, 1979; Heyderman, 1979). The immunoperoxidase technique is an immunological method which may be used for the demonstration of various substances in tissue sections and which utilizes labelled or unlabelled antibodies and the stable enzyme, horseradish peroxidase. The most widely used substrate, diaminobenzidine, polymerizes in the presence of peroxidase and hydrogen peroxidase to form an insoluble brown polymer which is deposited at the site of antigen–antibody reaction. The technique employed is the indirect (sandwich) method, in which the first antibody is unlabelled and the second antibody, which is directed against the immunoglobulin of the species in which the first antibody is raised, is conjugated to peroxidase. The sequence is summarized in Fig. 3.1 and has the advantage of

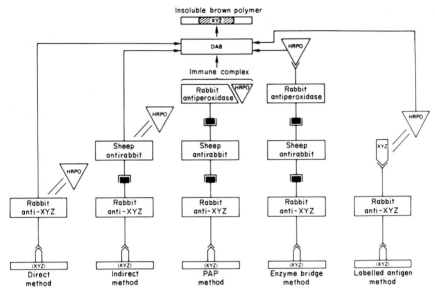

Fig. 3.1 Immunoperoxidase methods. The lowest line shows a slide on which there is a tissue section containing the antigen under test, XYZ. HRPO is the horse-radish peroxidase conjugate; DAB is the substrate, diaminobenzidine. (Reproduced from Heyderman 1979, *Journal of Clinical Pathology*, by kind permission of the editors.)

being permanent and suitable for conventional counterstaining, so that simultaneous histological diagnosis and the more precise identification of positive cells are thus possible. The immunoperoxidase technique is suitable for routinely fixed and paraffin-embedded material, as well as for cryostat sections. Therefore, retrospective as well as prospective studies are feasible. As for all immunological procedures, adequate controls are essential. These include the use of positive controls, tissues known to express the antigen being investigated, and negative controls using antisera whose activity has been completely abolished by absorption with the appropriate 'antigen' (Heyderman, 1979). We have found that more precise localization is achieved with affinity-purified antisera.

Tissue markers

There are several groups of potential markers relevant to testicular tumours.

1. Placental proteins. This group of markers includes human chorionic gonadotrophin (HCG) (Heyderman and Neville, 1976; Kurman *et al.*, 1977), pregnancy specific glycoprotein (SP_1) (Horne *et al.*, 1977; Rosen *et al.*, 1979), human placental lactogen (HPL) (Porteous *et al.*, 1968; Heyderman, 1979) and PP5 (Bohn, 1972; Obiekwe *et al.*, 1979).

2. Yolk-sac products. Included in this category are alphafetoprotein (Abelev *et al.*, 1967) and other yolk-sac products such as ferritin (Wahren, 1978), α_1-antitrypsin (Palmer *et al.*, 1976) and albumin and prealbumin (Shirai *et al.*, 1976; Tsuchida *et al.*, 1978).

3. Carcinoembryonic antigen (CEA) (Gold and Freedman, 1965; Talerman *et al.*, 1977; Wahren, 1978).

4. Steroid and steroid receptors (Javadpour, 1979; Kurman *et al.*, 1978) particularly in sex cord mesenchyme tumours.

5. New markers such as F9 antigen, a surface marker common to human sperm and embryonal carcinoma and pre-implantation mouse embryos (Artzt *et al.*, 1973; Hogan *et al.*, 1977; Holden *et al.*, 1977); fibronectin (cold insoluble globulin), found in the serum and in the extracellular tissues of various organs (Yamada and Olden, 1978); β_2-microglobulin and the HLA antigens (De Wolf *et al.*, 1979).

Placental hormones

Soon after Ascheim and Zondek described their pregnancy test, there were reports of positive results in men with trophoblastic tumours (Zondek, 1930). The early normal placenta as well as choriocarcinomas of the uterus, ovary and testis contain an outer syncytiotrophoblast layer which secretes placental hormones (Heyderman and Neville, 1976) and an inner generative cytotrophoblast layer. Human chorionic gonadotrophin is readily demonstrable in the syncytiotrophoblast of the normal placenta as well as in gestational, ovarian and testicular choriocarcinomas (Fig. 3.2). However, it was considered that raised levels of HCG were associated only with conventional trophoblastic differentiation (Pugh, 1976). Heyderman and Neville (1976) showed that the HCG could be demonstrated by the immunoperoxidase technique in isolated giant cells with syncytiotrophoblastic cytological features. This was confirmed subsequently by Kurman *et al.* (1977) and Hedinger *et al.* (1979). Moreover, these cells were associated frequently with raised serum levels of HCG pre-orchidectomy or in the presence of metastases. Failure to demonstrate syncytiotrophoblast in association with cytotrophoblast in the tumours of such patients is thus not necessarily due to sampling error as suggested by Hobson (1965). Over 50 per cent of teratomas classified either as malignant teratoma intermediate (MTI) or malignant teratoma undifferentiated (MTU) contained HCG-positive cells (Heyderman, 1978).

These HCG-positive cells correspond to the 'pseudotrophoblasts' of Collins and Pugh (1964): they are large, usually multinucleate, giant cells with eosinophilic vacuolated cytoplasm. Frequently they are seen to form a syncytium apparently lining the walls of vascular channels. Similar HCG-positive cells can be found in some seminomas (Fig. 3.3) and may be associated with raised

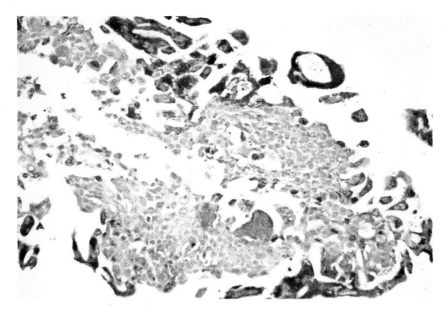

Fig. 3.2 Choriocarcinoma of the testis (MTT) stained with an antiserum to beta-HCG. The syncytiotrophoblast is strongly positive, while the cytotrophoblast is negative. Occasional positive mononuclear intermediate cells are present. Indirect immunoperoxidase ×80.

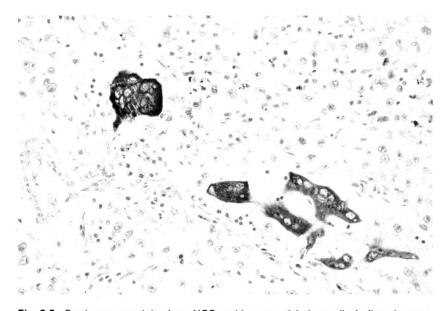

Fig. 3.3. Seminoma containing beta-HCG positive syncytial giant cells. Indirect immunoperoxidase ×80.

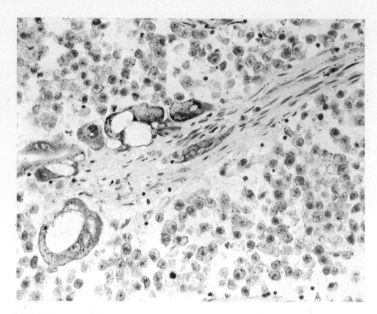

Fig. 3.4 Seminoma from patient with gynaecomastia showing bizarre giant cells stained for HPL. Indirect immunoperoxidase ×80.

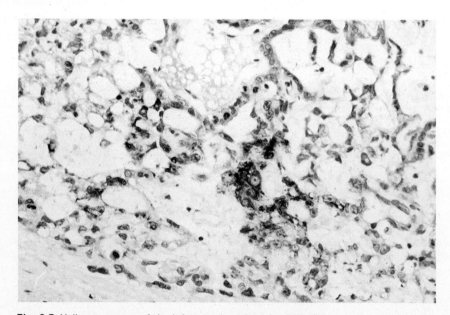

Fig. 3.5 Yolk-sac tumour of the infant testis stained for AFP. The reaction product is in the cells lining the vitelline cysts. Indirect immunoperoxidase ×80.

serum HCG levels. In such cases, therefore, there may be no need to postulate the presence of occult teratomatous elements. A study of 67 Stage 1 teratomas failed to show a statistically significant difference in prognosis between tumours with and without these syncytial giant cells and, although a worse prognosis has been suggested for seminoma with such cells (Friedman and Pearlman, 1970; Mostofi, 1980), no immunocytochemical studies have yet been published.

Other placental hormones
Human placental lactogen (HPL) has been demonstrated by immunofluorescence in testicular tumours (Porteous *et al.*, 1968) and by the immunoperoxidase technique in about 80 per cent of HCG-positive teratomas (Heyderman, 1978) and was found in cells similar to those containing HCG. Early studies using antisera to PP_5 indicate that syncytial giant cells secrete this placental protein (unpublished data). The presence of HPL may be one explanation for gynaecomastia in men with testicular tumours, both in those with or without evidence of raised HCG levels.

Raised levels of pregnancy-specific glycoprotein (SP_1) were found in 3 out of 6 men with malignant teratoma trophoblastic (MTT), 5 out of 17 with differentiated teratomas (TD) or malignant teratoma intermediate (MTI), and 5 out of 50 with malignant teratoma undifferentiated (MTU) (Rosen *et al.*, 1979). This placental protein has been demonstrated also in tissue sections of placenta and trophoblastic tumours (Horne *et al.*, 1977).

Alphafetoprotein (AFP)
The histological basis for synthesis in gonadal and extragonadal germ-cell tumours has been presented by many authors (Ballas, 1972; Wilkinson *et al.*, 1973; Itoh *et al.*, 1974; Talerman and Haije, 1974; Teilum *et al.*, 1974; Norgaard-Pedersen *et al.*, 1975; Tsuchida *et al.*, 1975). Increased serum AFP levels have been found in patients with tumours having vitelline (yolk-sac) components of various patterns. Positive staining for AFP has been found in the littoral cells of the endodermal sinuses of yolk-sac tumours (Fig. 3.4) and in the intra- and extracytoplasmic PAS-positive globules (Itoh *et al.*, 1974; Teilum *et al.*, 1974). However, there are testicular tumours associated with raised AFP levels where no morphological evidence of classical vitelline elements can be detected (Grigor *et al.*, 1977).

Others have claimed that AFP is present in single cells in embryonal carcinoma (Kurman *et al.*, 1977) and in undifferentiated somatic elements (Beilby *et al.*, 1979). It is clear that we do not yet recognize all the types of cell capable of synthesizing AFP. However, while many workers have demonstrated alphafetoprotein using immunofluorescent techniques (e.g. Teilum *et al.*, 1975; Tsuchida *et al.*, 1978) it has been difficult to obtain satisfactory results using the immunoperoxidase method. While this may in part be a reflection of the quality of reagents employed, it has been found also that formalin 'denatures' AFP and may thus contribute to a lack of reproducibility of staining, particularly in tissues with few AFP-producing cells (Raghavan *et al.*, unpublished). However, more success has been achieved with tissues fixed in Zenker's (Fig. 3.5) and Bouin's solutions and it may be necessary to explore other fixatives.

Albumin, prealbumin and α_1-antitrypsin have been localized also in the yolk-sac elements of some tumours (Palmer *et al.*, 1976; Shirai *et al.*, 1976; Tsuchida *et al.*, 1978).

Where we have localized both AFP and HCG in the same tumour the positive cells are morphologically distinct. A differential response to therapy of tumour with these markers may be explained readily on the basis of differing sensitivities of the two cell populations.

It is currently thought that raised serum AFP levels are associated only with teratomas and not with seminomas. Recently we have studied a series of xenografts of human germ-cell tumours grown in immune-suppressed mice to characterize the relationships between histology and tumour-marker production (Raghavan, Gibbs, Nogueira Costa *et al.*, 1980; Raghavan, Gibbs, Neville and Peckham, 1980; Raghavan, Heyderman, Gibbs *et al.*, 1980). One of these tumour lines was derived from a lymph-node metastasis from a patient with a histological diagnosis of seminoma but with elevated AFP levels (Raghavan, Heyderman, Monaghan *et al.*, 1981). Serial passages of the tumour have shown cells with light and electron microscopic features of classical seminoma, of yolk-sac carcinoma, and a third cell type with features common to both seminoma and yolk-sac carcinoma, suggesting either a continuum of differentiation between seminoma and yolk-sac carcinoma or the existence of a solid yolk-sac carcinoma with light morphological features similar to seminoma. Alphafetoprotein has been demonstrated both in the xenografted tissue and in the circulation of these tumour-bearing mice. This model may explain the association of seminoma and AFP in some patients without the need to postulate occult teratoma (cf. HCG *vide supra*).

Other markers

It has been found that measurement of serum CEA levels has little or no place in the routine monitoring of patients with testicular tumours (Talerman *et al.*, 1977) because of the poor correlation of serum level and tumour mass. However, the demonstration of CEA and other markers of epithelial differentiation may be useful as an indication of the type of tumour differentiation. Heyderman (1979) demonstrated CEA in some teratomas with gastrointestinal-like differentiation and, in one patient with widespread disease, CEA levels terminally were 240 ng/ml (normal 40 ng/ml). The epithelial membrane antigen (EMA) can be demonstrated in tumours with differentiation to form secretory epithelia (Heyderman, 1979).

There are problems concerned with the localization in tissue sections of ferritin and lactoferrin. Although we have demonstrated these substances in testicular tumours, the presence of the former in macrophages and the latter in myeloid cells has introduced difficulty especially when, as is often the case, there are areas of necrosis and an associated inflammatory response.

Conclusions

The introduction of immunocytochemical methods has an important role in the accurate classification of germ-cell tumours. An immunoperoxidase stain for human chorionic gonadotrophin using antisera to the specific β-subunit of HCG already forms part of the routine work-up of all teratomas of the testis treated at St Thomas' and the Royal Marsden Hospitals in London. As techniques improve and new markers become available we envisage that these will be included in an immunoperoxidase profile to accompany each histology report. An immunostain for HCG has been shown by us to be of value in the identification of small foci of trophoblastic differentiation. Conventional and isolated syncytial cell types may be recognized much more readily in a section stained for HCG or other placental proteins than in a routine haemotoxylin and eosin preparation. We have shown that such demonstration of HCG correlated well with raised serum levels in patients with metastases, although we have not shown that HCG-positive cells in the primary tumour carry the same poor prognostic significance as the presence of HCG in carcinomas of the colon (Buckley and Fox, 1979) or breast (Horne *et al.*, 1977; Walker, 1978). There is a need to study larger numbers of patients to assess this more fully. Extra-embryonic elements have been reported to be associated with a worse prognosis (Talerman, 1975; Parkinson and Beilby, 1977). The presence of yolk-sac elements should always be indicated in routine histopathological reports and when we are better able to recognize atypical AFP-producing cells these patterns will also need to be documented.

There is a need to find new markers for those tumours which do not produce HCG or AFP. The recently introduced, monoclonal antibody technology (Kohler and Milstein, 1975) used to produce antisera to other testicular tumour antigens may have great importance in this context. An alternative approach is to screen sections of tumours with antisera to a variety of cell products— hormones, immunoglobulins, fetal antigens, etc.—to look for further suitable markers, since teratomas may show a wide diversity of somatic differentiation.

In testicular neoplasia, as in all tumour pathology, there is a pressing need to improve the precision of classification using functional as well as morpho-logical criteria. More meaningful classification and improved understanding of testicular tumour biology may thus be achieved.

References

Abelev, G. I., Assecritowa, I. V., Kraevsky, N. A., Perova, S. D. and Perevodchikova, N. I. (1967). *International Journal of Cancer* **2**, 551.

Artzt, K. Dubois, P., Bennett, D., Condamine, H., Babinet, C. and Jacob, F. (1973). *Proceedings of the National Academy of Science (USA)* **70**, 2988.

Ballas, M. (1972). *American Journal of Clinical Pathology* **57**, 511.

Beilby, J. O. W., Horne, C. H. W., Milne, G. D. and Parkinson, C. (1979). *Journal of Clinical Pathology* **32**, 455.

Bohn, H. (1972). *Blüt* **24**, 292.

Braunstein, G. D., McIntire, K. R. and Waldmann, T. A. (1973). *Cancer* **31**, 1065.

Braunstein, G. D., Rasor, J. and Wade, M. E. (1975). *New England Journal of Medicine* **293**, 1339.

Braunstein, G. D., Vaitukaitis, J. L., Carbone, P. P. and Ross, G. T. (1973). *Annals of Internal Medicine* **78**, 39.

Buckley, C. H. and Fox, H. (1979). *Journal of Clinical Pathology* **32**, 368.

Collins, D. H. and Pugh, R. C. B. (1964). *British Journal of Urology*, Suppl. **36**, 1.

De Wolf, W. C., Lange, P. H., Einarson, M. E. and Yunis, E. J. (1979). *Nature* **277**, 216.

Engelhardt, N. V., Poltoranina, V. S. and Yazowa, A. K. (1971). *International Journal of Cancer* **11**, 448.

Friedman, M. and Pearlman, A. W. (1970). *Cancer* **26**, 46.

Gold, P. and Freedman, S. O. (1965). *Journal of Experimental Medicine* **122**, 467.

Grigor, K. M., Detre, S. I., Kohn, J. and Neville, A. M. (1977). *British Journal of Cancer* **35**, 52.

Hedinger, C. H. R., von Hochstetter, A. R. and Egloff, B. (1979). *Virchows Archives. A Pathology, Anatomy and Histology* **383**, 59.

Heyderman, E. (1978). *Scandinavian Journal of Immunology* **8**, Suppl. 8, 119.

Heyderman, E. (1979). *Journal of Clinical Pathology* **32**, 971.

Heyderman, E. and Neville, A. M. (1976). *Lancet* **ii**, 103.

Heyderman, E. and Neville, A. M. (1977). *Journal of Clinical Pathology* **30**, 138.

Heyderman, E., Steel, K. and Ormerod, M. G. (1979). *Journal of Clinical Pathology* **32**, 35.

Hobson, B. M. (1965). *Acta endocrinologica* **49**, 337.

Hogan, B., Fellows, M., Auner, P. and Jacob, F. (1977). *Nature* **270**, 515.

Holden, S., Bernard, O., Artzt, K., Whitmore, W. F. Jr. and Bennett, D. (1977). *Nature* **270**, 518.

Horne, C. H. W., Towler, C. M. and Milne, G. D. (1977). *Journal of Clinical Pathology* **30**, 19.

Itoh, T., Shirai, T., Nakan, A. and Matsumoto, S. (1974). *GANN Monograph on Cancer Research* **65**, 215.

Javadpour, N. (1979). *Human Pathology* **10**, 557.

Kohler, G. and Milstein, C. (1975). *Nature* **256**, 495.

Kurman, R. J., Andrade, D. Goebelsmann, V. and Taylor, C. R. (1978). *Cancer* **42**, 1772.

Kurman, R. J., Scardino, P. T., McIntire, K. R., Waldmann, T. A. and Javadpour, N. (1977). *Cancer* **40**, 2135.

de Lellis, R. A., Sternberger, L. A., Mann, R. B., Banks, P. M. and Nakane, P. K. (1979). *American Journal of Clinical Pathology* **71**, 483.

Mostofi, F. K. (1980). *Cancer* **45**, 1735.

Muggia, F. M., Rosen, S. W., Weintraub, B. D. and Hansen, H. H. (1975). *Cancer* **36**, 1327.

Norgaard-Pedersen, B., Albrechtsen, R. and Teilum, G. (1975). *Acta pathologica et microbiologica Scandinavica*, Sect. A. **83**, 573.

Obiekwe, B. C., Grudzinskas, J. G., Gordon, Y. B., Chard, T. and Bohn, H. (1979). In *Carcino-embryonic Proteins*, Vol. II, p. 629. Ed. by F. G. Lehmann. Elsevier/North Holland, Biomedical Press, Amsterdam.

Palmer, P. E., Safah, H. and Wolfe, H. (1976). *American Journal of Clinical Pathology* **65**, 575.

Parkinson, C. and Beilby, J. O. W. (1977). *Journal of Clinical Pathology* **30**, 113.

Porteous, I. B., Beck, J. S. and Pugh, R. C. B. (1968). *Journal of Pathology and Bacteriology* **95**, 527.

Pugh, R. C. B. (1976). *Scientific Foundations of Urology* **II**, 379.

Raghavan, D., Gibbs, J., Neville, A. M. and Peckham, M. J. (1980). *New England Journal of Medicine* **302**, 811.

Raghavan, D., Gibbs, J., Nogueira Costa, R., Kohn, J., Orr, A. H., Barrett, A. and Peckham, M. J. (1980). *British Journal of Cancer* **41**, Suppl. IV, 191.

Raghavan, D., Heyderman, E., Gibbs, J., Neville, A. M. and Peckham, M. J. (1981). In *Thymusaplastic Nude Mice and Rats in Clinical Oncology*, pp. 200–203. Ed. by G. Bastert, H. Schmidt-Matthiesson and H. P. Fortmeyer. Fischer-Verlag, Berlin.

Raghavan, D., Heyderman, E., Monaghan, P., Gibbs, J., Ruoslahti, E., Peckham, M. J. and Neville, A. M. (1981). *Journal of Clinical Pathology* **34**, pp. 123–128.

Rosen, S. W., Javadpour, N., Calbert, I. and Kaminska, J. (1979). *Journal of the National Cancer Institute* **62**, 1439.

Shirai, T., Itoh, T., Yoshiki, T., Noro, T., Tomino, Y. and Hayasaka, T. (1976). *Cancer* **38**, 1661.

Talerman, A. (1975). *Cancer* **36**, 211.

Talerman, A. and Haije, W. G. (1974). *Cancer* **34**, 1722.

Talerman, A., Pompe, W. B. van der, Haije, W. G., Baggerman, L. and Boeksstein-Tjahjadi, H. M. (1977). *British Journal of Cancer* **35**, 288.

Teilum, G., Albrechtsen, R. and Norgaard-Pedersen, B. (1974). *Acta pathologica et microbiologica Scandinavica*, Sect. A, **82**, 586.

Teilum, G., Albrechtsen, R. and Norgaard-Pedersen, B. (1975). *Acta pathologica et microbiologica Scandinavica*, Sect. A, **83**, 80.

Tsuchida, Y., Endo, Y., Urano, Y. and Ishida, M. (1975). *Annals of the New York Academy of Sciences* **259**, 221.

Tsuchida, Y. Kaneko, M., Saito, S., Endo, Y., Urano, Y., Ohmi, K. and Asaka, T. (1978). *Scandinavian Journal of Immunology* **8**, Suppl. 8, 137.

Tsuchida, Y., Kaneko, M., Yokomori, K., Saito, S., Urano, Y., Endo, Y., Asaka, T. and Takeuchi, T. (1978). *Journal of Pediatric Surgery* **13**, 25.

Wahren, B. (1978). *Scandinavian Journal of Immunology* **8**, Suppl. 8, 131.

Walker, R. A. (1978). *Journal of Clinical Pathology* **31**, 245.

Wilkinson, E. J., Hosty, T. A. and Friedrich, E. G. (1973). *American Journal of Obstetrics and Gynecology* **116**, 711.

Yamada, K. M. and Olden, K. (1978). *Nature* **275**, 179.

Zondek, B. (1930). *Der Chirurg* **2**, 1072.

4

Tumour markers in malignant germ-cell tumours

Joachim Kohn and Derek Raghavan

Introduction

The value of tumour markers in the diagnosis and management of germ-cell tumours of the testis is now well established. The clinical application of serum markers in non-seminomatous tumours is discussed further in Chapters 13 and 15. During the past few years, an extensive literature has developed in this field (indicated in the references by asterisks, pp 67–69). A current resumé and recommendations on the clinical use of alphafetoprotein (AFP) and human chorionic gonadotrophin (HCG) in testicular tumours has been published recently by an international panel of investigators (Norgaard-Pedersen *et al.*, 1978).

Table 4.1 Causes of elevated alphafetoprotein (AFP) and human chorionic gonadotrophin (HCG)

AFP	HCG
Physiological	**Physiological**
Pregnancy	Pregnancy
Early infancy	Early infancy
Neoplastic disease	**Neoplasia**
Hepatocellular carcinoma	(see Table 4.2)
Malignant teratoma	
Other gastrointestinal malignant disease	
Colon	
Pancreas	
Stomach	
Non-neoplastic disease	**Non-neoplastic disease**
(Liver)	Peptic ulcer
Cirrhosis	Cirrhosis
Hepatitis	Inflammatory bowel disease
Liver toxins	
Partial hepatectomy	
Benign diseases of childhood	
Biliary atresia	
Neonatal hepatitis	
Congenital abnormalities	
Ataxia telangiectasia	
Hereditary tyrosinaemia	
Neural tube defects	

In the 'ideal' situation, a tumour marker should:

i. be diagnostic of the presence of active tumour;
ii. bear a reliable quantitative relationship to tumour mass;
iii. be highly sensitive and specific;
iv. be readily and reproducibly assayed.

Although not ideal, AFP and HCG are the two most significant and most extensively studied tumour markers in testicular malignant disease. Since the introduction of sensitive and specific immunoassays, a large proportion of patients with malignant teratoma have been shown to have detectable AFP, HCG, or both, in their blood. Elevated levels of these tumour markers reliably indicate the presence of active malignant teratoma. Of the two, with the exception of malignant trophoblastic teratoma (MTT or choriocarcinoma), AFP is somewhat more specific and more frequently detected in malignant germ-cell tumours. When other sources of increased AFP or HCG have been excluded—and these are uncommon and easily identified (see Tables 4.1 and 4.2)—no false positives have been encountered in our experience of more than

Table 4.2 Incidence of immunoreactive HCG (beta subunit) in sera of patients with documented tumours (Vaitukaitis, 1979a)

Tumour	Number examined	Number positive	Percentage
Breast	162	34	21
Lung	161	18	11
Gastrointestinal	366	68	19
Oesophagus	12	0	0
Stomach	74	17	23
Small intestine	23	3	13
Pancreas	43	14	33
Biliary tract	9	1	11
Liver	93	19	20
Colon	112	14	13
Ovary (adenocarcinoma)	47	18	38
Miscellaneous	581	22	4

Table 4.3 Elevated marker levels in patients with active malignant teratoma (Stages II–IV)

Series	AFP only	(%)	HCG only	(%)	AFP or HCG	(%)	AFP and HCG	(%)
Royal Marsden	42/153	(27)	17/153	(11)	112/153	(73)	53/153	(35)
Scardino et al., (NCI) (1977)	5/36	(14)	12/36	(33)	33/36	(92)	16/36	(44)
Anderson et al. (NCI) (1979)	16/100	(16)	14/100	(14)	89/100	(89)	59/100	(59)
Lange and Fraley (1977)	19/59	(32)	10/59	(17)	54/59	(92)	25/59	(42)
Schultz, Sell et al., (1978)	7/34	(21)	8/34	(24)	20/34*	(59)	5/34	(15)
Mann et al. (1979)	17/64	(27)	9/64	(14)	56/64	(88)	30/64	(47)

* Higher incidence in patients with distant metastases.

200 cases. The simultaneous assay of the two markers increases the incidence of 'marker positive' cases, i.e. patients with elevated titres (Table 4.3; Braunstein, Vaitukaitis *et al.*, 1973; Newlands *et al.*, 1976; Perlin *et al.*, 1976; Lange and Fraley, 1977; Scardino *et al.*, 1977; Lange, 1978; Schultz, Sell *et al.*, 1978; Mann *et al.*, 1979).

Several potential markers of germ-cell tumours are being evaluated clinically and in particular in those tumours that are not associated with AFP or HCG production (*vide infra*).

Alphafetoprotein

Alphafetoprotein, a glycoprotein with a molecular weight of approximately 66 000 to 72 000 daltons, has an electrophoretic mobility of alpha$_1$-globulin. It consists of a single polypeptide chain in which no detectable subunits have been identified. Alphafetoprotein is synthesized by the fetal liver and organs derived from the yolk sac; the synthesis of AFP reported in some human placental tissues may be due to yolk sac elements. The AFP synthesized by malignant tumours, for example hepatoma and teratoma, is immunologically identical to fetal AFP. It has been shown that liver and yolk-sac AFP have some structural differences in carbohydrate content (Ruoslahti and Adamson, 1978).

Alphafetoprotein may be found in serum, amniotic fluid, urine, CSF and extracellular fluid. It is synthesized, normally in very large amounts, early in fetal life. Its synthesis has been detected as early as the sixth to the eighth week, the highest levels occurring at the twelfth to fourteenth week of gestation. The production rate stabilizes and the increasing fetal-serum pool in the mid-gestation period results in falling concentrations towards delivery, with levels of 10–15 mg/l at birth and then a rapid decline. After birth, AFP synthesis may not be switched off entirely and during the first year of life the serum levels are variable, falling in a non-linear fashion to reach adult levels between 6 to 12 months (Tsuchida, Endo *et al.*, 1978). Alphafetoprotein synthesis only becomes reactivated in certain pathological conditions, primarily in malignancies such as hepatocellular carcinoma and teratoma.

There is no doubt that low levels of AFP persist in normal adults, detectable only by sensitive immunoassay methods, and a normal range of 1–16 μg/l has been reported in healthy adults (Seppala and Ruoslahti, 1972; Sizaret, 1979). This has been confirmed, with small variations, by other laboratories. The upper limit of the normal range will depend on the laboratory performing the assay and the clinical purpose for which the assay is requested. In our studies, an upper level of 25 μg/l has been adopted for normal patients over the age of 1 year (Kohn, 1976). In malignant teratoma, serum levels cover a wide range from 'normal' up to greater than 200 000 μg/l.

The reported value of the normal plasma half-life of AFP varies from 3.5 to 6.2 days (Gitlin and Boesman, 1966; Hirai *et al.*, 1972); most workers regard 5 days as an acceptable figure and our studies agree with this. The discrepancies are due to the technique employed (elimination rate of injected labelled AFP, or serial assays following complete surgical ablation of tumour) and/or imprecise recording of specimen collection time.

The biological function of AFP is unknown. Its appearance in early fetal life, its rapid production rate and its very high concentration during the period of differentiation and growth perhaps reflect one of its roles. The following functions have been proposed but remain unconfirmed.

1. A homeostatic relationship to albumin. There is a reciprocal ratio of serum concentrations. It has been postulated that AFP functions in the same way as albumin in the fetus, acting as a carrier protein and maintaining osmotic gradients. The structures of albumin and AFP are similar.

2. Binding of oestrogenic hormones in the rat has been demonstrated and a protective role from maternal oestrogens has been suggested. It is not clear whether similar binding occurs in man.

3. Immunosuppression (and blocking of maternal rejection of the fetus in particular).

4. Growth control.

5. A tissue-organizing signal during the developmental fetal stage.

Human chorionic gonadotrophin

Human chorionic gonadotrophin is a most useful and highly sensitive tumour marker. The classical example of its clinical application is gestational chorio-carcinoma, where the use of the HCG assay has contributed substantially to therapeutic success both as a monitor of the response to treatment and as a parameter of the end-point of therapy (Bagshawe, 1969).

Human chorionic gonadotrophin, a glycoprotein hormone, is synthesized by trophoblastic tissues. Like other glycoprotein hormones, it consists of two dissimilar subunits (alpha and beta), of which the alpha subunit (molecular weight 14 900) is common to follicle-stimulating hormone (FSH), luteinising hormone (LH) and HCG. The beta subunit (molecular weight 23 000) confers biological and immunological specificity. Radio-immunoassay systems based on antisera raised against native (intact) HCG and LH cannot discriminate between these two hormones. A reliable assay method is attained only by the use of specific antibodies raised against the beta subunit of HCG (Vaitukaitis et al., 1972; Vaitukaitis, 1979b). There has been some controversy as to the extent to which purified anti-β subunit antibodies cross-react with luteinizing hormone (Vaitukaitis et al., 1972 Rutanen and Seppala, 1978.) The radio-immunoassay for HCG, with an antiserum to the beta subunit, has a sensitivity of less than 1 μg/l. Using this assay, circulating HCG values in normal, healthy individuals and male patients with benign disorders are usually less than 1–2 μg/l[7] (noting that 1.0 ng of highly purified HCG = 5 miu of second International Standard Hormone by radio-immunoassay (Vaitukaitis, 1979b)).

Human chorionic gonadotrophin is normally only present in large amounts in pregnancy. Although predominantly present in placental or neoplastic tissue, HCG immunoreactivity has been demonstrated in testis, pituitary, liver and colon (Braunstein et al., 1975; Chen et al., 1976; Yoshiki et al., 1976). In patients who have undergone bilateral orchidectomy, circulating LH titres are markedly elevated and may cause low level HCG positivity with most assays; this can be resolved by the administration of testosterone and subsequent retesting (Vaitukaitis, personal communication). Markedly elevated HCG levels have been documented in tumours with no detectable trophoblastic elements (see Table 4.2; Vaitukaitis, 1979a; Vaitukaitis, 1979b).

The HCG molecule in non-neoplastic tissue contains little or no carbohydrate (in contrast to placental HCG) (Yoshimoto *et al.*, 1977) and it has been suggested that this is the basis of its low biological activity and rapid blood clearance (Kawamura *et al.*, 1978).

Human chorionic gonadotrophin is present in blood and extracellular fluid and may be detected in CSF in the presence of central nervous system metastatic disease, or as a result of passive diffusion when blood levels are markedly elevated.

The plasma half-life of native HCG is twenty-four to thirty-six hours (Vaitukaitis, 1979a). By contrast, the alpha subunit has a half-life of less than twenty minutes. A radio-immunoassay for alpha-HCG has been reported to be useful in the localization of metastases, using selective catherization of the veins draining the area concerned, searching for a localized increase in concentration of α-HCG (Javadpour, 1978; Javadpour and Bergman, 1978). The short half-life avoids the problem of prolonged elevation in the peripheral circulation masking the local increase in marker concentration (Javadpour, 1978).

Another innovation, reported from the National Cancer Institute, has been the use of a sensitive antibody to the carboxy-terminal end of HCG to detect the presence of the hormone in concentrated 24-hour urine specimens. It has been stated that this technique is more sensitive than the standard blood radio-immunoassay, but further trials will be required to justify the claims (Javadpour, 1978).

Other markers

Although several tumour-associated antigens are being evaluated as potential markers of germ-cell tumours, the data available suggest that they will be of use only in a small proportion of patients.

Carcinoembryonic antigen has been shown to be produced by teratomas with gut-like differentiation (Heyderman, 1978). However, it does not reliably correlate with changes of tumour mass (Scardino *et al.*, 1977; Talerman, van der Pompe *et al.*, 1977; Wahren *et al.*, 1977) and its usefulness is thus limited.

A marker of placental tissue, SP_1 has been demonstrated immunocytochemically in teratomas (Heyderman, 1978) and has been shown to be present in elevated titres in the blood of up to 10 per cent of patients with malignant teratomas (Johnson *et al.*, 1977; Searle *et al.*, 1978; Rosen *et al.*, 1979). Of particular interest is the small proportion of patients with teratomas in whom circulating titres of SP_1 have been elevated in the absence of detectable HCG or AFP (Lange, personal communication).

Increased levels of serum ferritin (Wahren *et al.*, 1977) and lactate dehydrogenase (Von Eyben, 1978) have been shown to be associated with malignant teratomas, but have not yet been shown to be of major clinical value due to their lack of specificity. It may be that isoenzyme fractionation for both proteins will be needed to resolve this problem.

Placental alkaline phosphatase has been demonstrated in teratomas and in seminomas (Wahren, personal communication) and studies are required now to define its usefulness as a measure of tumour mass.

Although alpha$_1$-antitrypsin has been demonstrated in yolk-sac carcinomas, it has not yet been shown to occur in the absence of detectable alphafetoprotein (Talerman, Haije and Baggerman, 1977).

Methodology

Assay systems

Sensitive, accurate and reliable assay methods for tumour markers, particularly in the low ranges, are essential. Methods must be sufficiently sensitive to detect small but significant elevations of tumour markers, which in turn may allow the detection of minimal or subclinical tumour. The detection of tumour marker elevations, beginning to rise following a period of remission with normal levels, constitutes a valuable warning signal and can provide a useful diagnostic lead time. This in turn depends on the reliability and sensitivity of the technique used and an immunoassay suitable for monitoring progress and response to treatment must be capable of reliably estimating levels down to $<5\,\mu g/l$. Inter-laboratory and international quality control standards should be incorporated into reporting systems.

Current technology for AFP and HCG determination is based largely on radio-immunoassay methods, using the double antibody technique, solid phase or the polyethyleneglycol (PEG) precipitation assay. Recently, the enzyme-linked immunoassay has shown great promise. The more reliable the assay within these lower ranges, the more valuable the information obtained.

In teratomas, the interpretation of AFP levels is more complex than in cases of hepatocellular carcinoma, in which there is very little overlap with normal ranges; a considerable proportion of malignant teratomas is associated with relatively small increases of serum AFP, sometimes not exceeding $100\,\mu g/l$. Gel immunodiffusion techniques for AFP assay, with the exception of those using labelled antigens combined with autoradiography or enzyme activity estimation, are not suitable for the monitoring of malignant teratoma. They are not sufficiently sensitive to detect moderate elevations of marker levels which may well be a valuable warning signal. The type of assay used and the upper limit of the normal reference range adopted for the assay should be specified whenever results of an immunoassay are reported.

Frequency of sampling

Every patient with testicular tumour should have serial serum AFP and HCG assays performed at appropriate intervals, irrespective of the initial levels. Random specimens have only a very limited value for diagnosis and are of little use in management. Up to 50 per cent of marker-positive cases have been missed on single random assay, compared with those in which appropriately spaced multiple assays have been performed. Serum samples are more suitable than plasma. Correct labelling with exact and reliable dating are absolutely essential. A cumulative reporting system with a graphical display of both marker results is useful in monitoring the progress of disease and response to treatment. The first positive tumour marker result in any patient should always be checked and the assay repeated on a different sample to avoid clerical and laboratory errors. The same principle applies to obviously inconsistent results.

Sampling schedule

The details of the 'optimal' sampling schedule vary between centres, but the following general approach is now widely used.

1. Pre-operative specimens are essential to establish a baseline level—the collection of more than one specimen may help to assess the growth rate of the tumour. If a pre-operative serum sample is not available, an immediate postoperative specimen or one drawn during the operative procedure should be collected.

2. Following orchidectomy, samples should be collected twice weekly for at least two to three weeks in order to establish the rate of fall of the tumour markers and to assist in staging.

3. At the end of postoperative abdominal node irradiation or retroperitoneal node dissection, a sample should be collected to help to detect the presence of persistent metastases. If positive, the levels should be monitored regularly during further therapy. If negative, marker levels should be assayed nevertheless at each follow-up visit.

4. In patients receiving chemotherapy and/or further irradiation, levels should be checked prior to and during the course, at least once weekly up to the conclusion of the course, to monitor response.

5. Any rise of AFP or HCG in patients during remission requires an immediate check, and, if necessary, recommencement of more frequent serial assays, as above. The main objective should be to reduce the chance of missing small but significant rises which herald recurrence of the disease and thus provide a valuable lead-time.

Histology correlation

Synthesis of AFP occurs in the tumour cell itself, in the ribosomes of the rough endoplasmic reticulum (Urano et al., 1976). It has been confirmed also that pure yolk-sac tumours (endodermal sinus tumours) are associated usually with AFP synthesis and consequently with elevated serum AFP levels (Teilum et al., 1975; Grigor et al., 1977, Talerman, Haije and Baggerman, 1977; Tsuchida, Endo et al., 1978; Tsuchida, Kaneko et al., 1978). Teratomas frequently show differentiation into a variety of cell types, each of which may produce its own appropriate product. Tumours with classical choriocarcinomatous differentiation may secrete a range of placental hormones. Those with yolk sac elements may produce AFP and those with intestinal patterns of differentiation may produce CEA, or other membrane antigens (Heyderman, 1978).

Teratomas other than those containing classical vitelline (yolk-sac) elements may be capable also of producing AFP (Kurman et al., 1977). The levels will depend on the proportion of AFP-synthesizing elements within the tumour mass. If such regions are small, they may remain undetected, the minute amounts of the tumour marker produced being lost in the large plasma pool and escaping detection against the normal background level. Because of the polymorphic appearance of germ-cell tumours, elements which produce AFP may be present but not identified, due either to incomplete histological sampling, the histological criteria used, or lack of recognition of foci which may be small and scattered.

This may be the explanation for the occasional rare case of 'AFP-positive' seminomas which have been reported (Table 4.4). It must be stressed, however,

Table 4.4 Elevated markers in patients with seminoma

Series	AFP	(%)	HCG	(%)
Grigor et al. (1977)	0/016		—	
Lange*	0/37		6/31	(19)
Scardino et al. (1977)†	0/9		2/9	(22)
Javadpour, McIntire and Waldmann (1978)‡	0/130		10/130	(8)
Schultz, Sell et al. (1978) 1/33‡	(3)	0/33		
Mann, Lamerz et al. (1979)	0/137		21/137	(15)

* Personal communication.
† Note the discrepancies between small and large series from the same centre.
‡ Teratomatous focus not excluded.

that cases have been recorded in which, despite careful examination, no vitelline elements have been identified, although in most instances non-seminomatous metastases have been demonstrated subsequently. It has been postulated that multipotential undifferentiated cells may be capable of synthesizing AFP in these cases (Kohn et al., 1976). A third possibility is that some AFP-positive 'seminomas' represent histological variants of solid yolk-sac carcinoma.

Human chorionic gonadotrophin has been identified primarily within normal trophoblast and in choriocarcinomas. However, in a number of instances, elevations of HCG have been recorded in a variety of tumours in which no trophoblastic elements have been identified (Braunstein, Vaitukaitis et al., 1973; Table 4.4). 'HCG-positive' seminoma cases have been reported (Wilson and Woodhead, 1972; Heyderman, 1978) and although doubt has been expressed about the validity of the earlier cases (Cochran, 1976), Heyderman and Neville have shown the presence of HCG-positive giant cells within these tumours (Heyderman, 1978; see Chapter 3). It has been suggested also that some HCG-positive seminomas may represent a special type of tumour with a propensity to non-seminomatous transformation (Lange and Fraley, 1977).

The immunocytochemical demonstration of these tumour markers in the primary orchidectomy specimen is useful in the diagnosis and management of malignant testicular tumours. The demonstration of AFP or HCG positivity in tumour tissue can signal the most appropriate markers to follow clinically. Several prospective studies are underway to assess the prognostic significance of immunocytochemical positivity at diagnosis.

Another recently introduced technique permits the localization of AFP in tumour-tissue sections using 'radio-rocket' immuno-electrophoresis, particularly useful for cytological smears and tissue imprints (Norgaard-Pedersen, personal communication; Fig. 4.1).

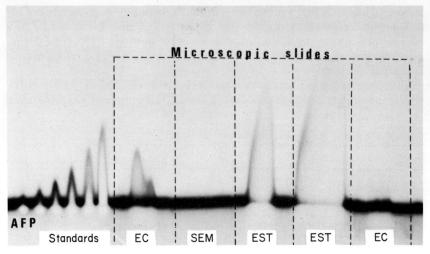

Fig. 4.1 Autoradiography of 'radiotissue immunoelectrophoresis' (RTIE) of 5μ-thick cryostat-cut tumour tissue specimens from patient with EC (embryonal carcinoma, MTU), SE (seminoma), EST (endodermal sinus tumour of infantile testis and sacrococcygeal region). Microscopic slides with the tissue specimens were placed directly upon a gel for radiorocket immunoelectrophoresis (Norgaard-Pedersen *et al.*, 1980).

Incidence of marker positivity

The incidence of elevation of levels of tumour markers reported in patients with malignant teratoma depends upon:

   i. the sensitivity of the assay technique;
   ii. the method and nature of the assay;
   iii. the frequency at which the assay is performed;
   iv. the time of sampling in relation to the course of the disease (i.e. pre-orchidectomy, pre-lymphadenectomy, etc.);
   v. the upper limit of normal range adopted;
   vi. the number of patients investigated;
   vii. the referral pattern and scope of the practice;
   viii. patient selection, i.e. patients with active disease versus the total numbers of patients seen.

Many reported studies have been performed at referral centres and their figures reflect marker values obtained only after removal of the primary tumour. Discrepancies in the figures reported by various authors (see Table 4.3) are due mainly to the factors listed above. Incidence figures for AFP and HCG positivity (i.e. the presence of elevated levels of these substances in the circulation) range from 35 to 70 per cent and, with the simultaneous measurement of both markers by radio-immunoassay, elevated levels have been reported in as many as 90 per cent of patients—this value reflecting advanced active disease (Lange and Fraley, 1977; Scardino *et al.*, 1977). In series where the distinction is made between active and inactive disease, marker positivity is much higher in the group with demonstrable disease. Similarly, in our practice and in reported series, patients with advanced disease appear to have a higher incidence of elevated marker levels (Scardino *et al.*, 1977; and see Chapter 15).

Stoichiometry

Although the ideal tumour marker should correlate with tumour bulk, in the clinical setting an exact tumour 'bulk:marker' ratio is usually difficult to define. The major problem is heterogeneity of tumour tissue—with varying proportions of stroma, necrotic tissue, cystic spaces and neoplastic tissue, this variability being a particular feature of malignant teratomas (Raghaven *et al.*, 1979).

In addition, it has been reported that the rate of production of tumour markers *in vitro* is dependent upon the stage of the cell cycle (Burk and Drewinko, 1976). Nevertheless, there is a striking relationship at the clinical level between tumour volume and serum marker levels (see Chapter 15).

It has been shown that in a tissue culture system the amount of HCG synthesized per cell varies with cell density (Kohler *et al.*, 1971). If the results of these tissue culture studies can be extrapolated to the clinical setting, they raise further problems in defining a true stoichiometric relationship.

Experiments in animal model systems and tissue culture have shown that marker production may be influenced directly by chemotherapeutic agents (see Chapter 5), which further complicates the issue.

Notwithstanding these problems, Bagshawe has attempted to define HCG output per unit mass of tumour in gestational choriocarcinoma (Bagshawe, 1969). In one study, blood HCG levels were related to the volume of excised tumour, and another series of experiments assessed HCG production by placental trophoblast and choriocarcinoma grown in tissue culture. Both methods gave values between 10^{-4} and 10^{-5} iu HCG/cell per day (although it should be noted that the results were obtained before the introduction of the beta-subunit radio-immunoassay technique). Thus a value of 5×10^{-5} iu HCG/day produced by each active cell would imply that a tumour producing 10 iu HCG/day contains 2×10^5 active cells (with an estimated volume of about 0.1 mm^3). The most useful concept to arise from these studies is that, in this situation, a patient with normal titres of HCG after treatment still may have several thousand occult tumour cells and that therapy should be continued beyond this time (Bagshawe, 1969). In cases where a clearly defined marker response has occurred, the curve of HCG decline can be extrapolated to define projected end-point of therapy. Although this concept is useful, it should be noted that gestational trophoblastic tumours are morphologically a more homogeneous group than are malignant teratomas and that the correlation is less well defined in the latter (Raghaven *et al.*, 1979).

Interpretation and clinical management

Germ-cell tumours, by the very nature of their origin, have a mixed cellular population that may be derived from each of the three germinal layers. Some tumours synthesize AFP or HCG, or both, but a proportion of them produce no known markers. Thus, marker protein assays reflect only the synthesizing capacity of the marker-producing elements and not the behaviour of the tumour as a whole. It appears that HCG and AFP are found in, and synthesized by, different cell types (Kurman *et al.*, 1977; Heyderman, 1978). These factors explain the clinical situation of a patient with static or advancing disease despite falling markers—the marker-producing elements in this case being responsive to therapy and the non-synthesizing cells being resistant (Raghaven *et al.*, 1979).

Similarly, the phenomenon of discordance (Braunstein, McIntire and Waldmann, 1973; Lange *et al.*, 1976; Raghaven *et al.*, 1979)—in which one tumour marker rises while the other falls or remains unchanged—can be explained on the basis of treatment affecting one cell population and not the other (Fig. 4.2). This aspect and attempts to assess the relative chemosensitivity of marker and non-marker producing elements are discussed in Chapter 15.

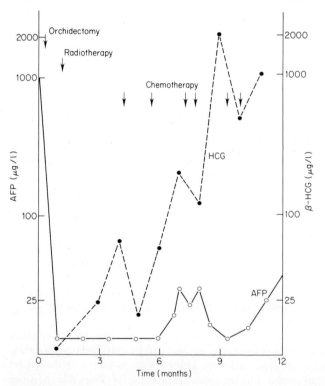

Fig. 4.2 Discrepancy between AFP and HCG levels in a patient with testicular teratoma after orchidectomy and during treatment. Note marked rise of HCG levels in spite of treatment.

As discussed above, because of the histological heterogeneity of malignant teratomas, no completely accurate assessment of tumour mass *per se* can be made from marker data.

Nevertheless, a general correlation between stage of disease and proportion of marker-positive patients has been demonstrated (Kohn *et al.*, 1976; Schultz, Sell *et al.*, 1978; and see Chapter 15).

Staging

Correct staging is a fundamental problem, as successful treatment of patients with malignant teratoma depends upon accurate staging before the choice of therapy.

Staging procedures usually are undertaken after orchidectomy (when the initial diagnosis of germ-cell malignancy is made) and are discussed in Chapters 7, 8 and 9

An area of controversy has been the relevance of marker proteins in the staging of disease and in particular with reference to 'Stage I' disease. By definition, Stage I refers to tumour clinically confined to the testis, implying the absence of tumour after orchidectomy. Thus, the persistence of elevated titres of AFP and/or HCG after orchidectomy implies either:

    i. a point on the natural elimination curve of the protein, consistent with its physiological half-life; or
    ii. the persistence of tumour after orchidectomy, altering the true stage from I to II, III or IV.

Many retrospective studies have analysed the significance of Stage I marker-positive teratomas without having restricted the definition to 'pre-orchidectomy marker-positivity' and thus have introduced a bias by including some cases that are in fact Stage II (at least).

It has been shown, however, that the error of conventional staging procedures can be reduced substantially by including routine marker determination to help to separate Stage I from more advanced stages of disease (Lange et al., 1977; Scardino et al., 1977; Anderson et al., 1979). These studies have been supported by the results of retroperitoneal node dissections, where retroperitoneal metastases have been found in cases in which the pre-operative marker levels were elevated but in which conventional staging investigations (including lymphography) were negative (Anderson et al., 1979).

A 'dissection' of clinical stage malignant teratomas which includes an analysis of marker pattern is described in Chapter 13.

It should be re-emphasized that normal marker levels do not exclude the presence of active disease, as non-synthesizing clones of cells may be present (Raghavan et al., 1979).

In addition to the application to initial staging, the measurement of marker status is important in defining the subsequent response to therapy and the status of disease upon completion of treatment. The persistence of elevated markers upon completion of abdominal irradiation or after retroperitoneal node dissection must be regarded as an indication of residual abdominal disease, or occult metastases, most commonly in the lungs, liver or supra-diaphragmatic nodes.

In our experience, no patient with a persistently elevated AFP titre has failed to show clinical evidence of active tumour, either at the time of the first marker elevation or subsequently.

In about 20 per cent of patients in clinical remission, clinically detectable recurrence may be preceded by a rise of marker levels from 4 to 36 weeks, with a mean of 15 weeks (Kohn, 1976; Grigor et al., 1977; Lange and Fralcy, 1977). However, we have also seen clinical recurrence preceding marker elevation.

It is our belief that persistently rising levels of either HCG or AFP constitute an indication for further therapy, even in the absence of measurable disease according to conventional criteria. Of course, in this context, other causes of marker elevation must be excluded.

Tissue fluids

The utility of marker protein estimations is not restricted to the blood. Elevations of AFP or HCG may be detected in pleural fluid, ascitic fluid and CSF (Yoshiki *et al.*, 1976; Kaye *et al.*, 1979) and often denote the presence of metastatic disease.

Human chorionic gonadotrophin has been of particular use in the management of central nervous system metastases in gestational choriocarcinoma. The two causes of elevated CSF gonadotrophin levels are (i) local disease; and (ii) passive diffusion resulting from grossly elevated blood levels (Bagshawe and Harland, 1976). A blood : CSF ratio can be calculated and values less than 40 suggest the presence of CNS disease. However, a ratio greater than 40 does not exclude the possibility of disease in the central nervous system and it may be necessary to initiate treatment and achieve normal blood levels before attempting to further define the ratio. The problems of interpretation that arise in this situation are the possible lowering of CSF gonadotrophin levels (with decreasing tumour bulk in the CNS) as a result of treatment, and the possible lag phase when diffusion of HCG out of the cerebrospinal fluid lags behind the rate of lowering of blood HCG in response to therapy.

Although these principles can be applied to malignant trophoblastic teratoma and occult brain metastases, the results appear somewhat less reliable, due primarily to the microscopical heterogeneity of these tumours.

Limited evidence available suggests that AFP is of less value in detecting or monitoring CNS metastatic disease as the correlation of increased CSF alphafetoprotein and the presence of malignant disease in the central nervous system is less reliable (Kaye *et al.*, 1979). However, only a small number of patients with cerebral metastases was reported and the series was weighted in favour of MTT histology (it should be noted that central nervous system metastases from teratoma occur most commonly in this histological subtype). The true role of alphafetoprotein in the management of nervous system metastases remains uncertain and will require a more extensive study of patients with tumour elements known to be associated with AFP production (such as yolk-sac tumour).

Marker patterns

Several patterns of behaviour of marker proteins have been noted in cases of germ-cell malignancy.

1. A large group in whom markers, according to current assay systems, remain consistently negative throughout the course of disease; it is in this group that efforts to define new tumour markers may be of particular value.

2. Patients in whom markers are initially positive and fall following surgery or another modality of treatment; these are particularly well suited to follow-

up screening in order to achieve early detection of recurrent disease. In these patients the rate of fall of marker levels is particularly important and will be discussed later.

3. A group of patients in whom marker proteins remain positive throughout the course of their disease. As a group, their prognosis is worse, correlating with continued tumour presence resulting in persistent marker detection.

4. A heterogenous set of patients in whom no clear pattern emerges—levels either fluctuate with therapy or are completely independent of outside intervention. Patients in whom marker levels remain persistently raised, notwithstanding fluctuations, eventually show evidence of recurrent disease. Occasionally, a transient rise in marker levels that subsides spontaneously is observed. This may represent either laboratory error, sampling problems or, rarely, spontaneous tumour regression.

5. Patients in whom marker estimations were initially negative, who subsequently develop elevated levels. The mechanism for this is not yet certain but may be related to the development of a new marker-secreting clone of cells, or may reflect changes in the kinetics or metabolism of the cell that allow marker production. The fact that this phenomenon occurs is one justification for continuing to screen patients in the first category above. Although the appearance of marker-producing clones *per se* has not been shown definitely to be of adverse prognostic significance, the appearance of a new line of cells (despite therapy) seems ominous.

6. A small group of patients who show a terminal rise in marker levels.

Summarizing, malignant testicular teratoma can produce elevated levels of AFP or HCG at any time during the course of the disease. Tumours which originally produce marker proteins may recur without an associated elevation in blood levels, and tumours which initially show no evidence of marker production may be accompanied by high serum levels when recurrence occurs. This lack of correlation may be explained by histological differences between primary tumour and metastases and reflects the different populations of cells dominating at any time. Although marker proteins are most useful as an adjunct to the monitoring of clinical progress, they cannot be used in isolation from clinical measurement and other diagnostic procedures.

Apparent half-life

In the management of these tumours, the absolute level of marker proteins is often not as important as the trends in levels on serial assays. A helpful concept in the management of testicular teratoma is the calculation of the apparent half-life (AHL) of a marker protein in the patient's blood (Kohn, 1979). This is an expression of the rate of elimination of that protein from the blood after a therapeutic procedure. Thus, if all the marker-producing bulk is destroyed by therapy, the serum marker protein level would be expected to decline exponentially according to the curve of its natural half-life. If, however, marker-producing elements remain upon completion of therapy, the curve of decline of marker protein is modified by continued production.

Alphafetoprotein, with its natural half-life of five days, is more useful in this context as it is less likely to be affected by external factors (such as exact sampling time) than is HCG (with a half-life of twenty-four to thirty-six hours). The AHL for alphafetoprotein is calculated from sequential assays by the formula:

$$AHL = \frac{-0.3 \times T}{\log_{10}(\text{conc. }T/\text{conc. }O)}$$

where T is the time interval between assays in days, conc. O is the initial concentration of AFP in $\mu g/l$, and conc. T is the concentration after time interval T. The AHL is expressed in days and is thus readily comparable with the true half-life value. A value of AHL greater than seven days implies the

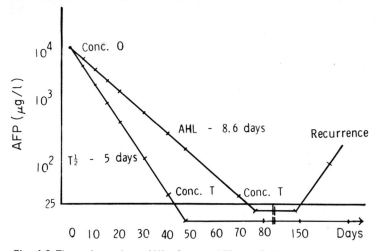

Fig. 4.3 The patient whose AHL of serum AFP was 5 days shows no recurrence to date. The other patient, with an AHL of 8.6 days, showed a recurrent elevation of serum AFP levels and a clinical relapse.

persistence of tumour and, in our preliminary studies, correlates with subsequent relapse (Raghavan *et al.*, 1979; Fig. 4.3). A similar formula has been derived from HCG (Lange and Fraley, 1977).

The reliability of the calculation is primarily dependent upon the correct recording of the collection time of the specimen and the accuracy of the assay system.

It is possible that the slope of the AHL curve provides more relevant information regarding progress of the disease and response to treatment than do the actual levels plotted on a graph. Increasingly abnormal AHL may be the first indication of treatment failure (and tumour proliferation), preceding both AFP rise and clinical tumour recurrence by several weeks (Kohn, 1979; Thompson and Haddow, 1979).

A similar concept has been reported to be helpful in assessing the prognosis of hepatocellular carcinoma (Mukojima *et al.*, 1973) and in the management of germ-cell tumours in children (Ratcliffe *et al.*, 1978).

The AHL determination can be made at any point during the course of treatment and, by extrapolation, may be useful in establishing the pre-operative AFP levels when pre-orchidectomy specimens are not available.

It has been reported that intensive therapy does not appear to be followed by significant elevations of AFP levels (Thompson and Haddow, 1979)—release phenomenon—in comparison to gestational choriocarcinoma. This issue is important, as any effect of therapy itself on the tumour marker levels (e.g. causing transient elevation) could influence the interpretation of the results.

Prognosis

The exact role of marker proteins in defining prognosis in malignant germ-cell neoplasms is not certain. It has been suggested that patients with elevated levels of AFP have a less favourable prognosis than those with normal levels (Talerman, 1975), but this could be due to the greater 'malignancy' of yolk-sac tumours compared with other histological types (Parkinson and Beilby, 1977) or, alternatively, may simply reflect greater tumour bulk. Similarly, HCG has been reported to correlate with poor prognosis and probably relates to the association of HCG and trophoblastic histology.

In our experience with 59 Stage I patients (see Chapter 13) in whom tissue was available for immunocytochemical staining, the presence of positive staining for HCG appeared to be of no prognostic significance. In this study, tissue staining for AFP was not performed (see Chapter 3) and it should be noted that no patients had trophoblastic (MTT) histology. By studying patients with Stage I disease, we attempted to separate tumour-marker positivity *per se* from tumour mass. Although in this series the presence of raised pre-orchidectomy HCG and AFP did not appear to be of major prognostic significance, there was unequivocal evidence that a delay in the rate of decline of the circulating levels of these proteins correlated with worse prognosis in terms of relapse and survival. Delay in the post-orchidectomy rate of decline of tumour markers in the blood implies occult metastatic disease and thus a worse prognosis.

Similar data have been produced from the National Cancer Institute (Scardino *et al.*, 1977), patients with elevated post-orchidectomy levels having a 67 per cent recurrence rate, as compared with 4 per cent in patients with normal levels, although decay rates of circulating markers were not taken into account.

With respect to seminoma, the presence of AFP at any point during the course of disease is taken usually to imply the presence of teratomatous elements, thus worsening the prognosis. However, the situation regarding HCG-positive seminomas is not clear and although there are reports that they are less responsive to treatment (Wilson and Woodhead, 1972), prospective trials are under way to evaluate this further. The question of whether one should regard HCG-positive seminomas functionally as teratomas remains unanswered at this time.

Future prospects

New markers

Although AFP and HCG titres correlate with the clinical course of most malignant teratomas, from 10 to 30 per cent of these tumours are 'silent'

(Raghaven *et al.*, 1979). This may reflect the cellular kinetics of these tumours, but it is also possible that the cells present do not carry genomes for the production of AFP or HCG.

There is a continuing search for new markers which may represent these non-secreting tumours. As noted previously, SP_1 (a marker of placental tissue) has been shown to be present in the sera of patients with testicular teratomas and some of these patients have not had detectable levels of AFP or HCG.

The study of the mouse teratocarcinoma has identified placental alkaline phosphatase as a possible marker for human germ-cell tumours, and this is under clinical evaluation.

Similarly, in the mouse teratocarcinoma model, surface markers such as the F9 antigen have been defined. F9 antigenic determinants have been demonstrated in human teratoma tissues (Hogan *et al.*, 1977; Holden *et al.*, 1977), but their possible roles as diagnostic or prognostic factors remain to be determined (see Chapter 5).

It is possible, nevertheless, that the use of those cell-surface markers in the management of human teratomas will be as useful as in leukaemia and lymphoma, particularly in tumours which are undifferentiated at the light microscope level.

Tumour localization

Goldenberg *et al.* (1978) have demonstrated in animal models and in human studies that it is possible to use labelled anti-CEA antibodies to localize deposits of CEA-producing tumours. The technique involves conjugation of the antibody with a radionucleide (such as ^{125}I) and the use of radiolabelled ^{131}I albumin and subtraction scanning procedures to eliminate the blood pool background on a computer print-out or screen.

Efforts are being directed now at the application of these methods to marker-producing germ-cell tumours in an effort to improve diagnosis of occult metastatic disease.

Therapy

In addition to the developments in the range and combinations of chemotherapeutic agents and other treatment modalities, there is increasing investigation of the mode of delivery of drugs to the sites of tumour. Antibodies against tumour cell-surface antigens have been used as carriers of cytotoxic agents in an attempt to increase their specificity (Ghose and Blair, 1978). However, many problems remain—for example, uncertainty with respect to therapeutically effective doses, cross-reactivity of antibodies, and possible inactivation of the drugs by the drug–antibody binding procedures.

Summary

Marker proteins provide a valuable aid in the management of testicular teratomas, as indicators of occult disease and monitors of response to therapy. Alphafetoprotein and human chorionic gonadotrophin are the two most useful available markers and may be found in up to 90 per cent of patients with these tumours. Although there is some evidence that the presence of marker proteins is of prognostic importance, the final definition of their role in this context will await the outcome of prospective trials currently in progress. Future developments in this field are likely to include the development of new diagnostic markers, the use of these proteins in tumour localization and possibly the clinical application of drug–antibody complexes in the therapy of malignant germ-cell tumours.

References

Asterisk indicates publications referred to on page 50

*Abelev, G. I. (1974). Transplantation Reviews 20, 3.

*Anderson, T., Waldmann, T. A. Javadpour, N. and Glatstein, E. (1979). Annals of Internal Medicine 90, 373.

Bagshawe, K. D. (1969). In Choriocarcinoma: the Clinical Biology of the Trophoblast and Its Tumours, p. 153. Edward Arnold, London.

*Bagshawe, K. D. and Harland, S. (1976). Cancer 38, 112.

*Bagshawe, K. D. and Searle, F. (1977). In Essays in Medical Biochemistry, p. 25. The Biochemical Society and the Association of Clinical Biochemists, London.

*Barzell, W. E. and Whitmore, W. F. Jr (1979). Seminars in Oncology 6, 48.

*Braunstein, G. D., McIntire, K. R. and Waldmann, T. A. (1973). Cancer 31, 1065.

Braunstein, G. D., Rasor, J. and Wade, M. E. (1975). New England Journal of Medicine 293, 1339.

*Braunstein, G. D., Vaitukaitis, J. L., Carbonne, P. P. and Ross, G. T. (1973). Annals of Internal Medicine 78, 39.

Burk, K. H. and Drewinko, B. (1976). Cancer Research 36, 3535.

Chen, H. C., Hodgen, G. D., Matsuura, S., Liu, L. J., Gross, E., Reichert, L. E. Jr., Birken, S., Canfield, R. E. and Ross, G. T. (1976). Proceedings of the National Academy of Science, (USA) 73, 2885.

Cochran, J. S. (1976). Journal of Urology 116, 465.

Ghose, T. and Blair, A. H. (1978). Journal of the National Cancer Institute 61, 657.

Gitlin, D. and Boesman, M. (1966). Journal of Clinical Investigation 45, 1826.

Goldenberg, D. M., De Land, F., Kim, E., Bennett, S., Primus, F. J., Van Nagell, J. R. Jr., Estes, N., Desimone, P. and Rayburn, P. (1978). New England Journal of Medicine 298, 1384.

Grigor, K. M., Detre, S. I., Kohn, J. and Neville, A. M. (1977). British Journal of Cancer 35, 52.

Heyderman, E. (1978). Scandinavian Journal of Immunology 8 (8), 119.

Hirai, H., Nishi, S. and Watabe, H. (1972). GANN Monograph of Cancer Research 14, 19.

Hogan, B., Fellous, M., Avner, P. and Jacob, F. (1977). Nature 270, 515.

Holden, S., Bernard, O., Artzt, K., Whitmore, W. F. Jr. and Bennett, D. (1977). Nature 270, 518.

*Javadpour, N. (1978). Journal of Urology 120, 651.

*Javadpour, N. and Bergman, S. (1978). Current Problems in Surgery 150, 1.

*Javadpour, N., McIntire, K. R. and Waldman, T. A. (1978). Cancer 42, 2768.

*Javadpour, N., McIntire, K. R., Waldmann, T. A., Scardino, P. T., Bergman, S. and Anderson, T. (1978). Journal of Urology 119, 759.

*Johnson, S. A. N., Grudzinskas, J. G., Gordon, Y. B. and Al-Ani, A. T. M. (1977). British Medical Journal 1, 951.

Kawamura, J., Machida, S., Yoshida, O., Oseko, F., Imura, H. and Hattori, M. (1978). Cancer 42, 2773.

*Kaye, S. B., Bagshawe, K. D., McElwain, T. J. and Peckham, M. J. (1979). British Journal of Cancer 39, 217.

Kohler, P. O., Bridson, W. E., Hammond, J. M., Weintraub, B., Kirschner, M. A. and Van Thiel, D. H. (1971). Acta Endocrinologica (Supplement) 153, 137.

*Kohn, J. (1976). In Onco-Developmental Gene Expression, p. 387. Ed. by W. H. Fishman and S. Sell. Academic Press, New York and London.

*Kohn, J. (1978). *Scandinavian Journal of Immunology* **8 (8)**, 103.

*Kohn, J. (1979). In *Carcino-Embryonic Proteins: Chemistry Biology, Clinical Application,* Vol. II, p. 383. Ed. by F. G. Lehmann. Elsevier/North Holland, Amsterdam.

*Kohn, J., Orr, A. H., McElwain, T. J., Bentall, M. and Peckham, M. J. (1976). *Lancet* **ii**, 433.

*Kurman, R. J., Scardino, P. T., McIntire, K. R., Waldmann, T. A. and Javadpour, N. (1977). *Cancer* **40**, 2136.

*Lange, P. H. (1978). *National Cancer Institute Monograph* **49**, 215.

*Lange, P. H. and Fraley, E. E. (1977). *Urological Clinics of North America* **4**, 393.

*Lange, P. H., McIntire, K. R., Waldmann, T. A., Hakala, T. R. and Fraley, E. E. (1976). *New England Journal of Medicine* **295**, 1237.

*Lange, P. H., McIntire, K. R., Waldmann, T. A., Hakala, T. R. and Fraley, E. E. (1977). *Journal of Urology* **118**, 593.

*Mann, K., Lamerz, R., Staehler, G., Lieven, H. V. and Karl, H. J. (1979). In *Carcino-Embryonic Proteins: Chemistry, Biology, Clinical Application,* Vol. II, p. 771. Ed. by F. G. Lehmann, Elsevier/North Holland, Amsterdam.

*Moore, M. R., Garrett, P. R., Walton, K. N., Waldmann, T. A., McIntire, K. R., Counts, P. and Vogel, C. L. (1978). *Surgery, Gynecology and Obstetrics* **147**, 167.

Mukojima, T., Hattori, N., Nakayama, N., Hasegawa, H., Ohkura, H. and Kitaoka, H. (1973). *Tumour Research* **8**, 194.

*Newlands, E. S., Dent, J., Kardana, A., Searle, F. and Bagshawe, K. D. (1976). *Lancet* **ii**, 744.

*Nørgaard-Pedersen, B. *et al.* (1978). *Lancet* **ii**, 1042.

Nørgaard-Pedersen, B., Toftager-Larsen, K., Nørregaard Hansen, K. and Albrechtsen, R. (1980). *Investigative Cell Pathology* **3**, 147–150.

Parkinson, C. and Beilby, J. O. W. (1977). *Journal of Clinical Pathology* **30**, 113.

*Perlin, E., Engeler, J. E., Edson, M., Karp, D., McIntire, K. R. and Waldmann, T. A. (1976). *Cancer* **37**, 215.

*Raghavan, D., Gibbs, J., Nogueira-Costa, R., Kohn, J., Orr, A. H., Barrett, A. and Peckham, M. J. (1980). *British Journal of Cancer* **41**, Supplement IV, pp. 191–194.

*Ratcliffe, J. G., Burt, R. W., Baird, G. M., Campbell, A. M., Barter, D. A. C. and Willoughby, M. L. N. (1978). *Scandinavian Journal of Immunology* **8 (8)**, 143.

*Rosen, S. W., Javadpour, N., Calvert, I. and Kaminska, J. (1979). *Journal of the National Cancer Institute* **62**, 1439.

Ruoslahti, E. and Adamson, E. (1978). *Biochemical and Biophysical Research Communications* **85**, 1622.

*Rutanen, E. M. and Seppala, M. (1978). *Cancer* **41**, 692.

*Scardino, P. T., Cox, H. D., Waldmann, T. A., McIntire, K. R., Mittemeyer, B. and Javadpour, N. (1977). *Journal of Urology* **118**, 994.

*Schultz, H., Arends, J., Brincker, H., Jensen, T. S., Norgaard-Pedersen, B., Sell, A. and Steenholdt, S. (1978). *Scandinavian Journal of Immunology* **8 (8)**.

*Schultz, H., Sell, A., Norgaard-Pedersen, B. and Arends, J. (1978). *Cancer* **42**, 2182.

*Searle, F., Leake, B. A., Bagshawe, K. D. and Dent, J. (1978). *Lancet* **i**, 579.

*Seppala, M. and Ruoslahti, E. (1972). *Lancet* **i**, 375.

Sizaret, P. (1979). *Clinica Chimica Acta* **96**, 59.

*Talerman, A. (1975). *Cancer* **36**, 211.

*Talerman, A., Haije, W. G. and Baggerman, L. (1977). *International Journal of Cancer* **19**, 741.

Talerman, A., Van der Pompe, W. B., Haije, W. H., Baggerman, L. and Boekestein-Tjahjadi, H. M. (1977). *British Journal of Cancer* **35**, 288.

Teilum, G., Albrechtsen, R. and Norgaard-Pedersen, B. (1975). *Acta Pathologica et Microbiologia Scandinavica* (Section A) **83**, 80.

*Thompson, D. K. and Haddow, J. E. (1979). *Cancer* **43**, 1820.

*Tsuchida, Y., Endo, Y., Saito, S., Kaneko, N., Shiraki, K. and Ohmi, K. (1978). *Journal of Pediatric Surgery* **13**, 155.

*Tsuchida, Y., Kaneko, M., Yokomori, K., Saito, S., Urano, Y., Endo, Y., Asaka, T. and Takeuchi, T. (1978). *Journal of Pediatric Surgery* **13**, 25.

*Urano, Y., Endo, Y. and Tsuchida, Y. (1976). In *Onco-Developmental Gene Expression,* p. 131. Ed. by W. H. Fishman and S. Sell. Academic Press, New York.

*Vaitukaitis, J. L. (1979a). In *Carcino-Embryonic Proteins: Chemistry, Biology, Clinical Application,* p. 447. Ed. by F. G. Lehmann. Elsevier/North Holland, Amsterdam.

*Vaitukaitis, J. L. (1979b). *New England Journal of Medicine* **301**, 324.
*Vaitukaitis, J. L., Braunstein, G. D. and Ross, G. T. (1972). *American Journal of Obstetrics and Gynecology* **112**, 751.
*Von Eyben, F. E. (1978). *Cancer* **41**, 648.
*Wahren, B., Alpert, E., Esposti, P. (1977). *Journal of the National Cancer Institute* **58**, 489.
*Wahren, B. and Edsmyr, F. (1974). *International Journal of Cancer* **14**, 207.
*Wahren, B. and Edsmyr, F. (1976). *International Journal of Radiation Oncology, Biology and Physics* **1**, 279.
*Wilson, J. M. and Woodhead, D. M. (1972). *Journal of Urology* **108**, 754.
Yoshiki, T., Itoh, T., Shirai, T., Noro, T., Tomino, Y., Hamajima, I. and Takeda, T. (1976). *Cancer* **37**, 2343.
Yoshimoto, Y., Wolfsen, A. R. and Odell, W. D. (1977). *Science* **197**, 575.

5

Testicular tumour xenografts and other experimental models

Derek Raghavan and Peter J. Selby

Introduction

Three models have been used to study the biology of human germ-cell tumours—animal teratomas, human tissue culture lines and human tumour xenografts in immune-deficient animals. In this chapter, we briefly review the features and uses of these systems, with an emphasis on the xenograft model.

Animal tumours

After the initial demonstration of spontaneous testicular teratomas occurring in the inbred mouse strain 129 with a frequency of about 1 per cent (Stevens and Little, 1954), a programme of research at the Jackson Laboratories, Maine, led to the development of the inbred strains 129/ter SV (Stevens, 1973) and LT/SV (Stevens and Varnum, 1974) with greater than 30 per cent incidence of spontaneous congenital testicular and ovarian teratomas respectively. The high incidence of tumours in these sublines may result from mutation of a single gene (Stevens, 1973).

In addition, teratomas have been induced artificially by the transplantation of genital ridges to the testes and epididymi in 129-strain mice (Stevens, 1964; Stevens, 1967a) and by the syngeneic transplantation of post-gastrulation embryos to extra-uterine sites in other strains of mice and in hamsters (Damjanov and Solter; 1974; Damjanov, 1978). Yolk-sac tumours have been induced in rats by fetectomy in which the fetal membranes are left trailing into the abdominal cavity after the procedure (Sakashita *et al.*, 1976; Sobis and Vandeputte, 1974; 1976; 1977; 1979) and by the injection of murine sarcoma virus into fetoplacental tissue (Sobis and Vandeputte, 1973). Finally, teratomas have been induced by the injection of metallic salts into the testes of cockerels during a period of artificial hormonal stimulation, or in the midst of the seasonal growth period (Carleton *et al.*, 1953; Damjanov, 1978; Michalowsky, 1979).

The establishment of reproducible animal models of germ-cell tumours has facilitated their study and characterization *in vivo* and *in vitro*. Marked similarities have been demonstrated between the undifferentiated cells of animal and human teratomas and between these tumour cells and normal, uncommitted embryonic cells. Primordial germ cells from 129-strain teratomas have been shown to be 'multipotent' (i.e. to be able to differentiate into cells of any of the

70

three germ layers) both *in vivo* (Pierce and Dixon, 1959a; Kleinsmith and Pierce, 1964) and *in vitro* (Kahan and Ephrussi, 1970; Rosenthal *et al.*, 1970; Martin and Evans, 1975), a property shared by uncommitted embryonic cells, although not all cells in a tumour have the same potential for differentiation (Pierce and Dixon, 1959a; Kahan and Ephrussi, 1970). In addition, phenotypically normal mice with a mosaic genetic structure have been produced by the injection of teratocarcinoma cells into normal blastocysts (Mintz and Illmensee, 1975) and normal embryoid bodies have been shown to be formed from malignant cells under the appropriate culture conditions (Martin and Evans, 1975). The important implications of these data are that the malignant change which teratocarcinoma cells have undergone is a reversible phenomenon and that the cells retain the capacity to differentiate normally.

Mouse embryonal carcinoma cells share common cell-surface antigenic determinants—the so-called F9 antigen (Artzt *et al.*, 1973) and perhaps others—with normal, uncommitted embryonic cells. The F9 antigen was found originally to be present on the surface of a cell line (the F9 line) derived from a 129-strain mouse teratocarcinoma. It can be recognized by antisera raised in normal adult 129-strain mice—which are thus not immunologically tolerant to it. However, F9 antigenic activity is present in male 129-strain mouse germ cells throughout adult life. It appears on mouse embryos soon after fertilization, but disappears from somatic cells after two weeks of intra-uterine life. The antigen is found also on human teratoma cells and normal human spermatozoa (see below).

Both embryonal carcinoma cells and uncommitted embryonic cells are able to produce biochemical substances such as alkaline phosphatase (Bernstine *et al.*, 1973) and alphafetoprotein (Kahan and Levine, 1971; Engelhardt *et al.*, 1973). Similarly, induced rat yolk-sac tumours have been shown to produce alphafetoprotein and other protein substances in common with normal embryos and murine teratomas (Sakashita *et al.*, 1976; Albrechtsen *et al.*, 1978; Endo *et al.*, 1978) and to share common surface antigens that have not yet been fully characterized (Van Hove *et al.*, 1978; Sobis *et al.*, 1979). The significance of these findings is somewhat puzzling, as mouse teratomas have been shown to be of germ-cell origin (Stevens, 1967b), whereas rat yolk-sac tumours appear to derive from visceral yolk-sac tissue rather than germ cells (Sobis and Vandeputte, 1976).

Perhaps of more direct relevance to cancer therapy have been preliminary studies of the effects of chemotherapy on mouse teratocarcinomas, which have demonstrated growth delay and changes in differentiation, both of which were highly variable in different tumours tested (Aldrich and Stevens, 1967; Mount *et al.*, 1970). 5-Fluorouracil was shown to prevent tumour growth when injected within twenty-four hours of genital-ridge grafting (Aldrich and Stevens, 1967), and in a comparison of a single agent (actinomycin-D) with a four-drug regimen (fluorouracil, vincristine, methotrexate and cyclophosphamide) it was shown that the combination produced a greater effect on the incidence, diameter and differentiation of tumour foci and that a course of single-agent injections produced a greater effect than a single dose (Mount *et al.*, 1970).

Human teratoma cell lines in tissue culture

Notwithstanding the extensive characterization of the animal teratoma models, there has been concern that they may not adequately represent the human disease state and attempts have been made to study human germ-cell tissues in culture systems.

The study of cell culture of normal placenta and normal yolk-sac have demonstrated histopathological and functional similarities between these tissues and their malignant equivalents, choriocarcinoma and yolk-sac tumours (Gey *et al.*, 1938; Patillo and Gey., 1968; Gitlin and Perricelli, 1970; Stromberg *et al.*, 1978), particularly with respect to the nature and sites of production of marker substances such as HCG and AFP. These markers have been shown to be important in the monitoring of germ-cell tumour therapy (see Chapter 4) and accordingly several lines of gestational choriocarcinoma have been established and studied *in vitro* in an effort to characterize tumour-marker production and the effects of chemotherapeutic agents on the marker-producing cell populations (Patillo and Gey, 1968; Kohler *et al.*, 1971; Bagshawe, 1973; Hussa *et al.*, 1973; Speeg *et al.*, 1976; Stromberg *et al.*, 1978). A stoichiometric relationship has been demonstrated in tissue culture between tumour cell mass of gestational choriocarcinoma and HCG production, with each cell producing an estimated 10^{-4} to 10^{-5} units of HCG per day, but varying with culture conditions and the kinetics of the cell populations (Bagshawe, 1973). Other workers have shown also that cell density and kinetics markedly alter cellular production of marker proteins in culture systems (Kohler *et al.*, 1971; Speeg *et al.*, 1976) and that chemotherapeutic agents themselves may increase cellular HCG production by choriocarcinoma cells—for example, actinomycin-D and methotrexate (Hussa *et al.*, 1973; Speeg *et al.*, 1976). However, this effect has not been demonstrated for normal trophoblastic cells in culture (Stromberg *et al.*, 1978).

Although the early attempts at tissue culture of teratoma cells were marred by inadequate characterization of the cell populations grown and, in some cases, failure to exclude contamination by fibroblasts (Bregman and Bregman, 1961; Kallen and Rohl, 1962), more recent studies have concentrated on greater definition of the cultured populations based predominantly on the histology, ultrastructure and tumour-marker production of the cells (Table 5.1; Fogh and Trempe, 1975; Hogan *et al.*, 1977; Jewett, 1977; Williams *et al.*, 1977; Albrechtsen *et al.*, 1978; Bronson *et al.*, 1978; Endo *et al.*, 1978; Tsuchida *et al.*, 1978; Bronson *et al.*, 1979; Cotte, unpublished data; Cotte *et al.*, unpublished data).

Marked similarities demonstrated among human teratoma cells in culture, animal teratomas and animal and human embryos include AFP and HCG production, histology of undifferentiated cells, ultrastructure and surface antigenic traits. The detection of shared cell-surface antigens (including F9—see above) among pre-implantation mouse embryos, human sperm and mouse and human embryonal carcinoma cells (Artzt *et al.*, 1973; Hogan *et al.*, 1977; Holden *et al.*, 1977; Edidin *et al.*, 1978; McIlhenny, 1979) suggests that these antigenic determinants are stable from an evolutional viewpoint and may have important functions in the differentiation of embryonic cells, uncommitted germ cells and of neoplastic tissue (Artzt, 1978). The development of the

Table 5.1 Tissue culture lines of human malignant germ-cell tumours

Designation	Histology	Medium	Markers	Xenografted	References
Tera I	E/T	McCoy's 5A + 15% FCS	No?	Yes	Fogh (1978)
Tera II	E/S	McCoy's 5A + 15% FCS	Yes	Yes	
833 K	C/E/T/S	RPMI 1640/15% FCS +10% tryptoserphosphate broth + L-glutamine	?	Yes	Bronson et al. (1978)
SuSa	E	Dulbecco's MEM + 10% FCS + 10% CS	Yes	No	Hogan, B. (personal communication)
Ludwig HX 39	E	Dulbecco's MEM	Yes	Yes	
Ludwig H Ter 1	E/C/T	Dulbecco's + 10% FCS	Yes	No	
Ludwig H Ter 3	E/Y	Dulbecco's + 10% FCS	Yes	No	Cotte, C. (unpublished data)
Ludwig H Ter 5	E/S/Y/T	Dulbecco's + 10% FCS	Yes	No	
Ludwig H Ter 7	E/Y	Dulbecco's + 10% FCS	Yes	No	
—	E	MEM/10% FCS	Yes	No	Sakashita et al. (1976)
—	E/Y	Eagle's MEM/20% FCS	Yes	No	
—	Y*	Eagle's MEM/20% FCS	Yes	No	Albrechtsen et al. (1978)
—	Y*	Eagle's MEM/20% FCS	Yes	No	
—	E/Y	Eagle's MEM/20% FCS	Yes	No	
—	Y	MEM/20% FCS	Yes	No?	Endo et al. (1978)
—	Y	MEM/20% FCS	Yes	No?	
PA 1	T*	MEM/10% FCS/L-glutamine	Yes	Yes	Zeuthen et al. (1980)

* Ovarian. E, embryonal cell carcinoma; MEM, minimal essential medium; FCS, fetal calf serum; C, choriocarcinoma; S, seminoma; T, teratoma.

techniques of monoclonal antibody production has led to the production of specific antisera to surface antigens on mouse and human embryonal carcinoma cells, which have been used to further characterize these cell populations (Goodfellow *et al.*, 1979; McIlhenny, 1979).

Another similarity between cultured teratoma cells and some embryonic tissues is the presence of retrovirus particles. Such particles have been demonstrated in the cell lines 833K and Tera I, and resemble those found in some human placentas and embryonic tissues (Kalter *et al.*, 1973; Bronson *et al.*, 1978; Bronson *et al.*, 1979) However, the significance of these findings remains uncertain.

The extensive tissue culture studies which have attempted to characterize the biology of germ cells have not been matched by the use of this model for drug-sensitivity testing. Although the effects of tumoricidal drugs on human tumour stem cells have been investigated *in vitro* (Salmon *et al.*, 1978), we know of no such data for normal or neoplastic human germinal tissue. One of the prerequisites for a quantifiable drug assay system is the ability to grow colonies from single-cell suspensions, and this has proved to be a limiting factor on the use of choriocarcinomas and yolk-sac tumours for this purpose.

Testicular tumour xenografts

The establishment and characterization of human testicular tumour xenografts in immune-deprived mice has been under investigation as part of an extensive programme of human tumour xenograft research being carried out in the Radiotherapy Research Unit at Sutton (Steel and Peckham, 1980; Peckham *et al.*, 1980). This includes studies in which xenografting is employed in conjunction with the in vitro agar assay of clonogenic tumour cells in order to quantitate the effects of cytotoxic therapy, and in the more basic study of clonal heterogeneity.

In this programme of work, young adult mice have been rendered immune deficient by thymectomy and total body irradiation. Initially, animals were reconstituted with autologous marrow which inevitably partly restored immune function. More recently, autologous marrow has been rendered unnecessary by employing a technique in which total body irradiation is preceded by a pulse of cytosine arabinoside. Animals prepared in this way are comparable, at least initially, to nude mice, although partial immune restoration occurs (Steel *et al.*, 1978).

A major objective of the xenograft programme is to separate functionally distinct elements using the cloning technique in order to establish monoclonal xenografts (Peckham *et al.*, 1980). So far it has proved difficult to clone testicular tumour xenografts in agar, a prerequisite both for studies of the clonal structure of these tumours and as a means of measuring the surviving fraction of clonogenic tumour cells after exposure to cytotoxic drugs or radiation.

The growth delay endpoint has been employed extensively in the experimental therapy of other tumours, including colorectal carcinoma (Nowak *et al.*, 1978), lung cancer (Shorthouse *et al.*, 1980) and melanoma (Selby *et al.*, 1980). To date, we have not exploited the testicular teratoma xenograft model for experimental tumour therapy extensively. The dose-response characteristics of seminoma exposed to radiation are of obvious interest, but it has proved impossible to establish a seminoma xenograft, although efforts are continuing.

Human tumours vary widely in the facility with which they are established as xenografts. Colonic and lung carcinomas are readily grown, whereas breast and prostatic carcinoma show low take-rates. Testicular tumours also have proved somewhat difficult to establish as xenografts.

As shown in Table 5.2, more than twenty human germ-cell xenograft lines have been reported, including six from our laboratory. In this latter group, efforts have been directed towards their characterization in terms of histology, ultrastructure, karyotype, marker production, cell-surface antigenicity and therapeutic response.

Table 5.2 Xenografted human malignant germ-cell tumour lines

Designation	Histology Donor	Xenograft	Host	Tissue culture	Marker production	References
PITT 61	E	E	HCP	No	No	
PITT 89	C	C	HCP	No	Yes	Pierce et al.
PITT 94	E	E	HCP	No	No	(1959a and b)
PITT 100	T/E	C	HCP	No	Yes	
Tera I	E/T	E/T	N	Yes	No?	Fogh (1978)
Tera II	E/S	E/S	N	Yes	Yes	
HX 36	C/E	C/E	Ix	No	Yes	Selby et al., (1979)
HX 39	E	E	Ix/N	Yes	Yes	
HX 53	S/Y	S/Y	Ix	No	Yes	
HX 57	Y	Y	Ix/N	No	Yes	Raghavan et al.,
HX 67	S/Y/T	S/Y/T	Ix	Yes	Yes	(1979, 1981)
HX 84	E	E	Ix	No	No	
833 K	C/E/T/S	E	N	Yes	?	Broson et al. (1979)
PA 1	E/T*	E/T	N	?	?	Lee et al. (1979)
TE	Y	Y	N	?	Yes	
OE	Y	Y	N	?	Yes	Yoshimura et al. (1978)
TT-1-JCK	Y	Y	N	?	Yes	
—	Y	Y	N	?	Yes	Shirai et al. (1977)
TC-1-JCK	A	A	N	?	?	Ueyama et al. (1977)
EST 1	Y	Y	N	?	Yes	Takeuchi et al. (1979)
EST 2	Y	Y	N	?	Yes	
SCH	C†	C	N	?	Yes	Kameya et al. (1976)
OCC-MM	C*	C	N	?	Yes	Kim et al. (1978)

* Ovarian primary tumour.
† Gastric primary tumour.
E, embryonal cell carcinoma; C, choriocarcinoma; T, teratoma; Y, yolk-sac tumour (or endodermal sinus tumour); S, seminoma; A, adenocarcinoma; HCP, hamster cheek pouch; N, nude; Ix, immune suppressed.

In general, malignant teratoma xenografts retain many of their histological features and growth characteristics in serial transplantation (Pierce *et al.*, 1958; Giovanella *et al.*, 1974; Stevens and Varnum, 1974; Shirai *et al.*, 1977; Ueyama *et al.*, 1977; Jewett, 1978; Mostofi, 1978; Sharkey *et al.*, 1978; Yoshimura *et al.*, 1978; Bronson *et al.*, 1979; Lee *et al.*, 1979; Raghavan *et al.*, 1979; Selby *et al.*, 1979).

However, we have reported also the xenograft HX 36, derived from a trophoblastic malignant teratoma, in which there was a progressive decrease in the proportion of HCG-synthesizing cells in serial transplants (Selby *et al.*, 1979). Using the immunoperoxidase method, HCG was demonstrated in xenografted tissue which also showed a high, although patchy, tritiated thymidine

(^{3}H-TdR) labelling index (Fig. 5.1). It appeared that HCG-positive cells did not incorporate ^{3}H-TdR and hence showed no evidence of proliferation. Human chorionic gonadotrophin also was demonstrated by radio-immunoassay in the blood of tumour-bearing mice and in tissue extracts from the xenografted tumour. Although the progressive decrease in HCG production may not be a general phenomenon, it emphasizes the need for careful and repeated assessment of serial xenograft passages.

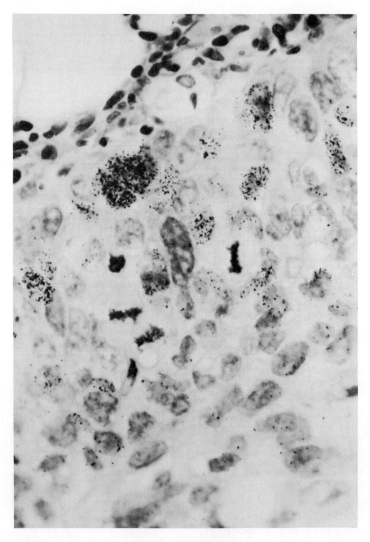

Fig. 5.1 Trophoblastic malignant teratoma xenograft (H×36). **(a)** Autoradiograph showing tumour cells labelled with tritiated thymidine.

Teratoma xenografts have been established most commonly by the subcutaneous implantation of tumour fragments or the intramuscular injection of cell suspensions derived from ascitic fluid. In our laboratory, transplantable teratomas have been established also by intraperitoneal injection of cell suspensions and intraperitoneal implantation of tumour fragments. These tumours grow as either solid or cystic masses with areas of haemorrhage and necrosis. Histologically, they are almost indistinguishable from human malignant teratomas, the only difference being occasional variation in the amounts of supporting tissue present. Distant metastases are not a feature of xenografted teratomas, although occasionally spread may occur along tissue planes—for example, within the subcutaneous layer or transperitoneally.

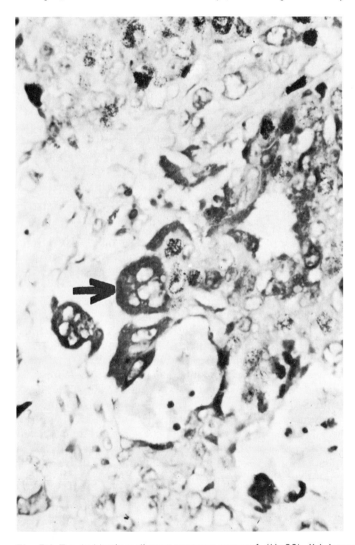

Fig. 5.1 Trophoblastic malignant teratoma xenograft (Hx 36). **(b)** Autoradiograph stained by the immunoperoxidase technique demonstrating human chorionic gonadotrophin in large unlabelled cells.

Most established xenograft lines have been derived directly from human biopsy material. Although established tissue culture lines of teratomas have proved to be difficult to grow in immune-suppressed animals (Hogan, 1979; Jewett, 1979), Jewett (1978) has successfully heterotransplanted Tera I and Tera II into nude mice and has shown stability of cellular morphology and human karyotype. We have demonstrated clumps of embryonal carcinoma (undifferentiated malignant teratoma) cells in fragments of gel foam implanted in immune-suppressed mice, and these also have retained the histological appearance of the original source of tumour.

For a variety of tumours, the xenograft model has been shown to function as a 'tissue amplifier', producing an unrestricted supply of tumour tissue for experimental use and higher titres of tumour-marker substances than in the original donor patients (Shirai et al., 1977; Yoshimura et al., 1978; Selby et al., 1979; Takeuchi et al., 1979; Raghavan et al., 1981). Yolk-sac tumours (endodermal sinus tumours) and choriocarcinomas (trophoblastic malignant teratomas), which comprise the majority of reported cell lines, have been of particular use in the study of tumour-marker production (Pierce et al., 1958; Shirai et al., 1977; Yoshimura et al., 1978; Raghavan et al., 1979; Selby et al., 1979; Takeuchi et al., 1979). In keeping with animal tissue culture and clinical data, yolk-sac tumour xenografts have been shown to produce a variety of proteins, including AFP (Shirai et al., 1977; Yoshimura et al., 1978; Raghavan et al., 1979; Takeuchi et al., 1979), alpha$_1$-antitrypsin (Raghavan and Norgaard-Pedersen, unpublished data; Shirai et al., 1977; Yoshimura et al., 1978; Takeuchi et al., 1979), hemopexin and transferrin (Yoshimura et al., 1978), LDH isoenzyme 1, alkaline phosphatase and carcinoembryonic antigen (Takeuchi et al., 1979), albumin (Yoshimura et al., 1978), pre-albumin (Raghavan and Norgaard-Pedersen, unpublished data; Yoshimura et al., 1978), beta-lipoprotein (Raghavan and Norgaard-Pedersen, unpublished data) and fibronectin (Ruoslahti and Raghavan, unpublished data). Similarly, choriocarcinoma xenografts have been shown to produce HCG (Pierce et al., 1958; Selby et al., 1979). We have established a direct relationship between circulating titres of AFP and AFP concentrations in fluid aspirated from those xenografts that grow as cysts (Raghavan et al., 1979).

Xenograft tissue has allowed us to demonstrate the presence of markers immunocytochemically and to relate this to the conventional histopathological diagnosis. Human chorionic gonadotrophin is produced in classical trophoblastic tissues, in syncytial giant cells and in mononuclear cells which appear to be embryonal carcinoma (MTU) by conventional histology (Selby et al., 1979). We have demonstrated AFP in cells showing classical yolk-sac differentiation, in undifferentiated tumour and in areas resembling pure seminoma (Raghavan, et al., 1981) suggesting either the existence of a solid variant of yolk-sac tumour or the presence of a continuum of differentiation between yolk-sac tumour and seminoma. These data, in combination with clinical studies, may lead ultimately to a functional reclassification of germ-cell tumour pathology.

As noted above, the effects of chemotherapy on tumour growth and marker production have not been studied extensively in testicular tumour xenografts. In general, circulating HCG titres have been shown to follow changes in tumour volume before and after treatment, although in some cases HCG production has been suppressed by the drugs in the absence of a demonstrable effect on tumour growth (Kameya *et al.*, 1976; Hayashi *et al.*, 1978; Kim *et al.*, 1978).

Lee and his co-workers have documented growth regression of malignant teratomas following high-dose infusion of thymidine (Lee *et al.*, 1979), and we have noted similar responses in preliminary experiments with cis-platinum, vinblastine, bleomycin and methyl-CCNU (Fig. 5.2). However, the interpretation of such data is made difficult by the drawbacks of the xenograft system: host responses differ from the human situation, particularly as the hosts are immune deficient; host responses may vary also with time (especially in thymectomised, irradiated mice); there is a difference in tumour : host size ratios; metabolic processes (such as drug metabolism) are markedly different; there is a continuing risk of cross-species interaction mediated by macrophages or natural 'killer' cells or by humoral factors.

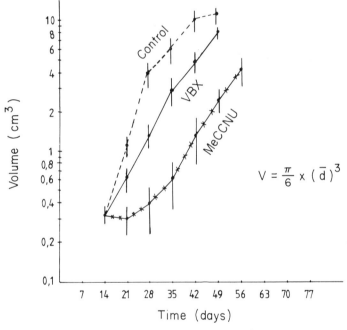

Fig. 5.2 Growth delay induced in xenograft Hx 39 following treatment with vinblastine (VBX) and methyl-CCNU (MeCCNU). The tumour volume is calculated according to the formula shown, where V represents tumour volume and d represents mean diameter.

The establishment of easily located, non-metastasizing, reproducible tumour xenografts has lent itself to attempts at radio-immunolocalization. Goldenberg *et al.* (1978) have shown specific uptake of radioactively labelled anti-CEA in CEA-producing colonic carcinoma xenografts in hamsters, and subsequently in clinical studies. Ballou *et al.* (1979) have demonstrated a degree of localization with 129-strain teratocarcinomas and ^{125}I-labelled monoclonal antibodies directed against surface antigens on the tumours. Our preliminary studies with three monoclonal antibodies directed against the cell surface of

HX 39 xenograft have documented specific uptake of ^{125}I-labelled monoclonal antibodies up to eight times greater than for ^{131}I-labelled non-specific gamma-globulin. Autoradiography has localized uptake to areas under the fibrous tumour capsule, tumour cell surfaces and occasionally in regions of tissue necrosis, but the significance of this is not yet clear.

Summary and conclusions

Three germ-cell tumour models have been developed. Animal teratomas, including the spontaneous and induced 129-strain mouse teratomas, and rat yolk-sac tumours have been studied extensively *in vivo* and *in vitro* and have been shown to share many morphological and functional properties in common with normal embryonic tissue and to be developmentally interchangeable with normal embryonic tissue.

The study of human teratoma cells in tissue culture has confirmed the similarities in structure and function of embryonic and neoplastic tissues from both human and animal sources. Tissue culture remains to be exploited in the quantitative study of radiation and drug sensitivity of germ-cell tumours and normal germinal tissues.

The establishment of germ-cell tumour xenografts and the use of techniques for assaying and identifying clonogenic cells in soft agar offers the exciting possibility of studying the clonal structure of these tumours in relation to marker production and therapeutic sensitivity. They may be useful also for the testing of new reagents for radio-immunolocalization of germ-cell tumours.

References

Albrechtsen, R., Hirai, H., Linder, D., Norgaard-Pedersen, B. and Wewer, U. (1978). *Scandinavian Journal of Immunology* **(8)**, 165.

Aldrich, J. T. and Stevens, L. C. (1967). *Cancer Research* **27**, 915.

Artzt, K. (1978). *Seminars in Oncology* **6**, 53.

Artzt, K., Dubois, P., Bennett, D., Condamine, H., Babinet, C. and Jacob, F., (1973). *Proceedings of the National Academy of Sciences (USA)* **70**, 2988.

Bagshawe, K. D. (1973). *Advances in Cancer Research* **18**, 231.

Ballou, B., Levine, G., Hakala, T. R. and Solter, D. (1979). *Science* **206**, 844.

Bernstine, E. G., Hooper, M. L., Grandchamp, S. and Ephrussi, B. (1973). *Proceedings of the National Academy of Sciences (USA)* **70**, 3899.

Bregman, R. U. and Bregman, E. T. (1961). *Journal of Urology* **86**, 642.

Bronson, D. L., Fraley, E. E., Fogh, J. and Kalter, S. S. (1979). *Journal of the National Cancer Institute* **63**, 337.

Bronson, D. L., Ritzi, D. M., Fraley, E. E. and Dalton, A. J. (1978). *Journal of the National Cancer Institute* **60**, 1305.

Carleton, R. L., Friedman, N. B. and Bomze, E. T. (1953). *Cancer* **6**, 464.

Damjanov, I. (1978). *Journal of the National Cancer Institute* **61**, 911.

Damjanov, I. and Solter, D. (1974). *Current Topics in Pathology* **59**, 69.

Edidin, M., Ostrand-Rosenberg, S. and Bartlett, P. F. (1978). *Cell Differentiation and Neoplasia*, p. 67. Ed. by G. F. Saunders. Raven Press, New York.

Endo, Y., Urano, Y., Tsuchida, Y., Asaka, T., Kaneko, Y., Kaneko, M., Sakashita, S., Tsukada, Y., Watabe, H., Hirai, H. and Oda, T. (1978). *Scandinavian Journal of Immunology* **(8)**, 171.

Engelhardt, N. V., Poltoranina, V. S. and Yazova, A. K. (1973). *International Journal of Cancer* **11**, 448.

Fogh, J. (1978). *National Cancer Institute Monograph* **49**, 5.

Fogh, J. and Trempe, G. (1975). *Human Tumor Cells In Vitro*, p. 115. Ed. by J. Fogh. Plenum Press, New York.

Gey, G. O., Seegar, G. E. and Hellman, L. M. (1938). *Science* **88**, 306.

Giovanella, B. C., Stehlin, J. S. and Williams, L. J. Jr. (1974). *Journal of the National Cancer Institute* **52**, 921.

Gitlin, D. and Perricelli, A. (1970). *Nature* **228**, 995.

Goldenberg, D. M., DeLand, F., Kim, E., Bennett, S., Primus, F. J., Van Nagell, J. R., Estes, N., DeSimone, P. and Rayburn, P. (1978). *New England Journal of Medicine* **298**, 1384.

Goodfellow, P. N., Levinson, J. R., Williams, V. E. and McDevitt, H. O. (1979). *Proceedings of the National Academy of Sciences (USA)* **76**, 377.

Hayashi, H., Kameya, T., Shimosato, Y. and Mukojima, T. (1978). *American Journal of Obstetrics and Gynecology* **131**, 548.

Hogan, B. (1979). Personal communication.

Hogan, B., Fellous, M., Avner, P. and Jacob, F. (1977). *Nature* **270**, 515.

Holden, S., Bernard, O., Artzt, K., Whitmore, W. F. Jr. and Bennett, D. (1977). *Nature* **270**, 518.

Hussa, R. O., Patillo, R. A., Delfs, E. and Mattingly, R. F. (1973). *Obstetrics and Gynecology* **42**, 651.

Jewett, M. A. S. (1977). *Urologic Clinics of North America* **4**, 495.

Jewett, M. A. S. (1978). *National Cancer Institute Monograph* **49**, 65.

Jewett, M. A. S. (1979). Personal communication.

Kahan, B. and Ephrussi, B. (1970). *Journal of the National Cancer Institute* **44**, 1015.

Kahan, B. and Levine, L. (1971). *Cancer Research* **31**, 930.

Kallen, B. and Rohl, L. (1962). *Journal of Urology* **87**, 906.

Kalter, S. S., Helmke, R. J. and Heberling, R. J. (1973). *Journal of the National Cancer Institute* **50**, 1081.

Kameya, T., Shimosato, Y., Tumuraya, M., Ohsawa, N. and Nomura, T. (1976). *Journal of the National Cancer Institute* **56**, 325.

Kim, W., Takahashi, T., Nisselbaum, J. S. and Lewis, J. L. (1978). *Gynecologic Oncology* **6**, 165.

Kleinsmith, L. J. and Pierce, G. B. (1964). *Cancer Research* 1544.

Kohler, P. O., Bridson, W. E., Hammond, J. M. and Weintraub, B. (1971). *Acta Endocrinologica Supplement* **153**, 137.

Lee, S. S., Giovanella, B. C., Stehlin, J. S. Jr. and Brunn, J. C. (1979). *Cancer Research* **39**, 2928.

Martin, G. R. and Evans, M. J. (1975). *Proceedings of the National Academy of Sciences (USA)* **72**, 1441.

McIlhenny, R. J. (1979). Unpublished data.

Michalowsky, I. (1979). *Virchows Archiv fur pathologische Anatomie und Physiologie und fur Klinische Medizin* **274**, 319.

Mintz, B. and Illmensee, K. (1975). *Proceedings of the National Academy of Sciences (USA)* **72**, 3585.

Mostofi, F. K. (1978). *National Cancer Institute Monograph* **49**, 74.

Mount, B. M., Stevens, L. C. and Whitmore, W. F. Jr. (1970). *Cancer* **26**, 570.

Nowak, K., Peckham, M. J. and Steel, G. G. (1978). *British Journal of Cancer* **37**, 578.

Patillo, R. A. and Gey, G. O. (1968). *Cancer Research* **28**, 1231.

Peckham, M. J., Selby, P. J. and Steel, G. G. (1980). In *Immunodeficient Animals in Cancer Research*, p. 227. Ed. by S. Sparrow. MacMillan, London.

Pierce, G. B. and Dixon, F. J. (1959a). *Cancer* **12**, 573.

Pierce, G. B. and Dixon, F. J. (1959b). *Cancer* **12**, 584.

Pierce, G. B., Dixon, F. J. and Verney, E. (1958). *Cancer Research* **18**, 204.

Raghavan, D., Gibbs, J., Nogueira Costa, R., Kohn, J., Orr, A. H., Barrett, A. and Peckham, M. J. (1979). *British Journal of Cancer* **41**, Suppl. IV, 191.

Raghavan, D., Heyderman, E., Gibbs, J., Neville, A. M. and Peckham, M. J. (1981). In *Thymusaplastic Nude Mice and Rats in Clinical Oncology*, p. 200. Ed. by G. Bastert, H. Schmidt-Matthiessen and H. P. Fortmeyer. Fischer-Verlag, Stuttgart.

Rosenthal, M. D., Wishnow, R. M. and Sato, G. H. (1970). *Journal of the National Cancer Institute* **44**, 1001.

Sakashita, S., Hirai, H., Nishi, S., Nakamura, K. and Tsuji, I. (1976). *Cancer Research* **36,** 4232.
Salmon, S. E. Hamburger, A. W., Soehnlen, B., Durie, B. G. M., Alberts, D. S. and Moon, T. E. (1978). *New England Journal of Medicine* **298,** 1321.
Salmon, S. E., Hamburger, A. W., Soehnlen, B., Durie, B. G. M., Alberts, D. S. and Moon, T. E. (1978). *New England Journal of Medicine* **298,** 1321.
Selby, P. J., Heyderman, E., Gibbs, J. and Peckham, M. J. (1979). *British Journal of Cancer* **39,** 578.
Selby, P. J., Courtney, V. D., McElwain, T. J., Peckham, M. J. and Steel, G. G. (1980). *British Journal of Cancer* **42,** 438.
Sharkey, F. E., Fogh, J. M., Hajdu, S. I., Fitzgerald, P. J. and Fogh, J. (1978). *The Nude Mouse in Experimental and Clinical Research*, p. 187. Ed. by J. Fogh and B. C. Giovanella. Academic Press, New York.
Shirai, T., Yoshiki, T. and Itoh, T. (1977). *GANN* **68,** 847.
Shorthouse, A. J., Peckham, M. J., Smyth, J. F. and Steel, G. G. (1980). *British Journal of Cancer* **41,** Suppl. IV, 142.
Sobis, H. and Vandeputte, M. (1973). *International Journal of Cancer* **11,** 543.
Sobis, H. and Vandeputte, M. (1974). *International Journal of Cancer* **13,** 444.
Sobis, H. and Vandeputte, M. (1976). *Developmental Biology* **51,** 320.
Sobis, H. and Vandeputte, M. (1977). *European Journal of Cancer* **13,** 1175.
Sobis, H. and Vandeputte, M. (1979). *European Journal of Cancer* **15,** 143.
Sobis, H., Van Hove, L., Delacourt, M., Park, B. and Vandeputte, M. (1979). In *Carcinoembryonic Proteins* Vol. II, p. 409. Ed. by F. G. Lehmann. Elsevier/North Holland Biomedical Press, Amsterdam.
Speeg, K. V. Jr., Aziakhan, J. C. and Stromberg, K. (1976). *Cancer Research* **36,** 4570.
Steel, G. G., Courtenay, V. D. and Rostom, A. Y. (1978). *British Journal of Cancer* **37,** 224.
Steel, G. G. and Peckham, M. J. (1980). *British Journal of Cancer* **41,** Suppl. IV, 133.
Stevens, L. C. (1964). *Proceedings of the National Academy of Science* **52,** 654.
Stevens, L. C. (1967a). *Advances in Morphogenesis* **6,** 1.
Stevens, L. C. (1967b). *Journal of the National Cancer Institute* **38,** 549.
Stevens, L. C. (1973). *Journal of the National Cancer Institute* **50,** 235.
Stevens, L. C. and Little, C. C. (1954). *Proceedings of the National Academy of Sciences (USA)* **40,** 1080.
Stevens, L. C. and Varnum, D. S. (1974). *Developmental Biology* **37,** 369.
Stromberg, K., Azizkhan, J. C. and Speeg, K. V. Jr. (1978). *In Vitro* **14,** 631.
Takeuchi, T., Nakayasu, M., Hirohashi, S., Kameya, T., Kaneko, M., Yokomori, K. and Tsuchida, Y. (1979). *Journal of Clinical Pathology* **32,** 693.
Tsuchida, Y., Kaneko, M., Saito, S., Endo, Y., Urano, Y., Ohmi, K. and Asaka, T. (1978). *Scandinavian Journal of Immunology* **(8),** 137.
Ueyama, Y., Yokoyama, M., Kondo, Y., Ohsawa, N. and Tamaoki, T. (1977). *GANN* **68,** 121.
Van Hove, L., Delacourt, M., Park, B., Sobis, H. and Vandeputte, M. (1978). *International Journal of Cancer* **21,** 731.
Williams, R. D., Bronson, D. L., Elliott, A. Y., Lange, P. H. and Fraley, E. E. (1977). *Urologic Clinics of North America* **4,** 529.
Yoshimura, S., Tamaoki, N., Ueyama, Y. and Hata, J. (1978). *Cancer Research* **38,** 3474.
Zeuthen, J., Norgaard, J. O. R., Avner, P., Fellous, M., Wartiovaara, J., Vaheri, A., Rosen, A. and Giovanella, B. C. (1980). *International Journal of Cancer* **25,** 19.

6

Diagnosis and management of the primary testicular tumour

W. F. Hendry

The young man with a swollen testicle presents a difficult problem to the doctor. It is often hard to believe that there is anything sinister in such a fit patient, and it is very tempting to make a provisional diagnosis of 'epididymo-orchitis', give some antibiotic and hope for the best. Yet the price for getting the diagnosis wrong can be very high indeed. If the swelling is due to torsion, the testis will be lost by delay, and if it is due to certain types of tumour, the interval may be long enough for distant metastases to become established. The relatively slow progress and good prognosis of some seminomas should not induce a complacent attitude to early diagnosis and management for, if the tumour is an anaplastic teratoma, every day lost will increase the chance of distant dissemination and increase in size of established subclinical deposits. The doctor who is consulted by a patient with a swollen testicle carries a heavy responsibility and there is unfortunately no easy way to make sure that the responsibility is discharged correctly every time.

Clinical history

Many patients wait a long time before seeking medical advice. Thompson *et al.* (1961) reported that 83 per cent of their series of patients delayed for over one month, 59 per cent for over three months and 37 per cent for more than six months. Unfortunately, the delay did not stop there. Even when these patients had gone to the doctor, 36 per cent of the 155 patients with testicular presentation were misdiagnosed: 19 as 'epididymo-orchitis', 16 as 'post-traumatic', 11 as simple hydrocele and 10 as hernia. Even in the well-supervised ranks of the British Army, the findings were similar. Stephen (1958) reported that the initial diagnosis was wrong in 56 of 100 cases and that the correct diagnosis was not established for over a year in 15 cases.

There are several reasons why the diagnosis of testicular tumours poses difficulties. Although they usually present as painless enlargement, the most common error is to mistake a tumour for 'epididymo-orchitis' because the swollen testicle is painful. In fact, Stephen (1958) reported that 13 of 92 cases with a swollen testicle complained of pain from the outset, and a further 18 subsequently developed pain which led them to seek medical advice (Table 6.1). Many of these testes were found to show haemorrhage within the tumour on pathological examination. Another problem is that the tumour-bearing testis may get *smaller* with antibiotic treatment, which tends to further mislead

Table 6.1 Findings recorded on examination of 100 testicular tumours (Stephen, 1958)

Feature	Consistency	Surface	Location	Sensation	Cord
Findings	Hard 80% Firm 18% Normal 2%	Irregular 60% Smooth 40%	Upper third 40% Lower third 35% Anterior 10% Hilum 15%	Absent 27% Partial 57% Dulled 10% Normal 6%	Normal 77% Thick 23%
Number of cases	82	65	45	77	100

the attending physician into believing that he is dealing with an inflammatory problem. We have seen this phenomenon as a disappointingly common cause of delay in patients referred to the Royal Marsden Hospital. Blandy *et al.* (1970) have suggested that the only safe course of action is to explore every apparent 'epididymitis' if there are neither pus cells nor bacteria in the urine.

The next major source of error lies in a history of trauma to the testicle. In many cases, there has been injury in the remote past, but much more dangerous is the testicle which has been swollen—or noticed to be swollen—only since a specific recent injury. This should not be allowed to mislead the physician, since a definite history of trauma was recorded in 17, 19 and 21 per cent of the large series described by Thomas and Bischoff (1954), Stephen (1958) and Thompson *et al.* (1961) respectively. In fact, the slightly enlarged testicle is slightly more vulnerable to injury and, if the enlargement has been insidious, attention is directed towards it only after it has had a knock. Once again, the safest action when in doubt is to explore the testis and, if necessary, evacuate haematoma or haematocele if no tumour is found.

Previous surgery to the testis or inguinal canal may make the findings more difficult to interpret. A history of previous hydrocele or hernia operation on the side of the tumour was recorded in 9 per cent of 178 cases by Thompson *et al.* (1961). Previous orchidopexy should be expected in about 6.5 per cent of tumours (from a collected analysis of 1865 cases) and in about 1 case in 5 (18.3 per cent) the malignancy will affect the opposite testicle (Hogan and Johnson, 1972). Interestingly, Gehring *et al.* (1974) reviewed 529 tumours and found that almost a third of 37 cryptorchid-associated tumours occurred in patients with a history of orchidopexy when they were between 6 and 12 years old; however, no tumour occurred in patients who had undergone orchidopexy before the age of 6 years. An association with subfertility is less well established, although tumours may develop in testes which are atrophic (Haines and Grabstald, 1950; Hausfeld and Schrandt, 1965).

The patient who has had a testicular tumour before, presents a particular problem. He has only one testicle and is usually acutely conscious of any changes that may occur in it. Testicular tumours occur bilaterally in up to 3.8 per cent of cases, usually sequentially but occasionally simultaneously; it has been estimated that the possibility of a second tumour developing in the remaining testis is about 500 times greater than in the normal population (Morris *et al.*, 1976). This is the main reason for our policy of following patients with testicular tumours indefinitely.

Gordon-Taylor and Wyndham (1947) pointed out that the course of the history may be variable, but usually falls into one of five patterns. It can be 'insidious but relentless', 'hurricane' leading to early death, 'chronic' with a long latent period, or 'pseudo-inflammatory' presenting diagnostic difficulties. The fifth clinical type presents with its metastases and comprises 4 to 14 per cent of all tumours (Kuhn and Johnson, 1972). Lymph-node metastases may produce backache, abdominal symptoms, hypertension or palpable lymphadenopathy in the supraclavicular fossa (or in the inguinal region after previous groin surgery). Blood-borne metastases may give pulmonary symptoms or bone pain, and bizarre metastases elsewhere have been recorded as presenting symptoms. Patients presenting with gynaecomastia usually, but not always, have metastases.

Perhaps the most difficult tumours of all are those that develop in undescended intra-abdominal testes. These may present acutely, with torsion or rupture, as an abdominal mass or, depressingly often, by their metastases. The poor prognosis associated with these tumours has led us to recommend orchidectomy for all postpubertal patients with unilateral abdominal cryptorchidism, and full explanation of the risks to bilateral cryptorchids who can now be offered satisfactory hormone replacement therapy if they agree to abdominal castration.

Physical examination

In examining the patient suspected of testicular tumour, particular attention should be paid to the testes, the groins, the abdominal node-bearing area and liver, the nipples and the neck.

It is worth starting the examination of the testes by looking at them with the patient lying and standing. A testis with a tumour usually lies lower than normal, whereas inflammatory lesions or torsion tend to raise the testis. The skin overlying the testes on each side should be inspected and the presence or absence of distended veins or varicocele noted.

Palpation most easily starts with the normal testis, which serves as a baseline. The entire outline of the body of the testis should be defined between the thumb, index and middle fingers and its overall consistency assessed by gently sliding the organ from one examining hand to the other. The position, consistency and any tenderness of the epididymis and cord are noted and particular attention is paid to the groove between the epididymis and the body of the testis. Finally, the body of the testis is squeezed *gently* to assess sensation. Attention is then turned to the suspect testicle and examination is repeated, taking care to proceed carefully and systematically, as outlined above. A tumour is identifiable firstly because it is firm or hard, secondly because it enlarges the testicle and thirdly because it causes the testicle to lose its normal sensation on squeezing. Although these criteria apply to most tumours, they do not apply to all, and outlined in Table 6.1 are the findings recorded in 100 cases by Stephen (1958). Abnormal firmness is the most reliable finding and this should always alert the examiner. The most difficult point is to define whether the firmness involves the body of the testis or the epididymis. The most common site for tumours to be missed is in the groove between testis and epididymis. It may be noted from Table 6.1 that 15 per cent of tumours occurred in the hilum, and these are most likely to be confused with epididymitis, especially tuberculous epididymitis. The surface of the testis may be smooth or irregular. Partial or complete loss of sensation is found commonly and I have found this a most useful sign. I believe that the diagnostic help derived from this test more than outweighs any possibility of disseminating the tumour by gently squeezing the testicle.

The cord and vas deferens should be palpated carefully on each side. If the vas is thickened or beaded on the affected side, a tumour is unlikely; however, as a testicular tumour becomes larger, the whole spermatic cord may become thickened due to cremasteric hypertrophy or venous dilatation.

A hydrocele may be present with 10 to 20 per cent of testicular tumours and it is usually small. Its presence should be confirmed by transillumination and, since tumour or other testicular disease is always a possibility in a young man, the hydrocele should *not* be aspirated. It is much better to explore the testicle, remove it if it is diseased or, if it is normal, perform an operation for radical cure of the hydrocele. If it is needled and the testis is benign, the hydrocele will refill; if the testis is malignant, the primary local defences will be breached.

Differential diagnosis

The diagnosis of testicular tumour is most likely to be confused with epididymo-orchitis, tuberculous epididymitis or gumma of the testis, torsion, hydrocele or hernia.

Epididymo-orchitis is the most common misdiagnosis. This diagnosis should be made only if the swelling is confined strictly to the epididymis and the urine contains pus or bacteria. It should be remembered that a testis involved by tumour can get smaller with antibiotics, and apparent response to this treatment does not exclude the diagnosis of tumour. Tuberculous epididymo-orchitis and gumma of the testis may be indistinguishable from tumour, but the testis will almost certainly be grossly disorganized and hence is better removed.

Torsion, of course, should be explored. Hydrocele in a young man should be treated surgically and hernia should be recognized and repaired.

It is clear, therefore, that there must be very good reasons for *not* exploring a testicle which is swollen, firm or painful. Instead of worrying about the very real possibility of missing a tumour in a doubtful case, it is far better to arrange for early exploration. There is little to be lost, except in the man with only one testicle. In that case, a special procedure should be followed, but the principle of early exploration still holds good.

The potentially useful role of serum alphafetoprotein and human chorionic gonadotrophin in differential diagnosis should not be overlooked, although there are few reliable data bearing on this point.

Surgical treatment

Once the suspicion of testicular tumour has been raised, the surgeon should arrange for immediate admission and early surgical exploration. Blood samples should be taken for AFP and HCG prior to exploration. In planning the surgical approach to the testicle, the surgeon *must* bear two factors in mind. The first concerns the pathways of spread of these tumours and the second is related to the patient's future fertility.

The dense membrane of the tunica albuginea will contain the tumour locally until it is far advanced, even though distant spread may be occurring via the lymphatics or bloodstream. Once this fibrous sheath is punctured, however, the local defences are breached and a scrotal recurrence is likely to occur (Dean, 1925; Stephen, 1962; Blandy et al., 1970). If the orchidectomy is done through an inguinal incision, however, and the testis is removed by gently withdrawing it intact through the neck of the scrotum, local recurrence is exceptionally rare. It follows that if the tunica albuginea has been punctured by needle aspiration or scrotal biopsy, or if the orchidectomyhas been done by a scrotal incision, it is necessary to irradiate the scrotum to prevent local recurrence, whereas this can be avoided if an inguinal incision has been used. Unless the contralateral testis is transposed to an extrascrotal position, for example the thigh, it is impossible to protect the opposite testicle adequately from radiation if the scrotum is treated. It follows that scrotal interference with a testicular tumour, by needle biopsy or scrotal incision, will lead inevitably to sterility, whereas fertility can be preserved after an inguinal incision (Smithers et al., 1973; Thomas et al., 1977).

The surgical approach, therefore, should be through a standard or skin-crease inguinal incision. The external oblique is opened, the cord is mobilized and clamped at the internal ring. If there is doubt about the diagnosis, a soft bowel clamp may be used. The testicle is then withdrawn from the scrotum, by gentle traction on the cord combined with scrotal counterpressure. It is freed of its scrotal connections and examined. If inspection and palpation confirm a firm area in the body of the testis, often associated with dilated overlying veins, then the cord is divided between clamps and the testis is removed. The cord is doubly ligated and the wound is closed in layers.

Biopsy is only necessary before the orchidectomy when there is only one testicle. Under these circumstances the testicle should be mobilized through an inguinal incision after applying a soft clamp to the cord. It is then bisected and a biopsy is taken from any firm areas to obtain histological confirmation of the diagnosis before removing the testis. If there is no tumour, the capsule can be closed and the testicle returned to the scrotum. Blandy et al. (1970) stress that this procedure—Chevassu's manœuvre—should very seldom be necessary, except when dealing with a solitary testicle.

Once the testicle has been removed, the patient should be referred for staging decision regarding further management as soon as the diagnosis of malignancy is made. By this time the tumour-marker results will also be available, and it is important to take at least two further blood samples during the first week after surgery. If the patient is referred from elsewhere and a scrotal incision has been used, a firm nodule is often left in the scrotum adjacent to the end of the cord and there may be considerable concern as to whether this is haema-toma or residual tumour. If there is real doubt, it is our policy to excise the stump of the cord through an inguinal incision, which is extended as a 'tennis-racquet incision' around the scrotum to excise the original scar and the under-lying nodule completely as a partial or hemi-scrotectomy. Markland et al. (1973) found residual tumour in 6 of 19 patients with non-seminomatous tumours treated by hemi-scrotectomy after primary scrotal biopsy or orchi-dectomy.

The rules for the successful management of the primary testicular tumour are clear. There should be no scrotal surgery of any sort and the tumour should be removed cleanly through an inguinal incision. This has been known for at least fifty years (Dean, 1925) and the consequences of ill-advised scrotal incision were described clearly over 200 years ago by Percival Pott in 1775. Nonetheless, almost one-third of the cases referred to the Royal Marsden Hospital have suffered scrotal interference and, if radiotherapy is employed, are thereby condemned to therapeutic sterilization.

References

Blandy, J. P., Hope-Stone, H. F. and Dayan, A. D. (1970). *Tumours of the Testicle*, Heinemann, London.

Dean, A. L. (1925). *Journal of Urology* **13**, 149.

Gehring, G. G., Rodriguez, F. R. and Woodhead, D. M. (1974). *Journal of Urology* **112**, 354.

Gordon-Taylor, G. and Wyndham, N. R. (1947). *British Journal of Surgery* **35**, 6.

Haines, J. S. and Grabstald, H. (1950). *Archives of Surgery* **60**, 857.

Hausfeld, K. F. and Schrandt, D. (1965). *Journal of Urology* **94**, 69.

Hogan, J. M. and Johnson, D. E. (1972). Etiology of Testicular Tumours. In *Testicular Tumours*, p. 31. Ed. by D. E. Johnson. Kimpton, London.

Kuhn, C. R. and Johnson, D. E. (1972). Clinical Diagnosis. In *Testicular Tumours*, p. 47. Ed. by D. E. Johnson. Kimpton, London.

Markland, C., Kedia, K. and Fraley, E. E. (1973). *Journal of the American Medical Association* **224**, 1025.

Morris, S. A., Vaughan, E. D. and Constable, W. C. (1976). *Journal of Urology* **115**, 566.

Pott, P. (1775). In *Chirurgical Observations* pp. 63–68. L. Hawes, W. Clarke and R. Collins, London.

Smithers, D. W., Wallace, D. M. and Austin, D. E. (1973). *British Medical Journal* **4**, 77.

Stephen, R. A. (1958). *Annals of the Royal College of Surgeons of England* **23**, 71.

Stephen, R. A. (1962). *British Journal of Urology* **34**, 448.

Thomas, G. and Bischoff, A. J. (1954). *Journal of Urology* **72**, 411.

Thomas, P. R. M., Mansfield, M. D., Hendry, W. F. and Peckham, M. J. (1977). *British Journal of Surgery* **64**, 352.

Thompson, I. M., Wear, J., Almond, C., Schewe, E. J. and Sala, J. (1961). *Journal of Urology* **85**, 173.

7
Investigation and staging: general aspects and staging classification
M. J. Peckham

The observations made in this section are directed predominantly towards the investigation of malignant teratoma, although the staging strategy described is applicable to childhood tumours and seminomas. The majority of patients, following orchidectomy, have no evidence of metastatic teratoma on clinical examination, although a minority present with rapidly progressive advanced disease and require immediate treatment. With the exception of this small group, a detailed evaluation of the patient must be carried out before treatment is initiated. The objective of staging is to determine the extent and sites of tumour spread. Furthermore, since the size of individual metastases exerts an important influence on the selection and effectiveness of treatment, an attempt must be made to measure tumour volume.

Clinical examination and history

Clinical examination and history are important. So far as the primary site and immediate draining lymph nodes are concerned, the type of operation performed is noted, a history of trans-scrotal needle biopsy sought and the patient questioned regarding previous orchidopexy for maldescent. These factors influence the radiotherapeutic approach, since there may be a risk of relapse in the scrotum and inguinal nodes. The contralateral testis is examined since synchronous bilateral malignancies occur, albeit rarely. Absence since childhood of one testis in the patient with a normal remaining testis, and evidence of metastatic tumour or an abdominal mass, should raise the possibility of malignancy in an intra-abdominal testis. Less commonly, a patient may present with symptoms caused by metastases. In exceptional cases both testes may be clinically normal even though metastases are present and one or both tumour markers elevated. In this situation a history of transient swelling and pain of one testis may be obtained and removal of this testis may reveal either an occult primary testicular tumour or an apparently spontaneously regressed primary tumour (see Chapter 1). At the Royal Marsden Hospital we have seen 23 patients who presented with metastatic disease and who either had occult impalpable primary testicular tumours, or small tumours that had been missed on clinical examination. Of this group, 20 presented with advanced bulky metastases and of 16 non-seminomas, 6 were trophoblastic malignant teratomas (3 pure choriocarcinomas) (Table 7.1).

In the absence of previous disturbance to the lymphatic drainage by

Table 7.1 Occult primary germ-cell tumours of the testis presenting with metastases

Stage	Histology				
	Seminoma	MTD	MTI	MTU	MTT or chorio*
II	4	1†	1‡	3	—
III	2	—	1	—	2
IV	1	—	—	4§	4
Total (23)	7	1	2	7	6

* Three pure choriocarcinoma.
† Testis MTD, abdominal nodes seminoma.
‡ Testis MRD, abdominal nodes MTI.
§ One patient, testis MTD, lung MTU.

herniorrhaphy or orchidopexy, or extension of tumour through the tunica vaginalis into the scrotal sac, involvement of the inguinal nodes is rarely seen. Metastases in iliac or para-aortic nodes may be palpable and a history of diffuse lumbar backache is typical of bulky retroperitoneal nodal metastases. Ureteric obstruction with renal pain may occur if gross adenopathy is present.

The supraclavicular fossae are palpated for evidence of lymph node involvement, which if present almost invariably occurs at the termination of the thoracic duct in the left cervical region. Occasionally in patients with bifid or right-sided thoracic ducts, or those in whom spread has occurred from the mediastinum, right supraclavicular nodes may be involved.

The extranodal sites most commonly involved in teratoma testis are the lungs and liver. Breathlessness and haemoptysis are manifestations of advanced lung disease but, in most cases, the patient is asymptomatic. Involvement of other sites, such as bone and the central nervous system, is associated usually with widespread tumour dissemination.

Evidence of nipple and breast tenderness and breast enlargement is sought. Gynaecomastia in the teratoma patient is associated, usually but not invariably, with an elevated serum chorionic gonadotrophin titre.

Histological review and pathological staging

It is essential that the histology is reviewed before a treatment decision is made. If examination is limited to one or two sections, it is likely that the range of histological components will not be identified. This is particularly important in combined seminoma–teratoma, since the non-seminoma component may be small in size yet determine the prognosis. Immunoperoxidase staining methods may provide evidence of unsuspected yolk-sac and trophoblastic components (see Chapter 3). If possible, the whole operative specimen is obtained. A full pathological assessment includes an appreciation of the range of histologically distinct components and determines whether or not the tumour has extended through the tunica and whether the epididymis and cord are involved. The tunica provides an effective barrier to direct extension, and scrotal involvement in the absence of inappropriate surgery is uncommon. The pathological staging system proposed by the British Testicular Tumour Panel (Pugh and Cameron, 1976) is summarized below.

P_1 Tumour confined to the testis; epididymis and cord free.
P_2 Involvement of epididymis and/or lower cord; upper cord free.
P_3 Involvement of upper cord.

In the Panel series, 23 of 54 (42.6 per cent) teratoma patients with involvement of the upper cord (P_3) had metastases at the time of surgery, compared with 6 per cent of P_1 and 27 per cent of P_2 patients (see Chapter 15). The presence of vascular and lymphatic permeation by tumour should be noted. Vascular invasion almost certainly predisposes the patient to early extralymphatic dissemination (see Chapter 15).

Clinical staging in relation to patterns of tumour dissemination

Testicular tumours may spread by direct infiltration of adjacent structures, via the lymphatics and by the haematogenous route.

Lymphatic spread

Lymphatic spread occurs along a leash of four to eight efferent lymphatic vessels which pass from the mediastinum testis along the spermatic cord to the internal inguinal ring, continuing along the spermatic vessels to the point where these vessels cross the ureter. The lymphatics then fan out and enter the retroperitoneal lymph nodes in the para-aortic region. There are some differences in the termination of the right and left-sided vessels. Thus, lymphography carried out via the testicular lymphatics fills nodes at the L_1 to L_3 level on the left and L_2 on the right. Involvement of contralateral pelvic nodes is rare and spread occurs predominantly to the upper para-aortic region and less commonly to the pelvic nodes on the same side as the tumour (see Chapter 8). Valuable information describing the disposition of lymph-node metastases comes from patients undergoing bilateral radical node dissection. Ray et al. (1974) found that primary lymphatic spread from left-sided tumours was to the para-aortic, pre-aortic, left common iliac and left external iliac nodes, in that order of frequency, with subsequent extension to the interaorta-caval, precaval and paracaval region. Right-sided tumours spread to the interaorta-caval, precaval, para-aortic, paracaval, right common iliac and right external iliac nodes in that order, with subsequent extension to para-aortic, left common iliac and left external iliac nodes. If fact, where multiple nodal metastases were present from right-sided tumours, 20 per cent of patients showed contralateral spread to the left side. Spread to the left common iliac nodes only, occurred in one patient and this patient had multiple nodal metastases at other sites. No patient with a left-sided tumour showed spread to the precaval or paracaval area, although 20 per cent had metastases in the interaorta-caval region. Thus, of 61 patients with left-sided tumours and positive nodes, 60 had para-aortic node involvement, 4 had left common iliac and 1 had left external iliac; of 61 positive nodes in patients with right-sided tumours, 47 (77 per cent) had inter-aorta-caval metastases, 10 had right common iliac, 3 had right external iliac and 1 had left common iliac. These observations are summarized in Fig. 7.1.

As pointed out above, extension of tumour via the thoracic duct to the left cervical region may occur (Fig. 7.2). Hitherto, mediastinal node involvement has been recognized uncommonly but experience with CT scanning has

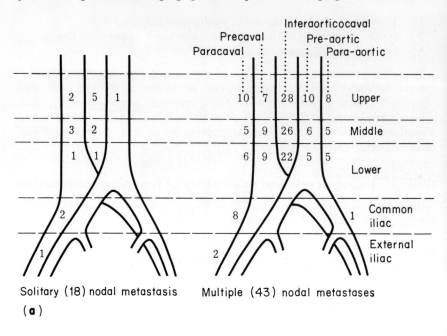

Solitary (18) nodal metastasis   Multiple (43) nodal metastases

(a)

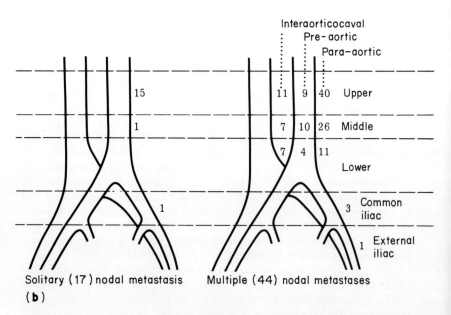

Solitary (17) nodal metastasis   Multiple (44) nodal metastases

(b)

Fig. 7.1 Topography of lymph node involvement in testicular teratoma. Radical node dissection data from Ray *et al.* (1974). **(a)** Nodal involvement in teratoma of the right testis; **(b)** nodal involvement in teratoma of the left testis.

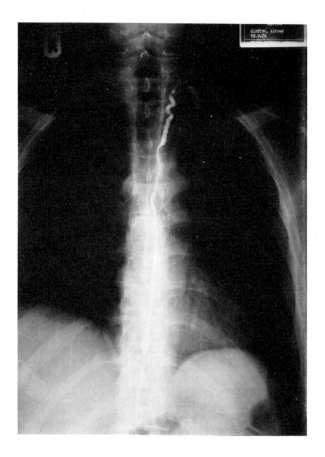

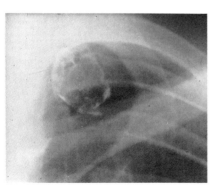 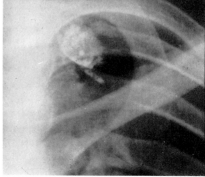

Fig. 7.2 Lymphatic extension via the thoracic duct in teratoma testis.
(a) Thoracic duct terminating in the left supraclavicular region; (b) an enlarging metastasis in a node at the termination of the thoracic duct.

indicated that tumour in this site has almost certainly been underdiagnosed (see Chapter 9).

Vascular spread

The primary site of vascular dissemination is the lungs. Data from thoracotomy excision of solitary metastases and from earlier experience employing lung irradiation indicate that in some patients tumour spread may be confined to the lungs. The next most commonly seen extralymphatic site of involvement is the liver. Liver involvement at diagnosis is relatively uncommon, which may in part reflect underdiagnosis with currently available staging procedures.

Staging protocol

The staging procedures in current use in the Testicular Tumour unit of the Royal Marsden Hospital are listed below and summarized in Fig. 7.3.

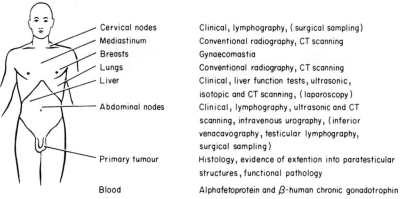

Cervical nodes	Clinical, lymphography, (surgical sampling)
Mediastinum	Conventional radiography, CT scanning
Breasts	Gynaecomastia
Lungs	Conventional radiography, CT scanning
Liver	Clinical, liver function tests, ultrasonic, isotopic and CT scanning, (laparoscopy)
Abdominal nodes	Clinical, lymphography, ultrasonic and CT scanning, intravenous urography, (inferior venacavography, testicular lymphography, surgical sampling)
Primary tumour	Histology, evidence of extention into paratesticular structures, functional pathology
Blood	Alphafetoprotein and β-human chronic gonadotrophin

Fig. 7.3 Schema for patient assessment in testicular teratoma. (Procedures not performed usually at the Royal Marsden Hospital are shown in parentheses.)

1. Chest radiograph.
2. Whole-lung tomography.
3. Computerized tomographic (CT) scan of lungs when 1. and 2. are clear, and in those patients with ≤ 3 identifiable metastases (see Chapter 9).
4. Bilateral lower limb lymphangiography (see Chapter 8).
5. Intravenous urography.
6. Ultrasonic scan of retroperitoneal area and liver.
7. CT scan of retroperitoneal area and liver (see Chapter 9).
8. Liver isotopic scan in patients with abnormal liver function tests or hepatomegaly when 6. and 7. are equivocal.
9. Serum alphafetoprotein (AFP) and beta-human chorionic gonadotrophin (β-HCG) levels (see Chapter 4).
10. Liver function tests.
11. Renal function tests (including creatinine clearance).
12. Full blood count.

Royal Marsden staging classification

The staging classification in current use in the Testicular Tumour unit is as follows and as summarized in Fig. 7.4.

    I. No evidence of disease outside the testis.

    II. Infradiaphragmatic node involvement

        This is subdivided according to the maximum diameter of metastases into the following substage categories:

        IIA. Maximum diameter of metastases <2 cm.

        IIB. Maximum diameter of metastases $2-5$ cm.

        IIC. Maximum diameter of metastases >5 cm.

    III. Supra- and infradiaphragmatic lymph node involvement.

        This is subdivided as follows:

        Abdominal nodes: A, B, C as for Stage II.

        Mediastinal nodes noted $M+$.

        Neck nodes noted $N+$.

        o = negative lymphogram.

    IV. Extension of tumour to extralymphatic sites.

        The following suffixes define the extent and volume of metastatic spread:

        O, A, B, C, for abdominal nodes as for Stages II and III.

        Mediastinal nodes noted $M+$.

        Neck nodes noted $N+$.

        Lung substage

        L_1 metastases $\leqslant 3$ in number.

        L_2 metastases >3 in number <2 cm maximum diameter.

        L_3 metastases >3 in number >2 cm maximum diameter.

        $H+$. Hepatic involvement.

        Other sites, e.g. bone and brain, are specified.

A staging system has been proposed by the UICC and this is shown below. Some of the features are similar to the system used at the Royal Marsden Hospital but the concept of tumour volume, which is an important prognostic feature, is stressed inadequately in the TNM system.

Fig. 7.4 Testicular tumours. Clinical staging categories. **(a)** Stage I: no evidence of disease outside the testis.

Fig. 7.4b Top. Stage II: infradiaphragmatic node involvement. This is subdivided according to the maximum diameter of metastases into the following substage categories. IIA, maximum diameter of metastases <2 cm; IIB, maximum diameter of metastases $2-5$ cm; IIC, maximum diameter of metastases >5 cm. **Bottom left.** An example of disease designated as IIA showing (arrowed) an involved node in the lower para-aortic region. **Bottom right.** An example of IIC disease showing a large mass of poorly opacified nodes displacing the ureter.

Fig. 7.4c Stage III. Supra- and infradiaphragmatic node involvement. This is subdivided as follows. Abdominal nodes: A, B and C as for State II; mediastinal node involvement: $M+$; neck nodes: $C+$.

Fig. 7.4d Top left. Stage IV. Extension of tumour to extralymphatic sites. The following suffices define the extent and volume of metastatic spread. Abdominal nodes: O = negative lymphogram; A, B, C as for Stages II and III. Mediastinal and neck nodes as for Stage III. Lungs: $L_1 \leqslant 3$ metastases; L_2 multiple metastases $\leqslant 2$ cm maximum diameter; L_3 multiple metastases >2 cm maximum diameter. Liver involvement is denoted $H+$. Other sites, e.g. bone and brain, are specified. **Top right.** An example of limited small-volume lung disease (L_1) demonstrated by CT scan. **Bottom left.** Multiple limited-volume lung metastases (L_2). **Bottom right.** Advanced pulmonary presentation (L_3).

Stage I

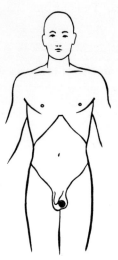

Fig 7.4 a

Stage II. Infradiaphragmatic node involvement

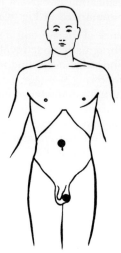

Fig 7.4b(i)

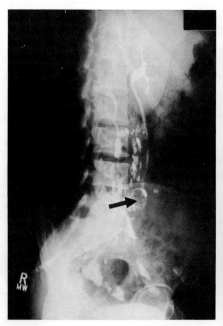

Fig 7.4b(ii)

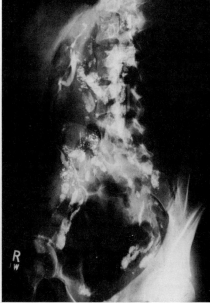

Fig 7.4b(iii)

Stage III. Supra and infradiaphragmatic
node involvement

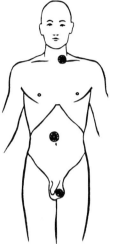

Fig 7.4c

Stage IV. Extension of tumour to
extralymphatic sites

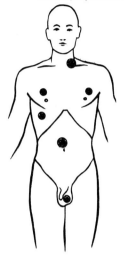

Fig 7.4d(i)

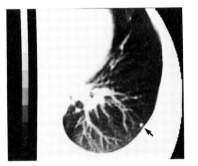

Fig 7.4d(ii)

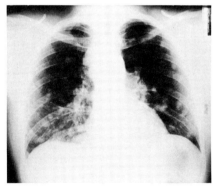

Fig 7.4d(iii)

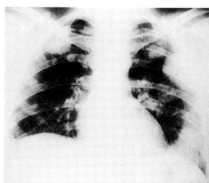

Fig 7.4d(iv)

UICC TNM classification for testicular tumours

T_1. Tumour confined to the body of the testis.
T_2. Tumour extending beyond the tunica.
T_3. Tumour involving rete testis or epididymis.
T_4. Tumour invading spermatic cord and/or scrotal wall.
   T_4a. Tumour invading spermatic cord.
   T_4b. Tumour invading scrotal wall.
N_0. No evidence of regional lymph nodes.
N_1. Involvement of a single homolateral regional lymph node which, if inguinal, is mobile.
N_2. Involvement of contralateral or bilateral or multiple regional nodes which, if inguinal, are mobile.
N_3. Palpable abdominal mass is present or there are fixed inguinal nodes.
N_4. Involvement of juxtaregional lymph nodes.
M_0. No evidence of distant metastases.
M_1. Distant metastases present.
   M_1a. Evidence of occult metastases based on biochemical and/or other tests.
   M_1b. Single metastasis in a single organ site.
   M_1c. Multiple metastases in a single organ site.
   M_1d. Metastases in multiple organ sites.

Stage distribution at presentation

The large majority of seminoma patients present in Stage I (Table 7.2 and Fig. 7.5). The stage distribution of non-seminomatous tumours cannot be assessed adequately from the selected patient population referred to specialist centres. It appears, however, that 50 to 60 per cent of patients present with clinical Stage I disease. Thus, in the Danish national study, 55 per cent of non-seminoma patients presented with clinical Stage I disease and less then 20 per cent in Stage IV (Schultz, H., personal communication). However, as discussed in Chapters 9, 13 and 15, the use of more accurate staging methods such as CT scanning in conjunction with an analysis of tumour markers should enable the

Table 7.2 Incidence of Stage I disease in seminoma testis (for references see Chapter 10)

	Total seminomas	Stage I
Ytredel and Bradfield (1972)	80	71
Saxena (1973)	77	75
Castro and Gonzalez (1971)	96	58
Van der Werf Messing (1976)	257	153*
Maier et al. (1968)	80	78
Kademian et al. (1976)	52	36
Calman et al. (1979)	191	121
Total	833	592 (71%)

* This includes 95 patients designated N_x in the absence of lymphography.

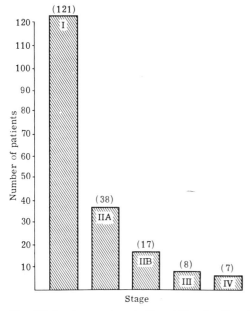

Fig. 7.5 Seminoma of testis (Royal Marsden Hospital, 1962–1975). Stage distribution at presentation of 191 previously untreated patients.

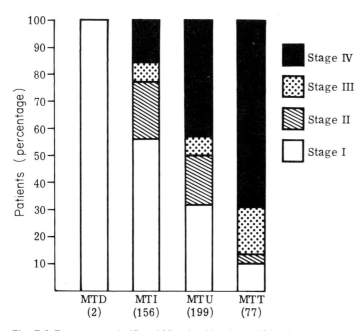

Fig. 7.6 Teratoma testis (Royal Marsden Hospital, 1963–1979). Histology and Stage distribution.

Table 7.3 Modified stage distribution of testicular teratoma patients undergoing CT scanning following orchidectomy

Stage prior to CT scan	Total no. of patients	Percentage stage distribution after CT scanning			
		I	II	III	IV
I	21	76	5	—	19
II	22	—	73	4	23
III	12	—	—	42	58
IV	25	—	—	—	100

different clinical stage categories to be defined with considerably more precision.

The extent to which CT scanning has modified stage distribution in our own experience is summarized in Table 7.3 and further discussed in Chapter 9. As shown, almost one-fifth of clinical Stage I patients had small lung metastases. The implications of this in the analysis of Stage I management are discussed in detail in Chapter 13.

Histology and spread pattern

Undifferentiated (MTU) and trophoblastic teratoma (MTT) behave in a more aggressive fashion than intermediate malignant teratoma (MTI). Thus, in the Testicular Tumour Panel experience, extension into the epididymis and spermatic cord was less common in MTI primary tumours (Table 7.4).

Similarly, histology of primary tumour and clinical stage shows that the majority of differentiated teratomas (TD) and MTI patients present with early stage disease, whereas MTU and MTT increasingly predominate in Stage IV (Fig. 7.6). This aspect is discussed in relation to the analysis of prognostic factors in Stage I disease in Chapter 13.

Table 7.4 Histology of primary testicular teratomas in relation to local extent of disease (data from Pugh, 1976)

Extent of primary tumour	Percentage distribution by histology		
	MTI (123)	MTU (102)	MTT (11)
P₁ (confined to testis or rete)	67	32	55
P₂ involvement epididymis and/or lower cord	18	33	36
P₃ involvement of upper cord	15	34	9

References

Calman, F. M. B., Peckham, M. J. and Hendry, W. F. (1979). *British Journal of Urology* **51**, 154.

Castro, J. R. and Gonzalez, M. (1971). *American Journal of Roentgenology* **111**, 355.

Kademian, M. T., Bosch, A. and Caldwell, W. L. (1976). *International Journal of Radiation Oncology Biology Physics* **1**, 1075.

Maier, J. G., Sulak, M. H. and Mittemeyer, B. T. (1968). *American Journal of Roentgenology* **102**, 596.

Pugh, R. C. B. and Cameron, K. M. (1976). *In Pathology of the Testis*, p. 199. Ed. by R. C. B. Pugh. Blackwell Scientific, London.

Ray, B., Hajdu, S. I. and Whitmore, W. F. (1974). *Cancer* **33**, 340.

Saxena, V. S. (1973). *American Journal of Roentgenology* **117**, 643.

Van der Werf Messing, B. (1976). *International Journal of Radiation Oncology Biology Physics* **1**, 235.

Ytredal, D. O. and Bradfield, J. S. (1972). *Cancer* **30**, 628.

8
Lymphography in testicular tumours

J. S. Macdonald

Since the early 1960s, lymphography has played an important part in the assessment and management of testicular tumours. These tumours spread from the testicle to the retroperitoneal lymph nodes, from there to the mediastinal or the supraclavicular nodes and to the lungs. In a proportion of cases, direct haematogenous spread also occurs, the spread pattern depending upon histopathological subtype. Lymphography opacifies the para-aortic and pelvic nodes and enables these to be assessed long before they beome suspect clinically. It has the advantage of being a direct examination, the lymphatic system itself is opacified, which enables smaller deposits to be detected than with indirect examinations which rely on increase in bulk of nodes and displacement of normal structures. When there is large bulky disease, lymphography becomes relatively less accurate in assessing the volume of tumour present.

Technique and complications

The technique used is basically that described by Kinmonth *et al.* (1955), with minor modifications. Nearly all lymphograms in this group can be done under local anaesthesia and as out-patients. The marker dye used is patent blue violet (2.5 per cent) mixed with lignocaine (2 per cent lignocaine hydrochloride plain) and normally only one small subcutaneous depot is needed lateral to the base of the great toe. The dorsum of the foot is infiltrated with local anaesthetic and a small longitudinal incision is preferred. This heals more easily and with less of a scar than a transverse incision and makes repeat lymphography easier. A lymphatic is brought to the surface and cleaned, then cannulated with a 30 swg needle (St Thomas' Hospital pattern lymphangiography set) and this is tied in place. The injection can be made with any automatic pump which will deliver the contrast medium (Lipiodol ultra fluid) at the rate of about 1 ml/10 minutes. The injection is stopped when the contrast medium reaches the level of the fourth lumbar vertebral body; it is always best to use the patient as his own control in this way, thus individualizing the investigation. When the injection is complete, the needle is removed, the wound stitched and the patient asked to exercise for ten minutes or so before the immediate radiographs are taken. These will show the lymphatics (the lymphangiogram) and the radiographs on the following day will show the nodes (lymphadenogram), together these make the lymphogram. It is policy at this hospital to combine the lymphadenogram with an intravenous urogram (IVU),
102

Table 8.1 Radiographs taken during and after lymphography

Timing	Radiographs	Purpose
Preliminary	PA chest	Assessment of suitability for lymphography
During the injection	Site of injection; then as required	Control of injection and safety
Shortly after injection completed (the lymphangiogram)	Abdomen and pelvis	To show the course of the lymphatics
Usually twenty-four hours after injection completed (the lymphadenogram)	Penetrated low kV. Chest; abdomen and pelvis; full-length IVU; series with oblique views	To show opacified mediastinal or supraclavicular nodes; assessment of opacified retroperitoneal nodes; position and size of kidneys and any displacement of urinary tract

which includes oblique views. The IVU is important for two reasons. In the first place, any displacement of the renal tract helps to assess the bulk of tumour present and, in the second place, it is necessary to know where the renal tissue is since so many of these patients will be going on to radiotherapy (Table 8.1).

Whenever foreign substances are injected into the body, allergic reactions are to be expected. Lymphography is no exception and during the course of the investigation several substances are injected: local anaesthetic, the marker dye, iodized oil and then intravenous contrast medium for the intravenous urogram. Reactions occur infrequently and are dealt with in the usual way. There are, however, certain complications which are peculiar to lymphography. Most of the blue dye is excreted rapidly by the kidneys and the patient should be warned that the urine will be coloured blue or green following lymphography. The site of injection of the blue dye may remain discoloured for many weeks and the patients should be warned that this will only disappear gradually.

The most important difference between lymphography and most other contrast investigations is that when Lipiodol is injected in diagnostic quantities, contrast which is not taken up by the nodes is discharged into the venous system, resulting in pulmonary oil embolism. This impairs lung function (Gold *et al.*, 1965) and most of the severe complications of lymphography are due to too much oil reaching the lungs. To prevent this, there should be x-ray control of the injection and lymphography is contra-indicated in patients who already have severely impaired lung function. It would also seem prudent to avoid lymphography in patients with acute venous thrombosis. Preferably the patient should not have a general anaesthetic for four days after lymphography. If large globules of oil reach the systemic circulation, there is a risk of cerebral oil embolism. This can happen if the normal lung is overloaded; overloading can be avoided by x-ray control and using the patient as his own control, i.e. stopping the injection when the contrast has reached the level of L4, no matter how little has been injected, and stopping the injection if a lymphaticovenous communication is seen.

There is also evidence to suggest that radiation in therapeutic doses damages the lung and allows larger globules to pass through (Davidson, 1969). A lymphogram should not be done while the patient is having radiotherapy to any part of the lung. Cardiac shunts and pulmonary arteriovenous malformations are also contra-indications. A proportion of patients, about 20 per cent, will have a mild pyrexia on the night of the lymphogram. The above is a summary of the complications and contra-indications; the subject has been dealt with more fully by Fischer (1969) and Macdonald (1976).

Lymphographic findings and philosophy of treatment

Treatment of testicular tumours is influenced by whether the lymphogram is negative (Stage I) or positive. In seminomas, irradiation in Stage I is confined to the abdominal nodes, but mediastinal and supraclavicular nodes are treated if the lymphogram is positive (see Chapter 10). In the teratomas, management may vary from watch policy to radical multimodality therapy, as discussed in Chapter 15. Radiation response depends upon the size of the deposits in the involved nodes (see Chapter 13). Chemotherapy response is influenced also by tumour volume (see Chapters 14 and 15). The lymphographic findings are seen, therefore, as central to the theme of treatment.

Lymph node drainage and anatomy (Fig. 8.1)

Lymph drainage of the testicle is to the para-aortic nodes and there is a

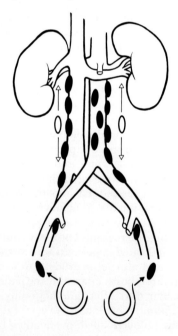

● Nodes normally opacified

Echelon nodes not normally opacified and variable in position

Fig. 8.1 Lymphatic drainage of the testicle and scrotum.

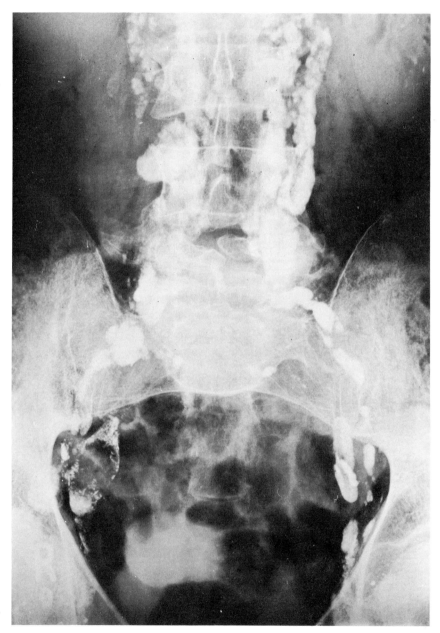

Fig. 8.2 Teratoma of right testicle with a deposit in a right upper external iliac lymph node. This was the only node shown to be involved.

relatively constant lymphatic which discharges into an upper external iliac node on the same side. Lymphography from the foot will show this and it is sometimes the only node seen to be involved (Fig. 8.2). The generally accepted anatomy is that there is an echelon node related to the hilum of the right kidney, but not on the left side (Rouviere, 1932). This, however, is open to doubt because, as was pointed out by Jackson (1972), standard textbook anatomy is based on a small number of cadaver dissections and this detailed antomy has been passed on from book to book. An echelon node on the left

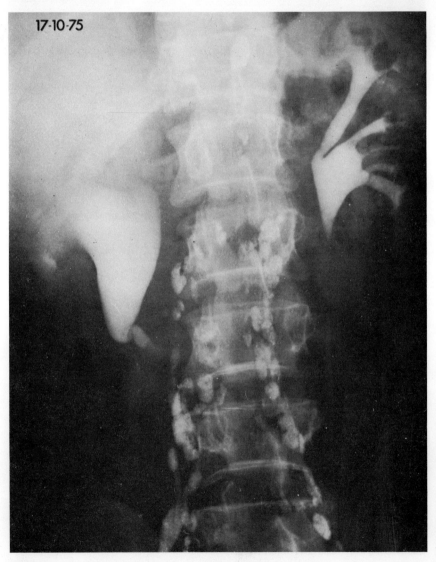

Fig. 8.3 Seminoma of the right testis. Normal lymphogram with evidence of a deposit in an echelon node at the level of L₃ involving the upper end of the right ureter.

side is probably less common and evidence for its existence was discussed by Fuchs (1969) and Macdonald and Paxton (1976). We have seen involvement of this node on the left side recently; it was detected on the intravenous urogram and confirmed by CT. Lymphography from the foot will not demonstrate these. An example of an involved echelon node on the right side is shown in Figs. 8.3 and 8.4. The position of these nodes is variable and they can occur as low as L3. It would be strange if this node were not seen on the left side,

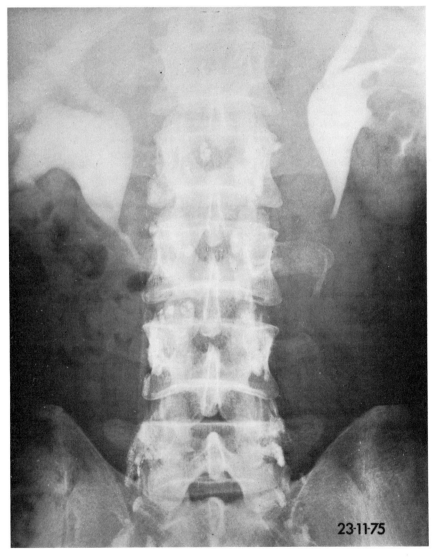

Fig. 8.4 Same patient as Fig. 8.3, towards the end of radiotherapy, showing a normal ureter.

because there is such variation in the lumbar lymphatics. The lumbar chains themselves are seen as a mirror image of the usual distribution in 25 per cent of patients (Jackson, 1974).

The anatomy of the para-aortic nodes is variable, but there is a rich plexus of lymphatic vessels in the area allowing easy crossover of deposits from one side to the other. The distribution of involved nodes in testicular tumours was found to be 71 per cent with involved nodes on the same side as the orchidectomy, 9 per cent with involvement of the contralateral side and 20 per cent with bilateral involvement (Wilkinson and Macdonald, 1975). There is also more likely to be crossover from right to left—56 per cent—than left to right—32 per cent—(Jackson, 1974). These findings have obvious implications when treatment is being considered.

Lymphography from the spermatic cord at the time of orchidectomy has been mentioned. This is the only lymphographic method whereby the echelon nodes may be opacified. There is a leash of lymphatics ascending from the testicle and injection of these has helped confirm the anatomy of lymphatic drainage of the testicle, but there is no guarantee that the lymphatic vessel draining the tumour is the one being cannulated, it is considered therefore that newer methods, such as CT scanning, are more appropriate.

Diagnostic criteria

It is important to define the criteria used in the interpretation of lymphograms. First, we should consider the behaviour of the normal node after lymphography. During the first twenty-four hours after injection of the oily contrast medium the normal node swells rapidly as it takes up the contrast (Steckel and Cameron, 1966), which then becomes evenly distributed throughout the node. This then gives the typical appearance of the normally opacified node. In the average patient the contrast medium will be retained in the nodes in diagnostic amounts for about one year and the normal node will be seen gradually to reduce in size over this period as it deals with the contrast, eventually returning to its prelymphogram size. This is a dynamic process and therefore any deviation from this, either in storage pattern (the nodes should be evenly opacified) or in behaviour (the node should gradually reduce in size) must be noted and looked upon with suspicion. At twenty-four hours, all contrast should have cleared from the lymphatics leaving only the nodes opacified.

Since the nodes retain the contrast medium over a long period, their behaviour can be watched as long as they contain enough contrast medium for the shape of the node to be assessed. All that is necessary for follow-up, in most cases, is a standard radiograph of the abdomen and chest. When the contrast medium has been absorbed, there is no reason why the lymphogram should not be repeated if it is required clinically. Thus, the behaviour of each opacified node can be studied on serial radiographs, thus introducing the concept of lymphography as a dynamic investigation. When used in this way it is possible to achieve:

    i. greater accuracy in the initial assessment;
    ii. a more complete picture of how the nodes are responding to treatment;
    iii. early warning of recurrence or spread of the tumour.

Deposits from testicular tumours normally do not take up contrast medium and therefore appear as filling defects within the opacified node (Figs. 8.2 and 8.5). Hence, we depend on what normal node tissue is left to surround and outline the deposit. A filling defect in a node may be due to fibro-fatty replacement from old infection, and the normal hilum of the node may also give this appearance. The normal hilum can be distinguished sometimes on the filling phase because efferent lymphatics will be seen to originate in this area. The filling defect caused by fibro-fatty replacement usually will have a

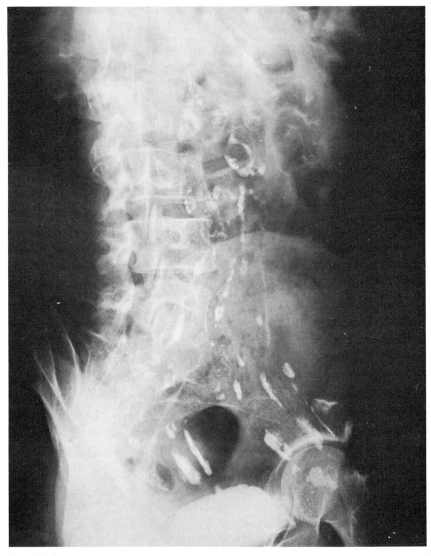

Fig. 8.5 Oblique view showing involved para-aortic node at the level of L_3. Note the rim of stretched, normal tissue surrounding the expanding lesion.

well-defined, serpiginous edge to it. These lesions are common, particularly in adults, and it is obviously important that they should be distinguished from deposits. It is for this reason that the concept of the filling defect in the opacified node must be taken further. When looking for deposits the question which should be asked is not 'Is there a filling defect present?' but rather 'Do any of the filling defects present in the opacified nodes give the impression of being expanding lesions?.' A deposit begins as a clump of cells which lodge in and grow in the node. As the deposit grows, its shape usually becomes spheroidal or ellipsoidal. As it enlarges it pushes a rim of normal node to the outside; it is this rim of compressed normal node which picks up the contrast medium and makes the unopacified deposit visible. Since the shape of the deposit is spheroidal or ellipsoidal, it has bulk and should appear as a more or less circular defect in more than one view. It is for this reason that additional oblique views as a routine are particularly useful (Fig. 8.5). Areas of fibro-fatty replacement do not give the impression of expanding lesions in several views, and a node containing a filling defect in one view and appearing flattened in an oblique view or a view taken at right angles to the first almost certainly does not contain a deposit.

There are nodes which contain very small filling defects and it is impossible to assess these on the 24-hour film because they are not yet disturbing the normal tissue around them. If we adhere to the concept of lymphography as a dynamic investigation and take follow-up radiographs as a routine, we can watch the behaviour of these filling defects and, if they progressively enlarge, then we are dealing with deposits; fibro-fatty areas and the normal hilum do not change in sequential views.

From what has been said, it will be apparent that only grossly involved nodes can be diagnosed with certainty at twenty-four hours. In all other cases, follow-up examinations are needed for a definite diagnosis to be made and confirmed. The only way to diagnose small deposits is to watch their behaviour, as deposits will behave in a different way from the normal nodes about them. This is another example of using the patient as his own control. It is vital that the diagnostic radiologist should know what treatment, if any, the patient is having. With no treatment there will be a differential enlargement of the deposit and with treatment a sensitive deposit will reduce in volume much faster than the surrounding normal nodes. It follows logically that there is no such thing as a negative lymphogram until it has been followed up adequately. The 24-hour films merely establish a baseline. Tumour deposits should be diagnosed as such only if they not only look like deposits but behave like deposits. Acute infection may mimic a deposit growing in part of a lymph node, but in such cases it is clinically obvious that there has been gross infection present for a node to behave like this. It is far more likely that infection will induce a picture of reactive change.

Follow-up films should be taken at two, four and eight weeks. It is obviously not necessary to hold up treatment until the diagnosis is certain, as long as the radiologist is told what treatment the patient is having and can assess the nodes accordingly. Some of these deposits can be very slow growing (Macdonald et al., 1968) and the histology of the primary tumour may not help, since a well-differentiated deposit may originate from an anaplastic teratoma.

In the case of testicular tumours, 10 per cent of positive lymphograms will

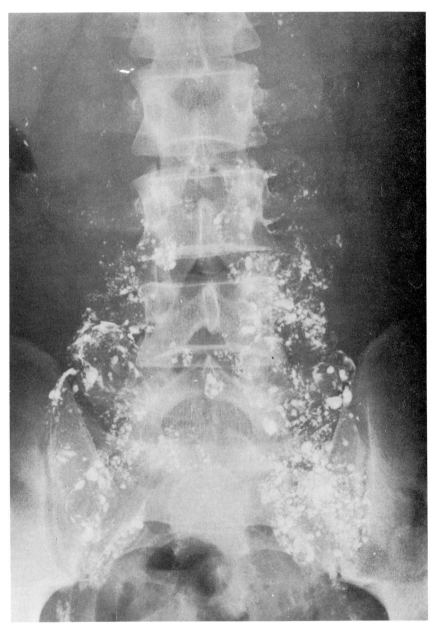

Fig. 8.6 Pseudolymphoma pattern on lymphography, with retrograde spread of tumour. Ten per cent of positive lymphograms in testicular tumour will show this pattern.

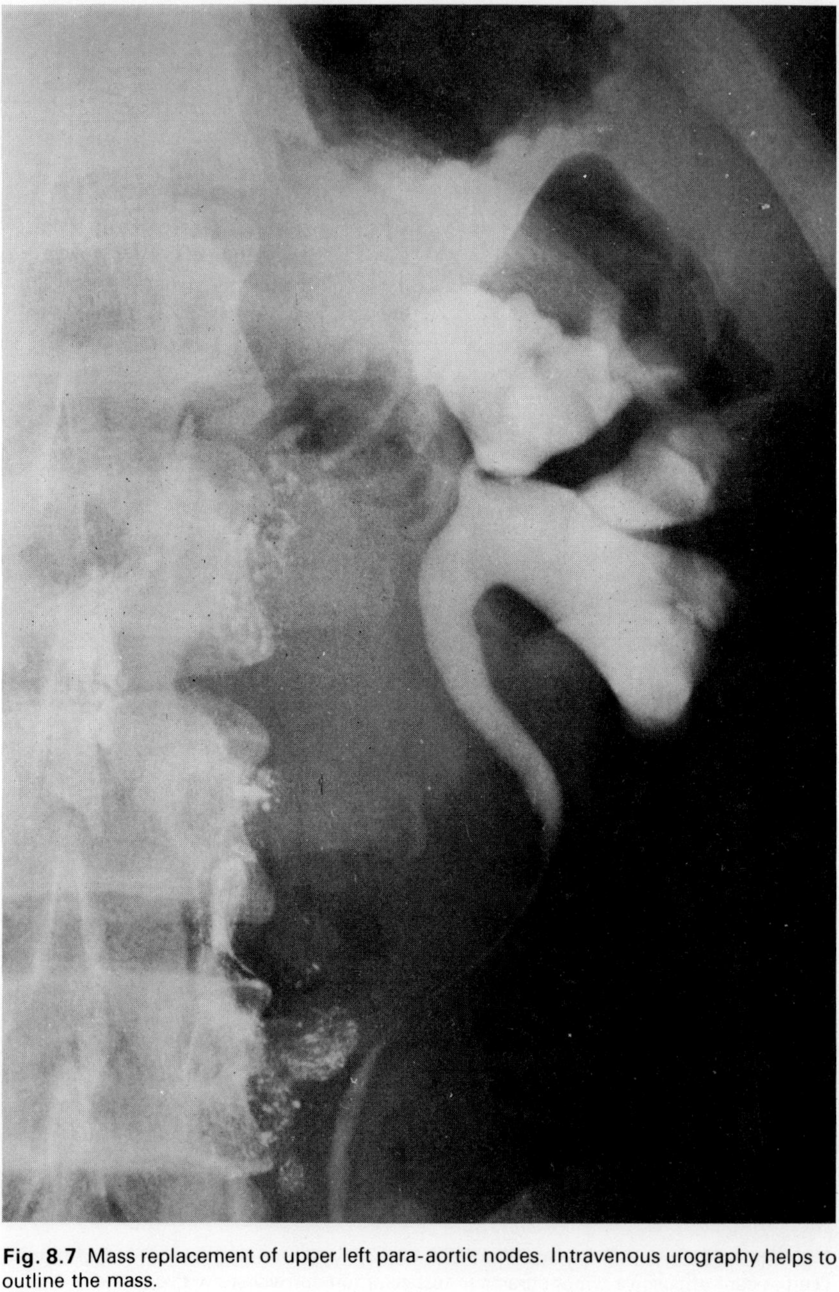

Fig. 8.7 Mass replacement of upper left para-aortic nodes. Intravenous urography helps to outline the mass.

show a pseudolymphoma appearance. This appearance, to all intents and purposes, is like the pattern seen in involved lymphomatous nodes. A gross example of this is seen in Fig. 8.6, which also shows retrograde spread to both side of the pelvis.

Retrograde involvement of nodes can happen when there is mass replacement of nodes by tumour. The afferent lymph vessels become obstructed and dilated, this leads first to stasis and then to incompetence of the valves. The way is then open for retrograde spread, the opening up of collateral channels and the possibility of lymphatico-venous anastomoses opening up. Since mass lesions cause these appearances, it is possible that smaller strategically situated deposits may do the same. This is why stasis, i.e. persistence of contrast medium in the lymphatic vessels at twenty-four hours, and the appearance of any abnormal collateral channels with opacification of unusual nodes supplied by these are looked upon with suspicion, and close attention should be paid to these areas on follow-up examinations. It is possible that these features may be congenital in origin, but equally well they may be caused by tumour deposits and, therefore, they must be carefully watched (Macdonald, 1978).

When the deposit has grown so large that it has burst outside the confines of the node, it is difficult to assess exactly how large it is, but often a clue to its size can be obtained by observing to what extent adjacent structures are displaced. These may be adjacent nodes or, for example, parts of the urinary tract (Fig. 8.7). It must be emphasized, however, that when deposits are as large as this, the exact size of the mass can only be guessed from the lymphogram. Another limitation of lymphography is that it will show the retroperitoneal nodes only as far as the origin of the thoracic duct. The intravenous urogram may help to define the size of large masses and may suggest also that there is involvement of an echelon node (see Figs. 8.3 and 8.4). It is because of these limitations of lymphography that a routine IVU and a well-penetrated view of the chest (to show any enlarged posterior mediastinal nodes) are advocated. It is precisely in these areas that ultrasound and computed axial tomography have been such a help in defining the bulk of tumour present.

Behaviour of nodes on refill lymphograms

Figures 8.8 and 8.9 show the lymphographic appearances of a patient with teratoma of the right testicle. Figure 8.8 is the appearance at twenty-four hours of the lymphogram done at the time of diagnosis of the tumour, shortly after orchidectomy, and Fig. 8.9 shows the appearances of a refill lymphogram eighteen months later. At the time of the first lymphogram, the nodes in both para-aortic regions are involved from the level of L1 to L5 and the pelvic nodes on both sides below this level are normal.

When normal nodes are irradiated their volume is reduced but they retain their shape and appearance. This is observed only very seldom during irradiation because the nodes become gradually smaller anyway as they lose the contrast medium, but it is seen immediately on a refill lymphogram (cf. pelvic nodes in Figs. 8.8, 8.9 and 8.10). If there has been no irradiation and the nodes are normal, then they can almost be superimposed on each other when a refill lymphogram is done.

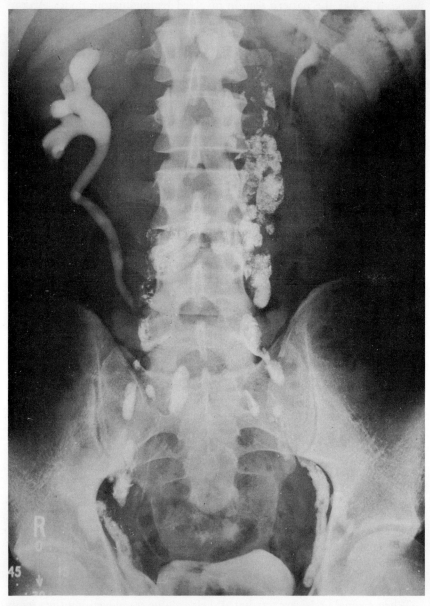

Fig. 8.8 Teratoma testis. Mass replacement of upper right para-aortic nodes with involvement, to a lesser extent, of the remaining para-aortic nodes and obstruction to the right ureter. The pelvic nodes are normal.

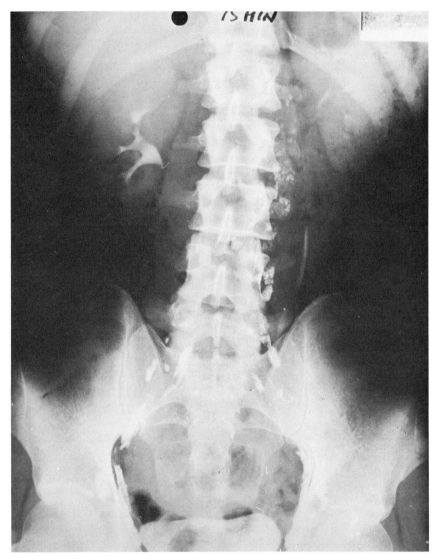

Fig. 8.9 Same patient as Fig. 8.8 Refill lymphogram eighteen months later, following radiotherapy. Note the normal nodes in the pelvis are smaller, but retain their shape and ability to take up contrast medium. The nodes seen to be involved in Fig. 8.8 are proportionally very much smaller than the normal nodes and there is less normal tissue left to take up the contrast. The back pressure on the right kidney has been relieved.

The involved nodes behave in a very different way. If there is mass replacement of the node by tumour, there will be no uptake of contrast medium in this area (upper right para-aortic region) and the presence of a mass can be deduced only by the displacement of the nodes which have opacified. When nodes are less heavily involved, the normal nodal tissue which is left will take up the contrast but, whereas irradiation will not change the shape of a normal node, it will cause considerable fibrosis and obliteration of an involved node. This effect is seen when the left para-aortic region is compared on the two radiographs. Also, there is a much greater proportional reduction in size of the involved nodes when compared with the normal ones.

As shown in Fig. 8.8, the node to the right of L4 is involving the ureter

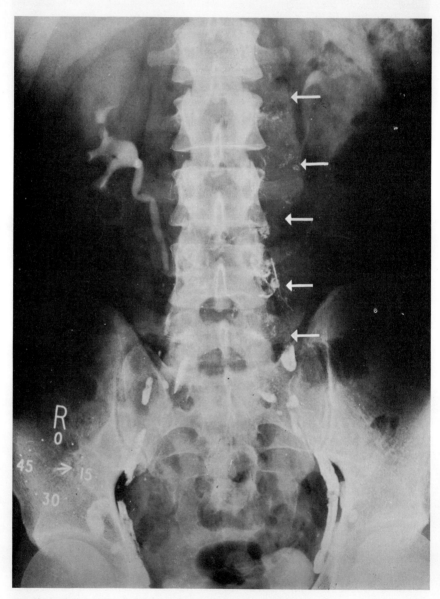

Fig. 8.10 Same patient as Figs. 8.8 and 8.9. Second refill lymphogram six months later. The para-aortic nodes are active again but are only faintly opacified (arrows indicate their size). The normal nodes in the pelvis retain their shape and ability to store contrast medium.

causing back pressure on the kidney, the appearances have returned to normal on the refill lymphogram.

When there are grossly abnormal nodes which only take up a little contrast medium, it is likely that they will remain opacified only for a short time and in the patient shown in Figs. 8.8 and 8.9 a further refill lymphogram was needed in six months when the markers were raised. The second refill lymphogram showed the nodes to be active again (Fig. 8.10). Involved nodes responding to chemotherapy will behave in the same way. Nodes that are only slightly involved will return to normal appearances after treatment and, in these cases, multiple repeat lymphograms and their follow up continue to yield useful information; but in patients who have heavily involved nodes the combined effect of tumour and treatment will obliterate what normal node tissue there is and the information provided by successive lymphograms will decrease. There will come a point when it is no longer profitable to repeat the lymphogram and other methods, such as CT, will have to be used. Lymphography should be used as long as it is providing the information, because once the nodes are opacified smaller abnormalities can be detected within them and a follow-up radiograph takes a matter of minutes, whereas repeated CT examinations will each take about one hour. This is an important factor when, for instance, numerous control films are needed during a course of chemotherapy.

Accuracy of lymphography

When used as described above, lymphography is a sensitive and accurate diagnostic examination. Accuracy, however, is a relative term and what is more important in a clinical setting is the question of how useful the investigation is. It is obvious that no radiological method will detect microscopic deposits and it is known that microscopic deposits are present in a proportion of lymphogram-negative (Stage I) patients. The evidence for this is from published series of para-aortic node dissections and from alphafetoprotein estimations and has been discussed elsewhere in this volume (see Chapter 13).

Conclusion

This chapter has examined the place of lymphography in testicular tumours. In 72 per cent of patients, lymphography will detect deposits otherwise unsuspected, and lymphography will be positive in 36 per cent of testicular tumours at the time of first diagnosis of the tumour (Table 8.2).

In experienced hands, lymphography is a safe investigation—safety depending on sensible patient selection, on an understanding of what complications may arise and on the radiological control of the injection.

The oily contrast medium remains in the nodes over long periods and this time should be used to monitor the behaviour of the nodes.

The lymphogram combined with follow up should be looked upon as a dynamic investigation. A deposit should be diagnosed only if it not only looks like one but behaves like one, and if it is not being treated it will behave as an expanding lesion. If it is being treated, it will contract more rapidly than the normal node. There are also secondary signs which are not diagnostic but help to increase the index of suspicion.

Table 8.2 Summary of positive lymphograms (Wilkinson and Macdonald, 1975)

Seminomas	30/116	26%
Teratoma	40/96	42%
Combined	20/38	53%
All	90/250	36%

Lymphography is the most accurate way of assessing those nodes which are opacified, but it must be remembered that the area above the origin of the thoracic duct and the echelon nodes on both sides are not and also, when there is mass disease present which has grown beyond the confines of the nodes, then the volume of disease can only be guessed at and other methods, such as CT, have to be used (see Chapter 9).

References

Davidson, J. W. (1969). *American Journal of Roentgenology* **105**, 763.

Fischer, H. W. (1969). *Lymphography in Cancer*, p. 24. Ed. by W. A. Fuchs, J. W. Davidson and H. W. Fischer. Heinemann Medical, London.

Fuchs, W. A. (1969). *Lymphography in Cancer*, p. 133. Ed. by W. A. Fuchs, J. W. Davidson and H. W. Fischer. Heinemann Medical, London.

Gold, W. M., Youker, J., Anderson, S. and Nadel, J. A. (1965). *New England Journal of Medicine* **273**, 519.

Jackson, B. T. (1972). *Thesis for Master of Surgery Degree*, University of London.

Jackson, B. T. (1974). *Annals of the Royal College of Surgeons of England* **54**, 3.

Kinmonth, J. B., Kemp-Harper, R. A. and Taylor, G. W. (1955). *Journal of the Faculty of Radiologists* **6**, 217.

Macdonald, J. S. (1976). *Complications of Diagnostic Radiology*, p. 301. Ed. by G. Ansell. Blackwell, Oxford.

Macdonald, J. S. (1978). *Circulation of the Blood*, p. 303. Ed. by D. G. James, Pitman, London.

Macdonald, J. S., Laugier, A.and Schlienger, M. (1968). *Clinical Radiology* **19**, 120.

Macdonald, J. S. and Paxton, R. M. (1976). *Scientific Foundations of Urology*, Vol. II, p. 226. Ed. by D. I. Williams and G. D. Chisholm. Heinemann Medical, London.

Rouviere, H. (1932). *Anatomie des Lymphatiques de l'homme*. Masson et Cie, Paris.

Steckel, R. J. and Cameron, T. P. (1966). *Radiology* **87**, 753.

Wilkinson, D. J. and Macdonald, J. S. (1975). *Clinical Radiology* **26**, 89.

9

Computed tomography in testicular tumours

Janet E. Husband

Computed tomography (CT) is an important imaging technique for the investigation of patients with malignant disease, because tumours can be demonstrated in almost every anatomical site. Apart from the obvious disadvantages of high cost and low patient throughput, the major limitations of the technique are the inability to demonstrate small metastases in those sites where there is insufficient contrast between the tumour and surrounding normal tissue, and the lack of tissue specificity. In testicular teratomas the predominant sites of metastatic spread are to the retroperitoneal and mediastinal lymph nodes, the lungs and the liver. These sites are among those best suited to examination by computed tomography and therefore the technique has gained particular significance in the assessment of this tumour.

In the evaluation of any new technique it is essential to compare the results with those obtained by conventional methods of investigation, but correlation with histopathology is frequently lacking. In patients with testicular teratomas, nodal dissection is employed only in selected patients following chemotherapy and radiotherapy (Peckham *et al.*, 1977). Thus, in the majority of patients the accuracy of CT scanning can be assessed only by changes in the scan appearances in response to treatment.

In this review the CT findings in patients with testicular teratoma will be described, followed by a discussion of the impact of CT on staging, monitoring therapeutic response and the detection of relapse. The physical principles of CT have been described in detail elsewhere (Hounsfield, 1973; Hill, 1974) and in this text only a brief outline is given.

Basic principles

Computed tomography uses x-radiation to produce an anatomical reconstruction of a thin slice of the patient. This is usually in the cross-sectional plane and the slice thickness is approximately 1 cm. The major advantage of the technique over conventional radiology is the ability to record fine anatomical detail, not otherwise visible, in the soft tissues, lungs and bones.

The original scanning system developed by Hounsfield (1973) uses a single source of x-rays and array of sodium-iodide detectors which are mounted on a scanning gantry. The source and detectors move across the body and then are rotated through a small angle and a further traverse is made (translate-rotate system). The process is repeated until the x-ray source has completed an arc of 180° around the patient. For mechanical reasons, this type of machine requires scan times of between fifteen and twenty seconds (Fig. 9.1). From this basic system, more sophisticated scanners have been developed in which scan times of less than five seconds have been achieved. Figure 9.2 illustrates the basic system of one type of fast scanner. The x-ray source rotates completely round the patient and a stationary ring of detectors is employed. The main advantage of these fast scanners is improved image quality. This is due partly

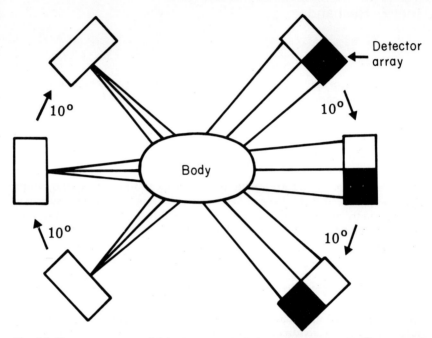

Fig. 9.1 The x-ray source and detectors are mounted on a scanning gantry. The x-ray tube and detectors traverse the patient, then rotate through a small angle and a further traverse is made.

to the inherent physics of the system and partly to a reduction in artefacts produced by patient movement.

The attenuation values (density) recorded by the detector array are analysed in a computer system and converted to an image which is then displayed on a video monitor. A scale of CT numbers has been introduced which relates the attenuation values of tissue to water. The CT number of water is zero and, using the EMI system of numbers, the scale ranges from +500 to −500. The value for air is approximately −500, the value for dense bone +200 to +500, for soft tissues +20 to +40 and for fat −30 to −50. This wide range of absorption values cannot be differentiated by the human eye simultaneously and therefore the viewing console is provided with a set of controls so that the observer can select a range of values for display. Thus, a low window level is used for examination of the lungs (Fig. 9.3), whereas a higher window level is used for examination of the soft tissues (Fig. 9.4). The range of density values

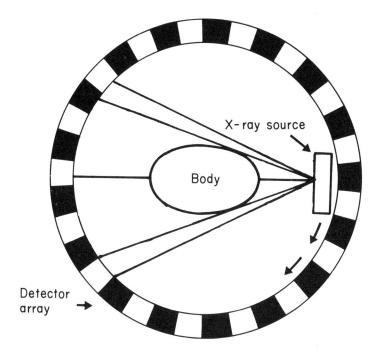

Fig. 9.2 The x-ray source rotates round the patient through 180°. There is a complete ring of stationary detectors.

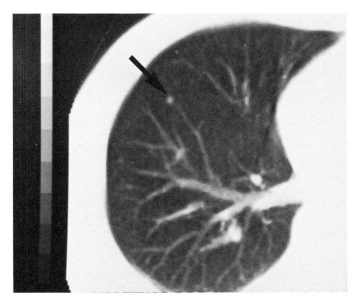

Fig. 9.3 CT scan through the chest (enlarged quadrant) showing a peripheral pulmonary metastasis in the right lung, approximately 4 mm in diameter (arrowed). A low window level is used (−258). The window width is 400.

displayed at a chosen window level can be varied also—this is known as the window width. Using a narrow window width, the contrast between different attenuation values is increased, thus permitting small differences in tissue density to be appreciated which may be missed if only a wide window width is used.

The examination

All the CT examinations discussed in this text have been obtained using the EMI (CT5005) General Purpose Scanner which has a scan time of twenty seconds and a slice thickness of 13 mm. Using this equipment, it is essential to

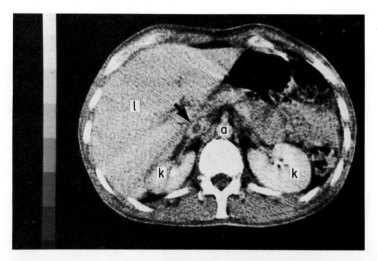

Fig. 9.4 CT scan through the abdomen. The soft tissues are viewed at a window level of +32. Intravenous contrast medium has been given by infusion into a vein in the foot to demonstrate the inferior vena cava. The lucency in the centre of the inferior vena cava (arrowed) represents tumour thrombosis. This thrombus was subsequently removed at surgery. a, Aorta; l, liver; k, kidney.

perform each scan during suspended respiration to avoid artefacts from respiratory movement. Artefacts are produced also by gas in moving bowel, but this problem is largely overcome by giving an anticholinergic agent before the abdominal scan. An oral contrast medium (sodium-meglumine diatrizoate—Gastrografin 300 ml, 5 per cent solution) is given also before the abdominal scan to delineate as much of the bowel as possible, because the absorption values of bowel and soft-tissue tumours are frequently similar. Intravenous contrast medium is required in two different situations. First, it is indicated in patients with suspected liver metastases; the intravenous contrast medium opacifies the normal parenchyma and increases the contrast between the metastasis and surrounding parenchyma. Second, scans obtained during or immediately after an intravenous injection of contrast medium demonstrate opacification of major vessels. This may be useful for distinguishing suspected lymphadenopathy from a large vessel or for the identification of tumour thrombus within the inferior vena cava (Fig. 9.4).

The chest and abdomen are examined in all patients with testicular teratomas, except in those with advanced lung disease when examination of the chest is considered unnecessary. Computed tomography sections are taken routinely through the lungs at 1-cm intervals and through the abdomen at 2-cm intervals. However, variation of this routine procedure is required occasionally in an attempt to resolve a particular clinical problem.

CT observations and results

Lungs

Pulmonary metastases appear as circular nodules, either in the lung parenchyma or arising from the pleural surface. Since the attenuation values of a metastasis are not significantly different from normal vessels, the lesion can be identified with confidence only if larger than the surrounding vascular structures (see Fig. 9.3). Small peripheral metastases, of the order of 3 to 4 mm in diameter, are shown easily but lesions of this size situated in the central part of the lungs may be missed. A malignant pulmonary nodule cannot be distinguished from a benign lesion (e.g. granuloma) on the basis of the CT scan appearances alone (Chang et al., 1979), but the demonstration of multiple pulmonary nodules is highly suspicious of metastatic disease. This may reflect the lower incidence of granulomatous disease in the United Kingdom compared to the United States of America. If a solitary nodule is identified, the scan should be repeated after an interval of three to four weeks in order to record any change in size of the lesion before definite diagnosis of lung involvement is made.

Computed tomography is more sensitive than conventional whole lung tomography for the detection of pulmonary nodules (Muhm et al., 1977; Schaner et al., 1978; Chang et al., 1979). In patients with testicular teratomas the yield appears to be particularly high. In a series of 77 patients investigated at the Royal Marsden Hospital, deposits were identified in the lungs reported as normal on conventional whole lung tomography in 14 patients. In a further 24 patients both techniques were positive.

Lymph nodes

Retroperitoneum

Although lymphography is a successful and accurate technique (Wallace, 1969; Wilkinson and Macdonald, 1975), lymph nodes in such sites as the upper para-aortic region, renal and splenic hila, porta hepatis and mesentery are not opacified with contrast medium. Furthermore, once the metastasis has broken out beyond the confines of the node, the size of the tumour cannot be assessed by lymphography and is only inferred from displacement of adjacent structures such as the kidneys and ureters. With CT, enlarged lymph nodes in the para-aortic region are easy to identify because usually they are surrounded by fat which has a low density, thus providing excellent contrast. Here even normal size nodes can be identified in patients with sufficient intra-abdominal fat (Fig. 9.5; Harell *et al.*, 1977). Enlarged nodes situated behind the crura of the

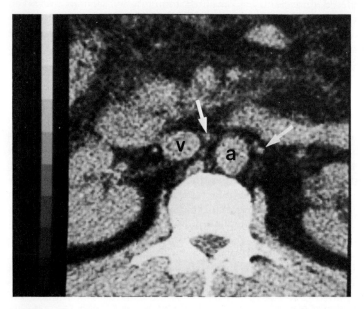

Fig. 9.5 CT scan at the level of the second lumbar vertebra. Enlarged quadrant showing normal size lymph nodes (arrowed). a, Aorta; v, inferior vena cava.

diaphragm are similarly well shown (Fig. 9.6; Callen *et al.*, 1977). Irrespective of the primary tumour, enlarged lymph nodes usually appear as well-defined structures with attenuation values similar to other soft tissues such as the pancreas, inferior vena cava and aorta (EMI units 20 to 30). However, in patients with testicular teratomas, lymph node metastases frequently have lower attenuation values (EMI units 10 to 20; Fig. 9.6; Husband, Peckham and Macdonald, 1980). There may be a number of discretely enlarged nodes or a conglomerate tumour mass when the individual nodes are no longer recognized (Figs. 9.7 and 9.8). These large tumours often obscure part or the whole of the margin of the aorta and/or inferior vena cava. One of the major disadvantages of CT for the detection of lymph node metastases is the inability to define the internal nodal architecture. Thus, metastases in normal size nodes

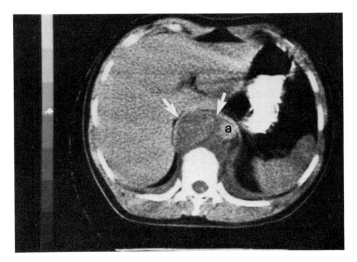

Fig. 9.6 CT scan to the twelfth thoracic vertebra showing enlarged retrocrural nodes (arrowed). Aorta (a) is more dense than the lymph node mass and is displaced anteriorly.

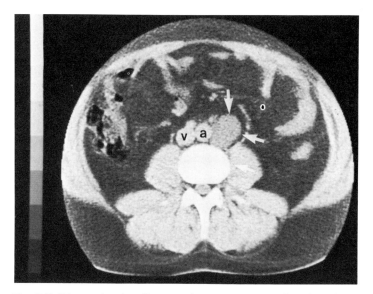

Fig. 9.7 CT scan showing discrete enlargement of a lymph node at the level of the lower border of the fourth lumbar vertebra (arrowed). a, Aorta; v, inferior vena cava.

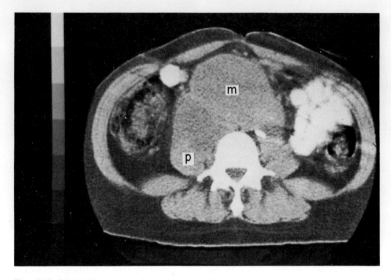

Fig. 9.8 CT scan at the level of the fourth lumbar vertebra showing a huge lymph node mass (m). The mass has completely obscured the margins of the aorta and inferior vena cava. It is inseparable from the psoas muscle on the right (p).

cannot be identified. In general, with CT, enlarged lymph nodes can be recognized down to the size of approximately 1.5 cm in diameter.

The results of a comparative study between CT and lymphography in 77 new patients investigated at the Royal Marsden Hospital are shown in Table 9.1. The findings illustrate several important points. First, CT is equally effective and may be slightly better than lymphography in detecting the presence of lymph node metastases. In this series, CT was unequivocally positive in 4 patients when the lymphogram was reported either negative or equivocal. In the 3 patients with negative lymphograms, the lymph node metastases were identified by CT high in the para-aortic region (2 patients)

Table 9.1 Comparison of CT with lymphography in testicular tera-tomas in 77 patients examined at presentation

Lymphogram	No of patients	CT findings	
		Negative	Positive
Negative	28	25	3*
Positive	44	1	43*
Equivocal	5	4	1*
Total	77	30	47

* Additional information obtained with CT.

Table 9.2 Comparison of lymphogram follow-up film with CT findings in testicular teratomas in 23 patients (40 scans)

Initial scan	No. of patients	Follow-up scans					
		LG+ No. of patients	CT+ No. of scans	LG− No. of patients	CT− No. of scans	LG− No. of patients	CT+ No. of scans
LG+ CT+	18	6	(11)	3	(3)	9	(13)
LG− CT−	5	—	—	5	(13)	—	—
Total	23	6	(11)	8	(16)	9	(13)

and at the renal hilum (1 patient). Computed tomography missed a lymph node metastasis in 1 patient, but the node was only minimally enlarged. In all patients with positive CT examinations, the precise extent of the tumour was defined more precisely by CT scanning than lymphography.

Follow-up abdominal radiographs are a well-established method of monitoring nodal response to therapy, but CT may show persisting lymph node masses after the lymphogram appearances have returned to normal. Table 9.2 shows that persisting abdominal tumour was demonstrated with CT in 9 out of 18 patients at a time when the abdominal radiograph showed no evidence of activity.

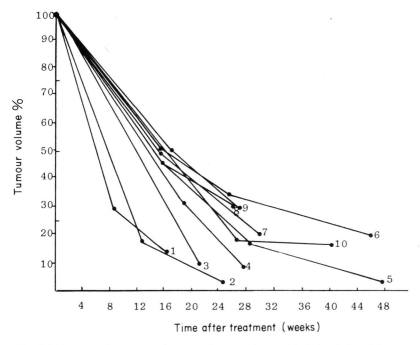

Fig. 9.9 Tumour volume regression rates in ten patients with abdominal nodal metastases with testicular teratoma treated by chemotherapy. Tumour volume has been expressed as a percentage of the initial absolute volume and error bars have not been shown for clearer representation. Absolute tumour volume estimations range from 4 to 1800 ml.

The ability to document tumour regression accurately has important significance both for therapy and for the study of human tumour biology. With CT, quantitation of tumour volume is carried out from calculations of the area of tumour on sequential CT sections throughout the tumour length using a computer programme (Husband *et al.*,1981). The tumour is outlined on each CT image using a precision touch-sensitive light pen and, although there are obvious errors due to the difficulty in defining tumour margins, the method does provide information which has previously been impossible to obtain. Figure 9.9 shows tumour volume regression of abdominal nodal masses in ten patients who were treated with chemotherapy.

Mediastinum

The major advantage of CT for examination of the mediastinum compared to conventional radiology is the ability to delineate mediastinal anatomy in the cross-sectional plane. Thus, small tumours which do not alter the mediastinal

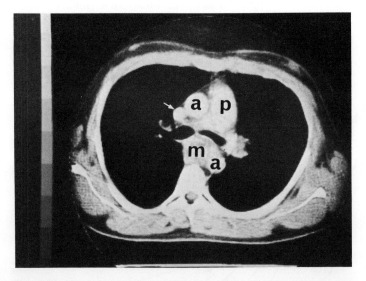

Fig. 9.10 CT scan at the level of the tracheal bifurcation showing the ascending and descending aorta (a), the pulmonary artery (p) and the superior vena cava (arrowed). There is a posterior mediastinal lymph node mass (m).

contour can be recognized (Fig. 9.10). Since the quantity of fat influences the ability to detect enlarged lymph nodes, evaluation of this area can be much more difficult than the retroperitoneum. When there is doubt, intravenous contrast medium is helpful for distinguishing vessels from suspected tumour. Out of a total of 78 patients, CT detected mediastinal lymphadenopathy in 6 when the conventional radiographs were reported as normal, and in a further

5 patients both techniques were abnormal. These CT findings have not been confirmed histologically, but continued patient observation during follow up has indicated that the CT results were correct.

Liver

Since the information from a single CT examination is not limited to one system, other abdominal organs such as the liver can be screened for the presence of metastases. The vast majority of space-occupying lesions, including metastases, have lower attenuation values than normal liver parenchyma and are seen therefore as areas of diminished density (Fig. 9.11; Petasnick and Clark, 1976). Usually, tumours can be identified when they reach the size of

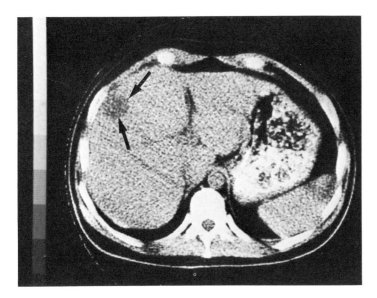

Fig. 9.11 CT scan at the level of the twelfth thoracic vertebra showing a solitary liver metastasis in the periphery of the right node (arrowed). The image is viewed at a narrow window width (75) in order to increase contrast between a normal liver parenchyma and the lesion.

1.5 to 2 cm in diameter, but often lesions smaller than this are missed (Stephens *et al.*, 1977). Opacification of the normal liver parenchyma with intravenous iodinated contrast medium increases the contrast between normal tissue and a suspected metastasis and is a useful manoeuvre if there is doubt about the presence of a lesion. The introduction of percutaneous CT-guided fine-needle aspiration techniques permits cytological confirmation if this is clinically indicated (Haaga *et al.*, 1977).

The results in our series of 195 patients (80 new patients, 115 previously treated before the first CT examination) indicate that CT is as effective as ultrasound in the detection of hepatic metastases. However, the incidence of liver involvement is low and figures regarding the relative accuracy of these techniques are therefore meaningless.

Bone

The vertebral bodies are examined at a high window level which shows the cortex and medullary trabecular pattern. The presence of lytic bone lesions can be indentified almost certainly before they are obvious on conventional radiology but isotope scanning is the method of choice as a screening procedure. The role of CT is probably to provide further information in patients with positive isotope scans but apparently normal radiographs. Although in the Royal Marsden series the bones have been examined in all patients with testicular teratoma, we have been unable to identify tumour which has not been obvious by conventional techniques.

Relationship of computed tomography to ultrasound

Ultrasound is a rapidly developing and expanding technique but, since it uses a different form of energy from CT (sound waves), completely different physical characteristics are measured and the advantages and limitations of the system frequently balance the disadvantages of CT (Kreel and Meire, 1977). For example, CT utilizes an automatic mechanism, but the capital outlay and running costs are much higher than ultrasound machines. At the present time ultrasound equipment is manually operated which means that the results obtained are highly dependent on the skill of the operator.

Although enlarged lymph nodes may be demonstrated with ultrasound, bowel gas lying anterior to the nodes frequently limits the investigation, particularly below the epigastrium. Tyrrell *et al.* (1977) reported successful ultrasound examinations of the para-aortic lymph nodes in 91 out of 95 patients, with an accuracy of 92 per cent, but these results are unlikely to be achieved in the majority of centres where a full-time ultrasonographer is not employed. Computed tomography is an excellent technique for demonstrating enlarged lymph nodes and is almost certainly the method of choice if the facilities are available.

In experienced hands, ultrasound is a highly successful and accurate technique for detecting focal liver disease (Cosgrove, 1978). Both CT and ultrasound can detect lesions as small as 1 to 2 cm in diameter and can provide information regarding composition (Meire and Husband, 1979). In the Royal Marsden series of patients with testicular teratoma, CT has been marginally more successful than ultrasound in detecting liver metastases. However, both techniques have missed hepatic involvement and at the present time it is probably best to employ both techniques rather than rely on the results of one.

Clinical applications

The employment of CT scanning in patients with testicular teratomas has

Table 9.3 Impact of CT on clinical staging in 80 patients

Conventional stage	No. of patients	CT stage			
		I	II	III	IV
I	21	16	1	—	4
II	22	—	16	1	5
III	12	—	—	5	7
IV	25	—	—	—	25
Total	80	16	17	6	41

demonstrated the superiority of this technique over conventional radiology in the lungs, mediastinum and retroperitoneum. The impact of these findings on staging is shown in Table 9.3. Sixteen patients were shown by CT scanning to have Stage IV disease (14 patients lung involvement; 2 patients liver metastases) which would otherwise have been undetected. Overall CT increased staging in 22 per cent out of a total of 80 patients.

Following initial staging, CT is used to monitor therapeutic response. Scans are repeated following four or six courses of chemotherapy (Stage IIB and C, Stage III and Stage IV). The lungs are scanned in those patients who presented with lung metastases but in whom conventional radiology has returned to normal, and abdominal scans are obtained in all patients who presented with an abdominal mass. In addition to measuring the extent of tumour regression or growth, the CT information is used for radiotherapy planning purposes. The technique of CT integrated radiotherapy treatment planning and results in various tumour types have been reported recently from the Royal Marsden Hospital (Hobday *et al.*, 1979). In those patients selected for abdominal nodal resection of abdominal residua, CT scans are obtained immediately before surgery. This provides valuable information to the surgeon regarding the presence of residual tumour, its precise location and relationship to important structures such as the renal arteries. Thus, operability and surgical approach are assessed on the basis of CT (Hendry *et al.*, 1980).

Apart from these protocol studies, CT scanning is used in patients who have been in clinical remission but in whom relapse is suspected either clinically or on the basis of serum-marker elevation. In a group of 16 patients with suspected relapse, CT was negative in 11 and positive in 5. One of the 11 patients with negative scans had persistently elevated serum markers and was treated on the

Table 9.4 Influence of CT on treatment policies in 126 patients

Treatment	Change	No. of patients
Chemotherapy	Introduced	10
	Continued	8
	Stopped	1
	Drugs changed	3
Surgery	Indicated by CT	2
	Contra-indicated	2
Radiotherapy	Introduced	1
No treatment		10
Total change		37

basis of this finding alone; the remainder of this group have remained well without treatment for a minimum period of six months.

The influence of CT on patient management has been analysed in a group of 126 patients. This group includes 80 patients who were staged by CT (see Table 9.3) and a further 46 patients who have been treated previously before the initial CT scan. The results are shown in Table 9.4 and indicate that CT has made a significant impact on treatment policy in 29 per cent of patients.

In conclusion, computed tomography has made a significant contribution to the management of patients with testicular teratomas at the Royal Marsden Hospital. However, the low patient throughput of approximately 10 to 12 patients precludes its use as the only radiological method of investigation. Thus, in our unit, whole lung tomography is still employed and CT scanning is undertaken in those patients with negative results. Lymphography is also routinely employed, not only to identify those patients with small volume nodal disease but also for follow-up purposes in the initial phases of treatment when only a single abdominal film is required to demonstrate response.

References

Callen, P. W., Korobkin, M. and Isherwood, I. (1977). *American Journal of Roentgenology* **129**, 907.

Chang, A. E., Schaner, E. G., Conkle, D. M., Flye, M. W., Doppman, J. L. and Rosenberg, S. A. (1979). *Cancer* **43**, 913.

Cosgrove, D. O. (1978). *Evaluation of Liver Tumours in Ultrasound in Tumour Diagnosis*, p. 104. Ed. by C. R. Hill, V. R. McCready and D. O. Cosgrove. Pitman Medical, London.

Haaga, J. R., Reich, N. E., Havrilla, T. R. and Alfidi, R. J. (1977). *Radiologic Clinics of North America* **15**, 449.

Harell, G. S., Breiman, R. S., Glatstein, E. J., Marshall, W. H. Jr. and Castellino, R. A. (1977). *Radiologic Clinics of North America* **15**, 391.

Hendry, W. F., Barrett, A., McElwain, T. J., Wallace, D. M. and Peckham, M. J. (1980). *British Journal of Urology* **52**, 38.

Hill, K. R. (1974). *British Journal of Hospital Medicine, Equipment Supplement* **11**, 5.

Hobday, P., Hodson, N. J., Husband, J., Parker, R. P. and Macdonald, J. S. (1979). *Radiology* **133**, 477.

Hounsfield, G. N. (1973). *British Journal of Radiology* **46**, 1016.

Husband, J. E., Peckham, M. J. and Macdonald, J. S. (1980). *Computerized Tomography* **4**, 1.

Husband, J. E., Cassell, K. J., Peckham, M. J. and Macdonald, J. S. (1981). *British Journal of Radiology*, Suppl. 15, pp 50–53.

Kreel, L. and Meire, H. B. (1977). *British Medical Journal* **2**, 809.

Meire, H. B. and Husband, J. E. (1979). Ultrasound and CT in the demonstration of focal liver disease. *Clinics in Diagnostic Ultrasound Vol. 1:* Diagnostic Ultrasound in Gastro-Intestinal Disease, p. 35. Ed. by K. W. F. Taylor. Churchill Livingstone, Edinburgh.

Muhm, J. R., Brown, L. R. and Crowe, J. K. (1977). *American Journal of Roentgenology* **128**, 267.

Peckham, M. J., Hendry, W. F., McElwain, T. J. and Calman, F. M. B. (1977). In *Adjuvant Therapy of Cancer*, p. 305. Ed. by S. E. Salmon and S. E. Jones. North Holland Publ. Co., Amsterdam, Oxford and New York.

Petasnick, J. P. and Clark, J. W. (1976). *Gastrointestinal Radiology* **1**, 201.

Schaner, E. G., Chang, A. E., Doppman, J. L., Conkle, D. M., Flye, M. W. and Rosenberg, S. A. (1978). *American Journal of Roentgenology* **131**, 51.

Stephens, D. H., Sheedy, P. F.II., Hattery, R. and MacCarthy, R. (1977). *American Journal of Roentgenology* **128**, 579.

Tyrrell, C. J., Cosgrove, D. O., McCready, V. R. and Peckham, M. J. (1977). *Clinical Radiology* **28**, 475.

Wallace, E. M. K. (1969). *Clinical Radiology* **20**, 453.

Wilkinson, D. J. and Macdonald, J. S. (1975). *Clinical Radiology* **26**, 89.

10

Seminoma testis

M. J. Peckham

Approximately 40 per cent of testicular tumours are seminomas. They are characterized by an exquisite sensitivity to radiation which, together with a predominance of early stage presentations, results in an excellent prognosis with overall cure rates exceeding 90 per cent.

Histogenesis and functional pathology

Seminomas arise from the germinal epithelium. In approximately 14 per cent of patients combined tumours, in which both seminoma and teratoma elements are combined, are present in the testis. The precise histogenetic relationship between seminoma and teratoma is unknown. As discussed below, a proportion of patients presenting with apparently pure advanced seminoma die with marker or histological evidence of non-seminoma (teratoma) elements. Whether this reflects an evolution of seminoma into teratoma or the expression of a small teratomatous component present initially is not known. Approximately 6 per cent of seminomas show histological evidence of giant cells (Thackray and Crane, 1976). These range in size from cells with two or three nuclei to irregular syncytial masses with many nuclei. As discussed in Chapter 3, the presence of human chorionic gonadotrophin may be identified by immunoperoxidase staining in a proportion of seminomas, although the significance, both biologically and prognostically, of this observation is unclear. A distinction should be made between the patient with a histologically pure seminoma, in which occasional giant cells are identified, and combined tumours, in which frank non-seminomatous components are present. The variant described as 'seminoma with trophocarcinoma' by Friedman and Pearlman (1970) should be considered as combined tumours and it is of interest that these authors observed unmasking of the syncytial non-seminoma cell population following destruction of the seminoma elements by a pre-operative dose of 1000 rads. The recent identification of a human testicular tumour xenograft which appears to have evolved from seminoma to an alphafetoprotein-producing tumour with some of the morphological features of yolk-sac malignancy, adds some support to the notion that seminoma can change into teratoma (see Chapter 5).

Subtypes of seminoma

Classical seminoma

The large majority, approximately 90 per cent, of seminomas are of *classical type* in which uniform, rounded tumour cells are arranged in sheets or columns. As noted above, 6 per cent show evidence of giant cells, areas of necrosis are present in approximately 50 per cent of cases, lymphocytic infiltration is commonly observed, which may be dense or in the form of follicles, and in about one-third of tumours granulomatous reactions are observed. As shown in Chapter 1, seminomas present approximately one decade later than teratomas and show a peak incidence at about 35 years of age. Classical seminoma is the most common tumour found in the cryptorchid testis in men and in the rare syndromes of testicular feminization and dysgenetic gonads (see Chapters 1 and 18).

Spermatocytic seminoma

This is a distinctive variant of pure seminoma of the testis. In contrast to classical seminoma, where the tumour cells are uniform in size with oval vesicular nuclei and pale vacuolated cytoplasm, the spermatocytic seminoma cells vary in size, have round nuclei and deeply staining cytoplasm. Some of the smaller cells may resemble spermatogonia and the larger spermatocytes. Spermatocytic seminomas tend to occur at an older age, the peak being between 45 and 50 years, with as many occurring above as below the age of 50. As shown in Table 10.1, 3.5 to 7.4 per cent of seminomas conform to the criteria for spermatocytic seminoma.

Table 10.1 Frequency of spermatocytic seminoma

References	Total seminomas	Number designated spermatocytic	Percentage
Scully (1961)	81	3	3.7
Jackson and Magner (1965)	42	5	11.9
Fox and Abell (1968)	170	6	3.5
Rosai et al. (1969)	81	6	7.4
Thackray and Crane (1976)	729	27	3.7

It is of interest that the incidence of bilateral tumours (6 per cent) is higher in spermatocytic seminoma than in other seminomas—2 per cent (Thackray and Crane, 1976).

So far as prognosis is concerned, most reports suggest that the metastatic potential of spermatocytic seminoma is low. Thus, there were no tumour deaths in the series of 27 reported by Thackray and Crane and, in a review of 52 patients, Weitzner (1976) could find no convincing evidence of metastases. Of the 5 patients reported by Jackson and Magner (1965), 4 died of tumour.

This is, however, an unusual experience and some doubt has been cast on the histological diagnosis of these 4 patients (Rossai *et al.*, 1969). In the United States Armed Forces series, Mostofi and Price (1973) found no example of metastatic spermatocytic seminoma.

From the reported experience of this uncommon variant, it appears that the probability of cure with orchidectomy alone is high and that, if the usual clinical staging procedures including lymphography are negative, a policy of close observation without elective lymph node irradiation is justifiable.

Anaplastic seminoma

This variant was defined by Mostofi (1973) as showing nuclear pleomorphism and more than three mitotic figures per high-power microscopic field. It has been held generally that anaplastic seminomas are a more aggressive variant than classical seminoma, although stage for stage there is little evidence to support this contention.

In a recent analysis of 77 patients with anaplastic seminoma from the Walter Reed Hospital, Percapio *et al.* (1979) reported a 96 per cent actuarial survival at ten years for 58 Stage I patients and 87 per cent for 19 Stage II patients. These results of orchidectomy and radiotherapy are comparable with those obtained in classical seminoma and are in keeping with the report of Maier *et al.* (1968), who had one death in 15 anaplastic seminoma Stage I patients. Johnson *et al.* (1975) reported that 3 of 5 Stage I and II patients were disease free at five or more years after radiotherapy.

Kademian *et al.* (1977) reported 8 patients with anaplastic seminoma in a total seminoma population of 66, treated between 1959 and 1976. The mean age was 40 years. Four patients had Stage I disease, 3 had Stage II and 1 had Stage IV. Two of the 4 Stage I patients developed widespread disease and died. Both Stage II patients were alive at the time of reporting, although one had recently completed treatment.

It is of interest that, in the Walter Reed series, 13 per cent of men developed this tumour in an undescended testis or after orchidopexy.

The comparability of diagnosis from one series to another needs to be taken into consideration when interpreting data from different centres. Thus, the series reported by Percapio *et al.* accounted for 20 per cent of the total seminoma population. In the series reported by Kademian, 8 out of 66 patients were considered to have anaplastic seminoma (12 per cent), whereas in the series of Thackray and Crane (1976), 3 per cent of seminomas were classified as atypical and these showed a worse prognosis. The histological diagnosis of anaplastic seminoma may be confused with undifferentiated teratoma or histiocytic lymphoma.

Ultrastructurally, Janssen and Johnston (1978) have reported that the features are essentially similar to classical seminoma.

In conclusion, there is no good evidence to suggest that anaplastic seminoma should be identified as a separate group for treatment purposes, since stage for stage the results of radiotherapy appear comparable to those obtained in classical seminoma.

Clinical stage at presentation

As shown in Table 10.2, more than 70 per cent of seminoma patients present with Stage I disease. Figure 10.1 shows the stage distribution of 190 previously untreated patients seen between 1963 and 1975 at the Royal Marsden Hospital and demonstrates the rarity (7 out of 190—3.7 per cent) of extralymphatic metastases at presentation. In a recent national study in Denmark (Schultz, H., personal communication), of 48 per cent consecutive cases of seminoma, 77.2 per cent were Stage I, 19.5 per cent Stage II, 2.0 per cent Stage III and 1.2 per cent Stage IV. Of the total group, 4.7 per cent were anaplastic seminomas and 2.2 per cent spermatocytic seminomas.

Table 10.2 Incidence of Stage I disease in seminoma testis

	Total seminomas	Stage I
Ytredal and Bradfield (1972)	80	71
Saxena (1973)	77	75
Castro and Gonzalez (1971)	96	58
Van der Werf Messing (1976)	257	153*
Maier et al. (1968)	80	78
Kademian et al. (1976)	52	36
Calman et al. (1979)	190	121
Total	832	592 (71%)

*This includes 95 patients designated N_x in the absence of lymphography.

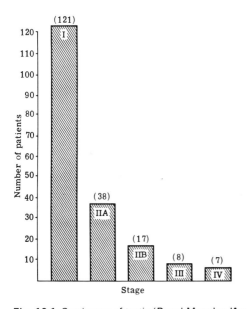

Fig. 10.1 Seminoma of testis (Royal Marsden Hospital, 1963–1975). Stage distribution at presentation of 190 previously untreated patients.

Investigation and staging

Because the majority of patients present with early stage disease and the overall prognosis is excellent with extralymphatic spread an uncommon feature, clinical staging procedures are limited to chest radiograph, intravenous urography and lymphography, routine renal and hepatic function tests and examination of the blood for alphafetoprotein and beta-human chorionic gonadotrophin. It is essential to examine the primary tumour with care to exclude the presence of a teratomatous component since, if a non-seminomatous element is identified, management should be as described for malignant teratoma. In selected patients, [67]Gallium scanning may prove useful in defining metastatic seminoma (Paterson *et al.*, 1976). In a small number of men with bulky abdominal metastases, laparotomy has been carried out to delineate the tumour accurately for radiation therapy as well as for staging purposes (see Fig. 13.4a). Since the advent of CT scanning, reliance has been placed on this procedure for providing information about the disposition and size of retroperitoneal lymph node metastases.

Staging classification

This is as described in Chapter 7. In an initial analysis of the pattern of spread and management of seminoma metastases, an arbitrary subdivision of Stage II was made on the basis of tumour size, using 5 cm as the dividing line. Patients with metastases <5 cm in maximum diameter correspond to Stages IIA and IIB, those with >5 cm to Stage IIC (see Chapter 7). There was a significant association between length of history and size of the retroperitoneal metastases. This is shown in Fig. 10.2, where it is seen that in Stage IIA/B (metastases $\leqslant 5$ cm in maximum diameter) the average delay in diagnosis was 10.9 months compared with 24.5 months in Stage IIC (>5 cm) patients.

Management

Stage I

Most patients will fall into this category. Following orchidectomy, routine radiotherapy is given to the para-aortic and ipsilateral pelvic lymph nodes, as described in Chapter 13. A midplane dose of 3000 rad (30 Gray) is given in three weeks, using daily fractionation and opposed anterior and posterior fields. If there is no history of orchidopexy, scrotal involvement or inappropriate surgery, the lower border of the treatment volume is placed at the midobturator foramen, the contralateral testis being protected by lead cups (see Chapter 13).

Stages IIA and IIB

In patients with limited disease in retroperitoneal nodes, radiotherapy is given as for Stage I. If involvement extends to the lower para-aortic chain and there is a risk of retrograde spread, the contralateral pelvic nodes are included. A midplane dose of 3500 rad (35 Gray) is given in three and a half weeks. Hitherto, it was Royal Marsden policy one month after completion of infradiaphragmatic treatment, to irradiate the mediastinum and supraclavicular fossae

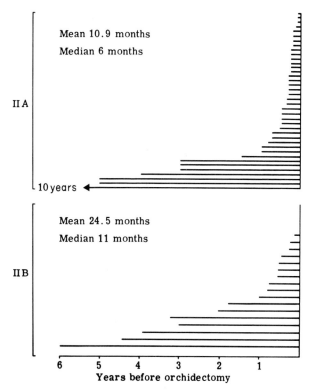

Fig. 10.2 Seminoma of testis (Royal Marsden Hospital, 1963–1975). Delay in diagnosis in relation to volume of metastatic abdominal tumour at the time of orchidectomy. The delay was significantly longer in patients with bulky nodes compared with those having smaller-volume disease (P<0.05).

to a dose of 3000 rad (30 Gray) in three weeks. The evidence for pursuing such a policy is scanty and, since it is clear that a proportion of Stage II patients will require chemotherapy, supradiaphragmatic irradiation has been abandoned for Stage II disease (*vide infra*).

Stage IIC

Hitherto, in patients with bulky disease radiotherapy was used alone and in patients with negative tumour markers, moderately good results were obtained (see below). If large-volume disease is present, it is current policy to employ chemotherapy as initial treatment to secure adequate volume reduction before proceeding to radiotherapy. Because metastic seminoma is uncommon, chemotherapy experience is relatively fragmentary. Limited experience suggests that chemotherapy regimes employed for teratoma are efficacious in the management of advanced seminoma and this aspect is discussed in more detail below.

Stage III

Previously, radiotherapy alone was employed. As for IIC, a policy of chemotherapy (vinblastine, bleomycin and cis-platinum) followed by radiotherapy is advocated.

Stage IV

Chemotherapy is the treatment of choice, although radiotherapy should be considered for sites of initial bulky disease.

Chemotherapy of Seminoma

Prior to the introduction of present combinations for testicular teratoma, alkylating agents were used widely to treat advanced seminoma. During this period it was clear that responses could be obtained, although relapse almost invariably occurred. For this reason an attempt was made to irradiate known sites of disease, even in advanced-staged disease. It is difficult to assess individual cytotoxic drugs in terms of response rate because of the sporadic nature of reported experience and the infrequency of advanced disease. In the Soviet Union, phenylalanine mustard (Sarcolysin) was employed extensively (Blokhin *et al.*, 1958). Subsequently, Chebotareva (1964) gave follow-up details on 42 seminoma patients, of whom 25 had died. Of the remaining 17, 6 had been followed for up to three years and 11 for more than three years. The disease

Table 10.3 Alkylating agent therapy of seminoma

References	Drug	Total no. of patients	Response	
Chebotareva (1964)	D-phenylalanine mustard (Sarcolysin)	42	'Remissions' in	38 (90%)
Mackenzie (1966)	Chlorambucil	4	Complete remission	2 (50%)
Snyder *et al.* (1964)	Cyclophosphamide	2	Complete remission	2 (100%)
*Calman *et al.* (1979)	Cyclophosphamide	19	Complete remission	6 (31.5%)
	Melphalan	1	Complete remission	0
	Chlorambucil	4	Complete remission	0

* Royal Marsden Hospital series.

Table 10.4 Combination chemotherapy for seminoma testis

References	Combination	Total no. of patients	Complete remission
Yagoda and Vugrin (1979)	Cyclo, cis-DDP	9	3
Samuels *et al.* (1976)	Bleomycin, cyclo, vincristine, 5-FU, methotrexate	11	4
Cheng *et al.* (1978)	Vinblastine, actinomycin D, bleomycin, cis-DDP, chlorambucil	1	0
Kardinal *et al.* (1976)	Bleomycin, adriamycin, vinblastine	2	0
Einhorn and Williams (1980)	Bleomycin, vinblastine, cis-DDP	19	12
Samson *et al.* (1979)	Bleomycin, vinblastine, cis-DDP	8	2
Royal Marsden Hospital	Bleomycin, vinblastine ±cis-DDP	9	5

status of the survivors was not stated. Mackenzie (1966) reported 6 patients with seminoma, 4 of whom received chlorambucil. All showed tumour regression, which was complete in 2 patients. Snyder *et al.* (1964) reported clearance of lung metastases in 2 patients treated with cyclophosphamide, with reappearance of tumour on cessation of chemotherapy. One of 2 patients treated with adriamycin obtained a partial response (Monfardini *et al.*, 1972). Data for alkylating agent therapy of seminoma are unimpressive and are summarized in Table 10.3.

The results of combination chemotherapy have been reported in limited series of patients (Table 10.4). It is too early to be able to assess the likely contribution of chemotherapeutic regimes usually employed for teratoma. It will be important to assess effect, not only in terms of response but of the durability of response, since relapse after alkylating agent chemotherapy was a common experience, despite initially good responses.

The results of treatment

Table 10.5 summarizes the results of treatment of 190 previously untreated patients with seminoma seen at the Royal Marsden Hospital between 1963 and 1975 (Calman *et al.*, 1979).

Stage I
Of 121 Stage I patients, only 1 has died of seminoma and this was due to metastases arising from a second testicular tumour. In all, 4 out of the 121 (3.3 per cent) patients relapsed, but 3 were satisfactorily controlled with further radiation therapy. It is of interest that 7 of the 121 (5.8 per cent) Stage I seminoma patients developed contralateral testicular tumours and 6 of these remain disease-free. Thirteen patients were lost to follow up, in all cases beyond the two-year follow-up period. All 13 were in complete remission at the previous follow-up examination. Thus, death from uncontrolled disease is an exceptional event in Stage I seminoma.

Stage II
Metastases to abdominal lymph nodes may be small in volume and demonstrable only by lymphography. At the other extreme, there may be massive nodal replacement with a large, palpable abdominal mass, as noted above. In an initial study from the Royal Marsden, we divided Stage II arbitrarily into two categories based on the size of abdominal node metastases.

   1. Stages IIA and IIB, maximum diameter of nodal mass $\leqslant 5$ cm.
   2. Stage IIC, maximum diameter of nodal mass > 5 cm.

Stages IIA and IIB
Between 1962 and 1975, 38 patients in this category were treated by irradiation, including treatment to the mediastinal and supraclavicular lymph nodes. Of this group, 32 (84 per cent) showed no evidence of relpase and 6 died of disseminated seminoma. Two patients developed recurrent disease, initially in the scrotal sac and inguinal nodes. Neither had received local irradiation as part of initial management, despite the presence of locally advanced primary tumours.

Table 10.5 The results of treatment by stage of 190 previously untreated patients with seminoma testis (Royal Marsden Hospital, 1963–1975)

	Total no. of patients	Lost to follow-up	Relapsed	Died of intercurrent disease	Died seminoma	Died teratoma	Developed second tumour
Stage I	121	13	4	4	1 (second tumour)	0	7
Stages IIA+IIB	38	1 (42 months)	6	4	6	0	0
Stage IIC	16	0	4	1	3	0	0
Stage III	8	1 (67 months)	1/1 NC	0	2	2	2 (both died teratoma)
Stage IV	7	1 (9 months)	0/4 NC	0	4	1	1 (died teratoma)

NC, never controlled by therapy.

Stage IIC
During the same time period, 16 IIC patients were treated with radiotherapy. One patient developed a second primary tumour (malignant teratoma) and died of disseminated disease. Three relapsed with seminoma and have died. Thirteen (81.3 per cent) patients showed no evidence of seminoma relapse, although one has subsequently died of intercurrent disease. Van der Werf Messing (1976), reporting on 46 patients with small-volume Stage II disease, recorded a 90 per cent cure rate, whereas for 21 patients with bulky Stage II disease the survival rate was approximately 60 per cent. This compares with a relapse rate of 15.8 per cent and 25 per cent for the Royal Marsden Hospital series of small and large volume Stage II patients respectively, and indicates that the patient with bulky intra-abdominal disease is at a higher risk from developing recurrent tumour. This aspect is considered below in the light of more recent data.

The causes of treatment failure are twofold: failure to include all tumour within the irradiated volume so that marginal recurrence occurs, and the subsequent appearance of extralymphatic metastases. Two measures can be taken to correct this deficiency: the more precise delineation of the tumour and the use of chemotherapy before irradiation to achieve tumour volume reduction and to eliminate subclinical metastases outside the treatment volume.

Stage III
Of 8 patients with Stage III disease, 2 died of seminoma and 2 of malignant teratoma metastasizing from second primary tumours.

Stage IV
Of 7 patients in this category, only 1 remains alive three years after initial therapy.

A progressive improvement in prognosis for testicular seminoma has been documented as radiotherapeutic facilities improved (Smithers, 1972). On the basis of the excellent overall survival figures, it has been a routine at the Royal Marsden Hospital for the past fifteen years to irradiate the para-aortic and ipsilateral pelvic nodes after orchidectomy for negative-lymphogram patients, and to irradiate the mediastinal and supraclavicular fossae in addition in patients with positive lymphograms. As noted above and discussed below, the latter practice has been abandoned. Using the diagnostic criteria developed for interpretation of lymphography at this centre, 70 per cent of patients with a seminoma have negative lymphograms. The proportion of patients within this group who have microscopic metastases is unknown, but is likely to be relatively low (Maier et al., 1968). There is no way in which the question can be resolved readily, apart from desisting from irradiation in Stage I patients or directly sampling retroperitoneal nodes. The latter would be unjustifiable and the former probably unwise since, in the first place, the therapeutic approach is virtually unassociated with morbidity and, secondly, the monitoring of the untreated patient would be both time consuming and inevitably would involve investigations which are at the present time not repeated after completion of radiotherapy.

Overall in the series, summarized in Table 10.5, 16 out of 190 patients have died of seminoma (8.4 per cent), 3 of teratoma (1.5 per cent) and 9 of intercurrent disease (4.7 per cent). In Stage I, where irradiation is directed towards the elimination of presumed micrometastases in the retroperitoneal nodes, the only death in 121 patients was associated with reseeding from a second seminoma into the previously irradiated retroperitoneal area. The control rate can be assumed to be 100 per cent.

In Stage II, the ability of radiation to eradicate overt nodal metastases can be assessed. Overall, 9 of 54 patients (16.7 per cent) died of seminoma; 7 of these patients died of widespread extranodal metastases. Tumour volume was associated with length of history and relapse rate (*vide infra*), but this did not exert a significant influence on prognosis. Thus, the ten-year survival of patients with bulky disease was 54 per cent and small volume disease 66 per cent. In calculating these figures, deaths from intercurrent disease have not been subtracted from the total number and it has been assumed that the survival experience of those lost to follow-up is the same as those patients still being followed. Long-term follow-up is necessary in these patients as, although most relapses occur early in the history of the patient, seminoma is a tumour renowned for its tendency to later relapse (Friedman and Purkayastha, 1960).

Of 8 Stage III patients, 2 died of seminoma. It may be concluded that nodal metastases can be controlled extremely well with radiation alone and that careful attention needs to be paid to accurate delineation of tumour and exclusion of teratomatous components histologically, by serum markers and immunocytochemical methods.

In this series, there have been 9 deaths from intercurrent disease in 183 patients with Stage I–III disease (Table 10.5). Of 54 Stage II patients where the mediastinum was electively irradiated, there have been 5 deaths from intercurrent disease; 2 of these (3.7 per cent) were due to cardiovascular disease. Bearing in mind that seminoma tends to occur a decade later than teratoma and follow-up now extends to fourteen years, these figures do not suggest that the treatment is associated with significant long-term morbidity.

Influence of tumour volume in Stage II seminoma

A more detailed analysis of patients with Stage II disease seen at the Royal Marsden Hospital between 1962 and April 1979 has been completed recently (Ball *et al.*, submitted for publication, 1981).

In this study, the results of radiotherapy were considered in relation to the size of the retroperitoneal lymph node metastases. The results are summarized in Table 10.6.

As shown in Table 10.7 and presented graphically in Fig. 10.3, there is a

Table 10.6 Results of treatment in Stage II seminoma testis (Royal Marsden Hospital, 1962–1979)

Stage	Size of retroperitoneal node metastases	Total no. of patients	Total relapsing		Dead of seminoma		Dead of intercurrent disease	
IIA	<2 cm	31	3	(9.7%)	2	(6.5%)	5	(16.1%)
IIB	5 cm	11	2	(18.2%)	1	(9.1%)	0	
IIC	>5 cm	21	8	(38.1%)	6	(28.6%)	3	(14.3%)
Total patients		63	13	(20.6%)	9	(14.3%)	8	(12.7%)

Table 10.7 Stage II seminoma testis: sites of initial relapse after radiotherapy (Royal Marsden Hospital, 1962–1979)

Stage	Size of retroperitoneal node metastases (cm)	Total no. of patients	Sites of first relapse					
			Lung ±mediastinum	Cervical	Scrotum or groin nodes*	Liver	Extradural	Multiple sites
IIA	<2	31	1	0	2	0	0	0
IIB	2–4.9	11	0	0	1	0	1	0
IIC	5–9.9	9	2	0	0	1	0	0
IID	>10	12	1	2	0	0	0	2
Total		63	4	2	3	1	1	2

* 2 of 3 patients who had scrotal interference prior to orchidectomy and who did not receive scrotal and groin node irradiation suffered local relapses.

striking relationship between tumour volume and probability of relapse following irradiation.

The sites of initial relapse in this group of patients are summarized in Table
10.7.

As shown in Table 10.7, all 13 first relapses were outside the abdominal
lymph-node chain. One patient developed mediastinal adenopathy in conjunction with pulmonary spread and two patients developed cervical nodes.
The remainder relapsed outside the lymphatic system. If the sites of second or
subsequent relapses are examined, then intra-abdominal disease in association
with treatment failure became apparent in 6 patients (Table 10.8). Since the

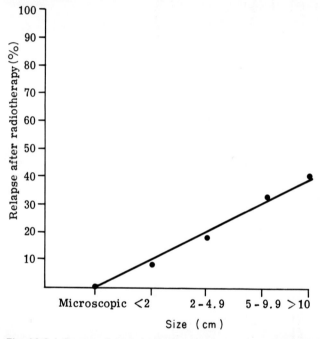

Fig. 10.3 Influence of the volume of abdominal lymph node metastases on the probability
of relapse following radiotherapy in seminoma testis (Royal Marsden Hospital, 1963–
1979).

restrospective analysis extends back to 1962, it is likely that the proportion of
treatment failures in the retroperitoneum may have been minimized. This is
suggested also by the documentation of intra-abdominal tumour later in the
course of the disease when it became more clinically obvious.

We may conclude from this analysis that a major factor predisposing to
treatment failure in seminoma is the volume of metastatic tumour, with 8 of 21
(38 per cent) patients with retroperitoneal metastases of >5 cm in diameter
relapsing after radiotherapy. Clearly, in the period during which patients
included in the above analysis were treated, clinical staging procedures improved markedly and the extent to which these improvements might contribute
to improved local control within the irradiated volume is unknown. Before the
introduction of CT scanning, staging laparotomies were carried out in a limited

Table 10.8 Stage II seminoma testis: sites of second or subsequent relapse following irradiation (Royal Marsden Hospital, 1962–1979)

Sites of relapse	No. of patients
Mediastinum	4
Lung	6
Cervical nodes	3
Abdomen	
ITV	2
OTV	4
Liver	4
Bone	1
Marrow	2

ITV, inside irradiated volume; OTV, outside irradiated volume.

number of patients to determine the extent of nodal involvement accurately and to exclude extralymphatic dissemination. As shown in Table 10.9, of 7 Stage IIC patients undergoing laparotomy prior to irradiation, 6 (86 per cent) are alive and disease free. This procedure has been abandoned in favour of routine CT scanning in seminoma patients with lymphographic evidence of metastases.

Table 10.9 Staging laparotomy prior to radiotherapy for bulky Stage II/III seminoma testis (Royal Marsden Hospital, 1972–1977)

Patient	Stage	Elective other treatment prior to irradiation	Outcome
1	II		NED 91
2	II		NED 74
3	II		NED 37
4	II		DOD 20
5	II	CY, VAM	NED 56
6	II		NED 40
7	II	Melphalan	NED 25
8	II	PVB	NED 20

VAM, vinblastine, actinomycin D and methotrexate; CY, cyclophosphamide; PVB, cis-platinum, vinblastine and bleomycin; NED, no evidence of disease; DOD, died of disease.

Time to relapse in seminoma

As shown in Fig. 10.4, 80 per cent of relapses occur within the first two years after treatment, although late relapse is a well-recognized occurrence in the occasional patient.

Tumour markers and seminoma

The occasional elevation of chorionic gonadotrophin in histologically pure seminoma is of interest. Recent work using an immunocytochemical approach

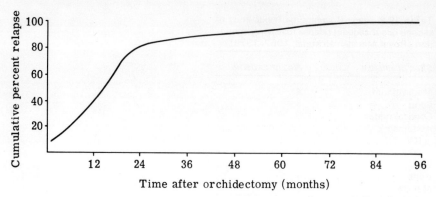

Fig. 10.4 Time to relapse in patients treated for seminoma testis with radiation therapy (Stages I, II and III). (Royal Marsden Hospital, 1963–1975.)

has demonstrated HCG-containing syncytial cells in some patients with testicular seminoma (Heyderman and Neville, 1976). The relationship of the presence of these cells to subsequent outcome is unclear at the present time, although there are no data to suggest that they are an adverse prognostic indicator.

Friedman and Pearlman (1970) have described a variant of seminoma called 'seminoma with trophocarcinoma', which is associated with elevated HCG levels, which is more aggressive and more radioresistant than classical seminoma and which these authors claimed to be distinct from combined tumours of the testis. In the earlier series of Royal Marsden patients with apparently pure seminoma primary tumours, 2 patients (9 per cent) showed histological evidence of non-seminomatous components at autopsy. One explanation for this evolution is to assume that metastasis has occurred from a small, undetected focus of teratoma present in the original tumour. However, the presence within one tumour of two histologically distinct components has not been explained satisfactorily in histogenetic terms. When found in combination with teratoma, the seminomatous component frequently forms discrete nodules of tumour, suggesting separate development (Dixon and Moore, 1953). It is conceivable that one element may precede the other in the process of tumour formation. If this is the case, then it might be postulated that seminoma could evolve into teratoma and that this might explain the presence of histologically confirmed teratoma identified in relapse in some patients with an apparently pure seminoma primary.

In the Royal Marsden series a seminoma patient with an elevated serum alphafetoprotein level has not been encountered. In those cases where there has been an elevated AFP level, a non-seminoma component has been demonstrated invariably at autopsy or by biopsy (Fig. 10.5). Gynaecomastia in testicular teratoma tends to be associated with an elevated HCG level, but it is of interest in the Royal Marsden series that gynaecomastia was detected in 5 seminoma patients in the absence of an elevated HCG level and was of no prognostic significance in 4.

Javadpour et al. (1978) reported elevation of serum HCG in 10 of 130 seminoma patients (7.6 per cent), but no patient had an elevated AFP level. In the latter series, stage of disease correlated with the probability of HCG

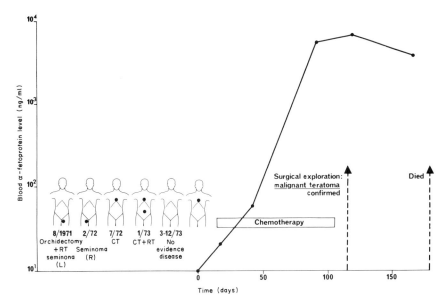

Fig. 10.5 Alphafetoprotein level and the appearance of malignant teratoma metastases in a patient with apparently pure bilateral testicular seminomas.

elevation (Table 10.10). Survival following radiotherapy of seminoma patients with elevated HCG levels is summarized in Table 10.11. The excellent survival figures in these small series indicate that slight to moderate elevations of β-HCG levels are not associated with an adverse prognosis. Serum levels are summarized in Table 10.12.

Table 10.10 Elevated HCG serum levels in seminoma testis (Javad-pour *et al.*, 1978)

Stage	Total no. of patients	Number with raised HCG levels	Percentage
I	109	4	3.7
II	18	7	39
III	3	0	
Total	130	11	8.5

Table 10.11 Survival after radiotherapy of patients with histologically pure seminoma testis and elevated serum HCG levels

References	Total no. of patients	Disease-free
Javadpour *et al.* (1978)	11*	11
Mauch *et al.* (1979)	6	6
Royal Marsden Hospital	9	9†

* One patient was treated by surgery alone.
† One patient had cyclophosphamide and one patient melphalan prior to irradiation.

Table 10.12 Serum beta-human chorionic gonadotrophin levels in histologically pure seminoma

Series	Total no. of patients	Serum β-HCG levels (ng/ml)		
		Range	Mean	Median
Royal Marsden Hospital	8	27–256	85	41
Javadpour et al. (1978)	10	2.3–438	51	4.5

Conclusions

Seminoma testis generally presents with Stage I disease and the prognosis with radiotherapy after orchidectomy is excellent. In patients with abdominal node metastases, careful attention needs to be paid to tumour localization and treatment planning. In patients with Stages IIA and IIB disease, abdominal node irradiation will secure control of almost 80 per cent of patients and chemotherapy is not indicated in this group, even if there is slight to moderate elevation of β-HCG serum levels. In patients with more bulky Stage II disease (>5 cm), the relapse rate is significantly higher, due predominantly to the increased probability of extranodal metastases. In this group, and in Stage III, chemotherapy is advocated followed by irradiation to sites of initial disease. The combination of cis-platinum, vinblastine and bleomycin (PVB) is producing encouraging results and there is no place for single-agent chemotherapy including alkylating agents. A similar chemotherapy approach is advocated in Stage IV patients with, if practicable, irradiation subsequently of bulky disease sites. It is our policy to employ four courses of PVB. There is no evidence to support a routine policy of supradiaphragmatic irradiation in Stage II patients, and it is advised that this should not be undertaken since, should subsequent chemotherapy become necessary, the extensive bone marrow irradiation renders this difficult and hazardous. Elevated serum HCG levels tend to occur in patients with bulky disease and, although this does not *per se* appear to be an adverse prognostic sign, these patients in any event should, as described above, receive sequential drug–radiation therapy. High levels of HCG and elevated AFP serum levels denote a non-seminoma component and management should be modified accordingly. The concept of anaplastic seminoma does not contribute to clinical management and stage-by-stage analysis does not indicate that a diagnosis of anaplastic seminoma is associated with an adverse prognosis.

References

Ball, D., Barrett, A. and Peckham, M. J. (1981).
   Submitted for publication.
Blokhin, N., Larionov, L., Perevodchikova, L., Chebotareva, L. and Merkulova, N. (1958).
   Annals of the New York Academy of Science **68**, 1128.
Calman, F. M. B., Peckham, M. J. and Hendry, W. F. (1979). *British Journal of Urology* **51**, 154.
Castro, J. R. and Gonzalez, M. (1971). *American Journal of Roentgenology* **111**, 355.
Chebotareva, L. I. (1964). *Acta Unio internationalis contra Cancrum* **20**, 380.
Cheng, E., Cvitkovic, E., Wittes, R. E. and Golbey, R. B. (1978). *Cancer* **42**, 2162.
Dixon, F. J. and Moore, R. A. (1953). *Cancer* **6**, 427.

Einhorn, L. H. and Williams, S. D. (1980). *Cancer Clinical Trials* **3**, 307.

Fox, J. E. and Abell, M. R. (1968). *Journal of Urology* **100**, 757.

Friedman, M. and Pearlman, A. W. (1970). *Cancer* **26**, 46.

Friedman, M. and Purkayastha, M. C. (1960). *American Journal of Roentgenology Radium Therapy and Nuclear Medicine* **83**, 25.

Heyderman, E. and Neville, A. M. (1976). *Lancet* **ii**, 103.

Jackson, J. R. and Magner, D. (1965). *Cancer* **18**, 751.

Janssen, M. and Johnston, W. H. (1978). *Cancer* **41**, 538.

Javadpour, N., McIntire, K. R. and Waldemann, T. A. (1978). *Cancer* **42**, 2768.

Johnson, D. E., Gomez, J. J. and Ayala, A. G. (1975). *Journal of Urology* **114**, 80.

Kademian, M. T., Bosch, A. and Caldwell, W. L. (1976). *International Journal of Radiation Oncology Biology Physics* **1**, 1075.

Kademian, M., Bosch, A., Caldwell, W. L. and Jaeschke, W. (1977). Cancer **40**, 3082.

Kardinal, C. G., Jacobs, E. M., Bull, F., Bateman, J. R. and Pajak, T. (1976). *Cancer Treatment Reports* **60**, 953.

Mackenzie, A. R. (1966). *Journal of Urology* **96**, 790.

Maier, J. G., Sulak, M. H. and Mittemeyer, B. T. (1968). *American Journal of Roentgenology* **102**, 596.

Mauch, P., Weichselbaum, R. and Botnick, L. (1979). *International Journal of Radiation Oncology Biology Physics* **5**, 887.

Monfardini, S., Bajetta, E., Musumeci, R. and Bonadonna, G. (1972). *Journal of Urology* **108**, 293.

Mostofi, F. K. (1973). *Cancer* **32**, 1186.

Mostofi, F. K. and Price, E. B. Jr. (1973). *Atlas of Tumor Pathology*, Series 2, Fascicle 7. Armed Forces Institute of Pathology, Washington, DC.

Paterson, A. H. G., Peckham, M. J. and McCready, V. R. (1976). *British Medical Journal* **1**, 1118.

Percapio, B., Clements, J. C., McCleod, D. G., Sorgen, S. D. and Cardinale, F. S. (1979). *Cancer* **43**, 2510.

Rosai, J., Silber, I. and Khodadoust, K. (1969). *Cancer* **24**, 92.

Samson, M. K., Stephens, R. L., Rivkin, S., Opipari, M., Maloney, T., Groppe, C. W. and Fisher, R. (1979). *Cancer Treatment Reports* **63**, 1663.

Samuels, M. L., Lanzotti, V. J., Holoye, P. Y., Boyle, L. E., Smith, T. L. and Johnson, D. E. (1976). *Cancer Treatment Reviews* **3**, 185.

Saxena, V. S. (1973). *American Journal of Roentgenology Radium Therapy and Nuclear Medicine* **17**, 643.

Scully, R. E. (1961). *Cancer* **14**, 788.

Smithers, Sir David (1972). *Journal of the Royal College of Surgeons of Edinburgh* **17**, 133.

Snyder, W., Rodensky, P. and Lieberman, B. (1964). *Cancer Chemotherapy Reports* **41**, 37.

Thackray, A. C. and Crane, W. A. J. (1976). In *Pathology of the Testis*, p. 164. Ed. by R. C. B. Pugh. Blackwell, Oxford and London.

Van der Werf Messing, B. (1976). *International Journal of Radiation Oncology Biology Physics* **1**, 235.

Weitzner, S. (1976). *Urology* **7**, 646.

Yagoda, A. and Vugrin, D. (1979). *Seminars in Oncology* **6**, 74.

Ytredal, D. O. and Bradfield, J. S. (1972). *Cancer* **30**, 628.

11

Treatment of non-seminomatous germ-cell tumours of the testis: general strategy

M. J. Peckham

Since the treatment of patients with malignant teratoma varies from one centre to another, some general observations will be made at this stage in an attempt to clarify existing differences of opinion. Historically in the United Kingdom, patients with early-stage disease have been managed by orchidectomy and lymph node irradiation. In the United States, in patients with no evidence of metastases beyond the abdominal nodes, radical node dissection is generally performed. In patients with distant metastases, single-agent chemotherapy was employed prior to 1970 but since that time a wide range of chemotherapeutic approaches has been explored. It has been recognized for many years that testicular teratomas are chemosensitive tumours and even before the development of effective chemotherapy a small proportion (5–10 per cent) of advanced stage patients were cured with single-agent treatment. The introduction of the combinations of vinblastine and bleomycin (VB) and cis-platinum, vinblastine and bleomycin (PVB) (see Chapters 14 and 15) has constituted a major advance. Clearly the advances in systemic therapy necessitate a reappraisal of overall treatment strategy. It is important to stress that both VB and the PVB regimes are toxic and hence should be deployed only where it is essential. The effectiveness and toxicity of these combinations argue for delay until clearly documented relapse has occurred in early-stage disease, since most of the patients in this group are cured by orchidectomy and radiation or node dissection. On the other hand, chemotherapy should be primary treatment in all advanced stage categories. The major argument against nodal ir-radiation as primary treatment for early-stage patients is that the consequent marrow suppression may compromise effective chemotherapy. Experience cited in Chapters 13 and 15 indicates that prior irradiation limited to infradiaphragmatic lymph node areas does not seriously compromise sub-sequent chemotherapy. Radical node dissection (see Chapter 12) provides essentially similar results to node irradiation. It is, however, a major procedure associated with retrograde ejaculation and infertility, both of which can be avoided with radiation therapy. The prospective identification of those patients with apparently early-stage disease who are destined to relapse following radiotherapy or surgery would allow this group to be treated from the outset with chemotherapy. Similarly, the identification of a group of patients cured by orchidectomy alone would mean that treatment directed at the draining lymph nodes could be omitted. These issues are discussed further in Chapter 15.

With these various considerations in mind, the current policy in use at the Royal Marsden Hospital is outlined below.

Stage I

The patient who has undergone an orchidectomy for removal of the primary tumour and in whom clinical staging has demonstrated no evidence of metastases presents a range of problems. A recent analysis aimed at defining the subgroups described below is presented in Chapter 13.

Patients cured by orchidectomy
The older literature reporting the results of orchidectomy as the only method of treatment demonstrates clearly that a proportion of patients is cured by this procedure.

Patients with negative lymphograms and occult node metastases
Correlation of lymphographic appearances with the histology of resected lymph nodes indicates that approximately 25 per cent of patients with Stage I disease harbour subclinical abdominal node metastases.

Patients harbouring occult extralymphatic metastases
The results of retroperitoneal lymph node irradiation for Stage I teratoma indicate that local recurrence is a rare event, but that relapse occurs in approximately 20 per cent of patients predominantly in the lungs and supradiaphragmatic nodes (see Chapter 13). From this observation we can deduce that subclinical pulmonary metastases are present *ab initio* in approximately 20 per cent of clinical Stage I patients. This aspect is considered in more detail in Chapter 13.

Patients with elevated serum markers and clinical Stage I disease
Serum alphafetoprotein (AFP) and/or beta-human chorionic gonadotrophin (β-HCG) levels may be elevated before removal of the primary tumour and, if this elevation is due to production by the testicular tumour, the levels will fall to normal promptly following orchidectomy. On the other hand, an elevated level persisting after orchidectomy is clear evidence in the Stage I patients of subclinical metastases.

Extent of the primary tumour and prognosis in Stage I
Stage I patients with involvement of the proximal spermatic cord (P_3) are at high risk of harbouring subclinical metastases. Similarly, it appears probable that the presence of vascular invasion is an adverse prognostic feature and associated with an increased risk of extralymphatic dissemination.

Implications for management of the Stage I patient

As described in Chapters 12 and 13, the results of radical node dissection and nodal irradiation for Stage I patients are similar. Until the various subgroups of patients included in the clinical Stage I category can be defined with more precision, and bearing in mind the effectiveness but toxicity of current chemotherapy, it could be argued that orchidectomy and either excision or irradiation of the abdominal nodes should be retained as initial management for Stage I disease, with the exception of patients with involvement of the proximal spermatic cord, although recent data on the fate of this group of patients are scanty. So far as the choice between radical node dissection and radiation therapy is concerned, it is argued that the latter is preferable since it avoids major surgery with its immediate morbidity and interference with sexual function, while at the same time not seriously compromising eventual chemotherapy should this become necessary (see Chapter 15).

On the other hand, it seems likely that the combined use of lymphography, ultrasonography and CT scanning, together with the sequential study of serum markers may allow the identification of two subgroups of 'Stage I' patients; those with occult extralymphatic metastases who require chemotherapy and those with a high probability of having been cured by orchidectomy and in whom a 'watch' policy can be employed justifiably (see Chapters 13 and 15).

Stage II

In this group of patients, where metastases are apparently limited to the abdominal lymph nodes, both radical node dissection and radiation therapy are associated with a significant treatment failure. So far as irradiation is concerned, small volume metastases (Stage IIA) can be eradicated and radiotherapy results in cure rates similar to those achieved in Stage I disease (see Chapter 13). In patients with bulkier metastases (IIB and IIC) management approaches vary widely. In the United States, chemotherapy preceded by or followed by surgery has been employed. Observations on chemotherapy response in relation to the size of metastases show that bulky disease is eradicated less readily than small aggregates of tumour (see Chapters 14 and 15). For this reason, in Stages IIB and IIC a sequential approach of chemotherapy–radiation and surgery is being explored (see Chapter 15).

Stage III

A purely surgical approach in patients with infra- and supradiaphragmatic node metastases obviously involves a major intervention and, although this type of approach has been reported, its avoidance is clearly desirable. The results in Stage III with radiation alone are poor (see Chapter 13), and a combination of chemotherapy with radiotherapy and surgery is advocated (see Chapter 15).

Stage IV

Extending the observations made on the influence of tumour size on drug and radiation response, a somewhat elaborate subclassification of Stage IV patients is employed at the Royal Marsden Hospital (see Chapter 7). This is based partly on metastatic site and partly on the size of metastases. If extranodal metastases appear to be confined to the lungs, experience has demonstrated that chemotherapy is effective, unless multiple, large deposits are present. In the latter group (IV L$_3$), initial responses to chemotherapy tend to be followed

Table 11.1 Treatment protocols employed at the Royal Marsden Hospital

Stage	Postorchidectomy treatment	Serum AFP and/or HCG levels		Proximal spermatic cord involved	Vascular invasion primary tumour
		Pre-orchidectomy	Postorchidectomy		
I	Watch policy	Negative	Negative	Negative	Positive†/negative
I	Watch policy	Positive	Negative*	Negative	Positive/negative
I	CT	Positive	Positive	Positive	
I	CT				
IIA, IIB, IIC,					
III, IV A, B, C L_1	CT±RT±S				
IV A, B, C L_2					
IV 0 L_1					
IV 0 L_2	CT				
IV L_3, IV H+					

*Falling to normal postorchidectomy with $T_{\frac{1}{2}}$ consistent with plasma clearance of AFP and HCG (see Chapters 4 and 13).
†Absence of conclusive data on the significance of vascular invasion warrants evaluation.
CT = chemotherapy; RT = radiotherapy.

by tumour regrowth in a disappointingly high proportion of patients. If the deposits are small in volume, the probability of eradication with chemotherapy is high and the presence in such patients of bulky nodal metastases, for example in the abdomen, is an indication for radiotherapy and/or surgery.

Therapeutic protocol

The treatment protocols employed for patients with testicular teratoma at the Royal Marsden Hospital are summarized in Table 11.1 and elaborated in Chapter 15.

12

Radical lymphadenectomy

W. F. Hendry

There has always been controversy about the best way to treat the lymphatic metastases of testicular tumours, ever since Most (1898) showed that the first nodes to be involved lay far away from the testis, high in the para-aortic region near the renal vessels. Roberts (1902) recognized that 'operations for malignant disease should usually include removal of the adjacent lymph nodes' and, after studying Dr Most's work, described an anterior, transperitoneal approach by which the lymph nodes from the renal vessels down to the aortic bifurcation could be removed, and he commented 'it is perhaps wise to excise glands on both sides'. Unfortunately, his patient developed a faecal fistula, and a safer but less radical retroperitoneal approach was used by Bland-Sutton (1909) and Chevassu (1910). This surgical approach was limited to the side of the tumour, and the dissection could not proceed safely above the renal pedicle—recognized by Chevassu as 'la zone critique'.

The limitations of surgical extirpation of these lymph nodes was pointed out by Jamieson and Dobson (1910), who commented: 'it cannot be allowed that either operation ... warrants the use of the term radical'. They showed that the only effective method would be to strip the aorta, vena cava, common iliac vessels, the upper part of the spermatic vessels on both sides and the trunk of the inferior mesenteric artery of all cellulo-fatty tissue on, around and between them from the level of the renal vessels downwards. However, anaesthetic and other limitations imposed on surgery ensured that the unilateral retroperitoneal approach continued to be used in the first half of the century (Hinman, 1919; Hinman et al., 1923; Lewis, 1948).

Careful pathological studies confirmed the fact that lymph node metastases did not remain ipsilateral, but crossed over to the other side in up to one-third of cases and sometimes extended above the level of the renal vessels (Lowry et al., 1946). With the advent of safe thoracic surgery, a thoraco-abdominal approach was described by Cooper et al. (1950) and in four cases greatly improved access to nodes lying above the renal pedicle was obtained, although bilateral node clearance was still difficult. In 1958, Mallis and Patton described in detail an anterior transperitoneal technique, remarkably similar in principle to that originally suggested by Roberts in 1902, which did allow direct access to all the nodes below the renal vessels and hence enabled the surgeon to attempt to clear the nodes on both sides from this level downwards. Tavel et al. (1963) used this approach to perform bilateral lymphadenectomy in cadavers, but found that even under these ideal circumstances about one-third of the nodes were still present on subsequent pathological examination, being situated mostly behind the aorta and vena cava. Kaswick *et al.* (1976) have shown that complete node clearance could be achieved in 11 of 12 cadavers, provided that all the lumbar vessels distal to the renal pedicles were ligated and divided to provide access to the posterior nodes. It was stated that concern over possible devascularization of the spinal cord was not warranted, provided no lumbar vessels above the renal pedicle were ligated.

Radical retroperitoneal lymphadenectomy has evolved slowly, and with present techniques a reasonably thorough clearance of the nodes can be achieved, bilaterally up to the renal vessels, and this can be extended to the diaphragm on one side by use of a thoraco-abdominal approach. The operation is not free from risk, however, and it produces significant morbidity. In about 10 per cent of cases explored, the nodes are found to be fixed or to extend too high and these are declared inoperable and may have been consigned to palliative treatment.

It is clear then, that this operation is a formidable technical undertaking and pathological studies have shown that, in a considerable proportion of cases, it may not eradicate all the nodes which are likely to be affected, because they are relatively inaccessible behind the great vessels or above the renal pedicle. It is therefore reasonable to examine alternative methods of treatment with care, in order to define with some precision those cases which can be treated effectively by other means and distinguish them from those who might benefit from this operation.

It is accepted universally now that seminomas are so radiosensitive that they can be cured nearly always by radiotherapy (see Chapter 10). The problem lies with the teratomas, and it is here that the great divergence of opinion has occurred, between Britain and Scandinavia, where radiotherapy has been favoured and continental Europe and the USA where routine retroperitoneal lymphadenectomy has generally been practised. In this chapter, we shall consider in detail the pathological distribution of lymphatic spread and the surgical techniques evolved to remove it. We shall look at the results in terms of complications and survival rate and compare them—as far as we can—with those achieved by radiotherapy. Finally, we shall examine the hypothesis that this operation may be needed only in a highly selected and well-defined subgroup of teratoma patients.

The pathology and radiology of lymphatic spread

The most detailed information on the frequency and sites of metastases has been provided by Ray *et al.* (1974), who described their findings in 283 radical lymphadenectomy specimens. The pattern of spread showed distinct differences depending on the side of the primary tumour. Right-sided tumours spread to the paracaval, precaval, interaorto-caval, pre-aortic, right common iliac and proximal external iliac nodes in that order. Ipsilateral nodes only were involved in 85 per cent of cases, ipsilateral and contralateral in 13 per cent and contralateral only in 1.6 per cent. On the left side, para-aortic, pre-aortic, left common iliac and left external iliac nodes were involved in that order, with subsequent extension to interaorto-caval, precaval and paracaval nodes. The spread was ipsilateral in 80 per cent and bilateral in 20 per cent. In no case was spread confined to the contralateral nodes.

As a result of these studies, Ray *et al.* (1974) recommended areas for lymphadenectomy as follows. For *right*-sided tumours, the aorta and vena cava should be cleared below the renal vessels (the upper 2–3 cm only below the renal vessels to the left of the aorta), preserving the inferior mesenteric artery, down to the aortic bifurcation distally, and including the right common iliac and proximal 2 cm of the right external iliac artery. On the *left* side, the dissection should include the anterior and left side of the cava, both sides of the aorta usually with the inferior mesenteric artery, and extending to the left common iliac and proximal 2 cm of the left external iliac artery.

Surgical/pathological correlation on node histology in this study was 91 per cent if the nodes were positive, and 92 per cent if negative. Clinically detectable metastases above the renal vessels were usually non-resectable, but in the forty-three patients in whom thoraco-abdominal dissection was done no metastases were found above the renal vessels.

It may be concluded that, if radical lymphadenectomy is done, it should be bilateral up to the level of the renal vessels in all cases. Extension of the dissection above the renal vessels up to the diaphragm may be required occasionally, but obviously this should be recognized before operation so that a thoraco-abdominal incision may be used.

Lymphography has proved to be relatively accurate in the detection and localization of metastases (see Chapter 8), although approximately 25 per cent of patients with negative lymphograms have occult metastases (see Chapter 13). Safer *et al.* (1975) found a 79 per cent overall correlation between lymphography and histology in 33 cases, while Kademian and Wirtanen (1977) showed that, although correlation was only 75 per cent in 16 negative lymphograms due to the presence of micrometastases, the correlation in 29 lymphographically positive cases was 97 per cent. The accuracy of this investigation undoubtedly improves with increasing experience, and it is our view that lymphography is an essential investigation for planning the therapeutic approach in testicular teratoma.

The surgical approach for radical lymphadenectomy

There are several possible routes to the retroperitoneal lymph nodes, and each approach has advantages and limitations.

Retroperitoneal
This operation was used originally as an extension of the orchidectomy, to permit the testicle, the cord, the testicular vessels and the lymph nodes to be removed as a monobloc dissection. The incision varied slightly (Hinman, 1919; Hinman *et al.*, 1923), but usually extended from the tenth or twelfth rib, obliquely downwards to the internal inguinal ring. After dividing the muscles of the abdominal wall, the peritoneum was reflected forwards to allow the dissection to be carried up to the renal pedicle. This was a very safe operation and Lewis reported no mortality in 169 cases in 1948, at a time when 8 patients in his series of 250 cases died of complications of radiotherapy. The node dissection was limited to the side of the tumour, and it was difficult to extend

the exposure if the nodes appeared to be extensively involved. Ten per cent of the 169 cases described by Lewis were found to be inoperable.

Thoraco-abdominal

This was developed from the retroperitoneal approach, by extending the incision through the bed of the tenth rib as far back as the posterior axillary line (Cooper *et al.*, 1950), in order to obtain clearance of ipsilateral nodes above the renal vessels. Skinner and Leadbetter (1971) have shown that a bilateral para-aortic node dissection also could be completed up to the renal vessels, with extension up to the diaphragm on the side of the incision, and they described fifty-eight cases without operative mortality.

Anterior transperitoneal

Once the abdomen has been opened by a long midline incision extending from xiphisternum to pubis, access to the para-aortic nodes is obtained by one of two methods. The first method was described by Mallis and Patton (1958). The transverse colon is placed on the chest between moist packs and the small bowel is put into a bowel bag. The posterior peritoneum is then incised between the aorta and the vena cava, and the incision is extended down to the bifurcation of the ipsilateral iliac artery and up to the level of the renal vessels. An alternate approach was described by Staubitz *et al.* (1969). The ascending colon and duodenum are mobilized and reflected to the left until both renal pedicles are exposed superiorly. The entire small bowel, ascending and transverse colon are then exteriorized to allow free access to the great vessels.

The ureters mark the lateral extent of the dissection on each side. The ipsilateral testicular artery and vein are always included in the dissection and traced down as far as the internal ring. The inferior mesenteric artery can be preserved sometimes, but it should be divided if it is surrounded by involved nodes. The dissection proceeds up as far as the renal pedicle, an most surgeons who use this approach consider the tumour to be inoperable if there are metastases present above this level.

Complications

The surgical excision of involved lymph nodes adjacent to the great vessels is difficult and dangerous, and significant complications have been reported including death from massive haemorrhage, ischaemic necrosis of aorta, renal vein thrombosis, nephrectomy, ureteric division or fibrosis requiring lysis, retroperitoneal lymphocyst, chylous ascites, pancreatitis, intestinal ischaemia or obstruction due to adhesions and wound infection, dehiscence or hernia. The overall complication rate in two large series has been reported as 11 per cent (Lindsey and Glenn, 1976) and 12 per cent (Staubitz *et al.*, 1974).

Ejaculatory impotence commonly occurs after bilateral lymphadenectomy. Bracken and Johnson (1976) reported a significant decrease in semen volume in 42 of 50 patients, although 7 of 12 patients who wanted to were able to produce pregnancies. Six of 44 patients reported diminished sex performance and 9 had decreased sex drive. In contrast, 29 patients irradiated for seminoma all reported little or no change in performance or drive and two-thirds of those who wanted to were able to produce pregnancies.

Leiter and Brendler (1967) considered that loss of ejaculation was due to interruption of lumbar sympathetic outflow, which passes via the presacral plexus to provide motor innervation to the vasa and vesicles. Damage usually occurs either at the level of the lumbar sympathetic ganglia or at the presacral (hypogastric) plexus. Although many patients report improvement with the passage of time, sometimes the disability may be permanent.

Results

It is important to look at the reported results of radical lymphadenectomy with care, for this is an area of great controversy. With modern radiotherapy techniques, complications and morbidity are minimal following high-dose irradiation treatment of the para-aortic nodes (see Chapter 13). If radical lymphadenectomy is to be recommended for these patients with apparently early disease, there must be good reasons for doing so in view of the morbidity and postoperative complications which may result from this procedure.

The first question that must be considered is whether improvements in the operative techniques and the introduction of bilateral lymphadenectomy have improved the results. Maier and Sulak (1973) reviewed the experience with 503 patients with testicular teratomas at the Walter Reed General Hospital over a 29-year period. Of these patients 196 (39 per cent) had lymphadenectomy; 111 of these had positive nodes and received postoperative radiotherapy. In 125 patients prior to 1953 unilateral dissection was done; 171 subsequent cases had bilateral lymphadenectomy. Only when the lymph nodes were negative was there improved survival for the bilateral operation—probably a reflection that all the retroperitoneal nodes were free of tumour and no contralateral micrometastases were missed. It may be concluded that if lymphadenectomy is done as a staging procedure to select cases for radiotherapy—as has been suggested in some American centres (Johnson, Bracken and Blight, 1976)—the dissection should be bilateral. Knowledge of the pathology of lymphatic spread would have predicted this conclusion. On the other hand, if the nodes are positive, there is no evidence that bilateral lymphadenectomy gives any better results than unilateral, if effective postoperative radiotherapy is given as well.

The most important question is whether there is any convincing evidence that radical lymphadenectomy is necessary at all in early cases. Differences in histological classification, and between operative and nonoperative staging, make valid comparisons between results obtained in different countries extremely difficult and there is no doubt that controlled trials are long overdue. Unfortunately, the protagonists of each technique believe in their own methods so completely that their positions are now deeply entrenched.

It is possible, however, to assemble the reported survival rates (for all teratomas) in several large, published series of patients treated by radical lymphadenectomy (Table 12.1). The fact that these cases were operable implies that there was no evidence of disease above the diaphragm or elsewhere, and hence they coincide with cases classified as Stages I and II at the Royal Marsden Hospital (see Chapter 7). Approximately 10 per cent of cases explored with a view to radical lymphadenectomy are found to be inoperable (Staubitz et al., 1974) and these advanced cases are excluded from the survival figures (whereas they remain included in any series treated by irradiation).

Table 12.1 Survival (minimum three years) in testicular teratoma patients after retroperitoneal node dissection

References	Histology	
	Negative nodes	Positive nodes
Whitmore (1968)	43/49	9/16
Bradfield et al. (1973)*	28/40	11/34
Culp et al. (1973)*	13/15	6/10
Skinner et al. (1971)*	27/30	15/27
Castro (1969)*	31/37	11/22
Maier et al. (1969)*	80/109	44/97
Walsh et al. (1971)	24/25	3/4
Staubitz et al. (1974)	42/45	15/20
Lindsey and Glenn (1976)*	20/23	13/27
	308/373	127/257
	(82.6%)	(49.4%)

* Some had supplementary radiotherapy.

It may be seen from Table 12.1 that the minimum three-year survival rates for patients treated by radical lymphadenectomy were 82.6 per cent if the nodes were histologically negative and 49.4 per cent if they were positive. The equivalent results for all teratoma patients treated by radiotherapy between 1962 and 1975 at the Royal Marsden Hospital were 82 per cent for lymphographic Stage I and 51 per cent for Stage II cases (see Chapter 13). In so far as these comparisons are valid, there seems to be little therapeutic justification for radical lymphadenectomy in early cases of testicular teratoma. This conclusion coincides with the view of Guinn (1972), who writes from a major American cancer centre 'the procedure often serves merely as a diagnostic tool for determining the advisability of employing immediate irradiation since the removal of all lymph nodes is unlikely'.

It may be noted also from Table 12.1 that pre- or postoperative radiotherapy was given in most published series of radical lymphadenectomy, which makes it difficult to assess the therapeutic value of this procedure. Recently, only Staubitz et al. (1974) are reporting results of radical surgery alone. With 42 out of 45 (93 per cent) Stage I and 15 out of 20 (75 per cent) Stage II cases alive at three years, the results appear to be exceptionally good—and unique.

In the author's view it is difficult to justify the use of this operation in the routine management of early cases. Examination of the sites of relapse in Stage I and IIA testicular teratoma patients treated by orchidectomy and nodal irradiation at the Royal Marsden Hospital shows that recurrence in the para-aortic node area is exceptionally uncommon. Johnson, Bracken and Blight (1976) believe that this operation is mandatory in early cases as a clinical staging procedure. We disagree with this, believing that the use of lymphography combined with ultrasound or CT scanning together with serum markers provides a sensitive clinical staging method (see Chapter 13).

Combined treatment policy

Careful analysis of the results of treatment of testicular teratomas by radiotherapy (see Chapter 13) or by radical node dissection (Skinner, 1976) shows that excellent results may be obtained by either therapeutic method, provided that nodal metastases are limited in extent (Stage IIa or B1 respectively). But the prognosis worsens markedly once the nodal metastases exceed 2 cm in diameter lymphographically (Stage IIb) or when more than six nodes are involved microscopically, or the capsule of the node is breached (B2). This is the group of patients in whom combined treatment policies have the most to offer. Skinner (1976) improved the results in B2 cases from 7 out of 12 (58 per cent) to 9 out of 10 (90 per cent) with minimum follow up of two years, by combining chemotherapy with radical node dissection (Table 12.2).

Table 12.2 Survival (minimum two years) in testicular teratoma patients after retroperitoneal node dissection ± chemotherapy (from Skinner, 1976)

Pathological stage	Survival rate surgery alone		Survival rate surgery + chemotherapy	
A	27/30	(90%)	12/13	(92%)
B1	5/6	(83%)	7/8	(88%)
B2	7/12	(58%)	9/10	(90%)
C	3/9	(33%)	5/8	(63%)
Total	42/57	(74%)	33/39	(85%)

Several other series have been reported in which extensive or initially unresectable lymph node metastases have been treated by a combination of chemotherapy, pre-operation radiotherapy and radical lymphadenectomy (Table 12.3). Although distant metastases were present initially in some of these cases, an encouraging number are still alive up to eighty-three months after treatment, and it should be noted that in many of the cases there was no evidence of malignancy—or only adult teratoma—in the tissue removed at operation.

Table 12.3 Results of combination therapy including surgery for advanced (initially unresectable) metastatic testicular teratoma

References	Treatment policy	No. with distant metastases	Pathology NEM	No. of survivors	Duration of survival (months)
Comisarow and Grabstald (1976)	Chemotherapy + DXT, surgery	2/11	4/11	7/11	6–48
Johnson, Bracken, Ayala et al. (1976)	Chemotherapy, surgery	7/10	7/10	8/10	2–48
Wettlaufer (1976)	Chemotherapy, surgery, ± DXT	3/11	4/11	7/11	24–83

Thirty-three patients in the Royal Marsden series (Table 12.4) with para-aortic metastases exceeding 2 cm in diameter have been treated with radio-therapy, chemotherapy (VB and PVB) or both (see Chapter 15), followed by

Table 12.4 Retroperitoneal node resection: tumour stage related to treatment group (Royal Marsden Hospital)

Group	Total no. of patients	Stage IIB	IIC	III	IV
Old series	13	8	2	3	—
Chemotherapy plus radiotherapy (protocol)	13	2	7	2	2
Chemotherapy only	7	—	4	—	3
Total	33	10	13	5	5

surgical excision of the residual para-aortic mass (Hendry *et al.*, 1980). Examples of the extent of disease tackled by this combined approach are shown in Figs. 12.1 and 12.2. Figure 12.1 shows extensive involvement of retroperitoneal nodes on both sides, demonstrated by lymphography which shows a pseudo-lymphomatous pattern. Following chemotherapy and radiation therapy, a residual mass was excised which showed no histological evidence of active tumour. As shown in Fig. 12.3, the reconstruction from CT scans of the residuum on a plain abdominal radiograph provides a useful guide to surgical approach.

Figure 12.2 shows a patient with a massive tumour (undifferentiated malignant teratoma and yolk-sac) in the left abdomen, responding partially to chemotherapy and subsequently proceeding directly to surgery. Foci of active tumour were identified histologically.

An anterior midline incision was used for most cases, but a thoraco-abdominal incision was needed on 6 occasions for very large tumours (Fig. 12.2). Removal of a poorly functioning ipsilateral kidney was necessary in 7 out of 33 patients (21 per cent), and a segment of vena cava was resected in 2 (12.5 per cent) of 16 patients with primary right-sided tumours (Fig. 12.4). Removal was incomplete in only 1 patient, who had femoral nerve root involvement, and he subsequently died of secondary haemorrhage (operative mortality 3 per cent).

The pathology of the testicular lesion compared with the pathology in the excised nodes can be seen in Tables 12.5 and 12.6. There was undifferentiated tumour in 8 (62 per cent) of 13 patients in Group 1 treated with radiotherapy (and, in some cases, ineffective chemotherapy) between 1968 and 1976. By contrast, active malignancy was only present in 2 (15 per cent) of 13 in Group 2 who had chemotherapy (VB or PVB) and radiotherapy. Four (57 per cent) of 7 patients in Group 3 had undifferentiated tumour after chemotherapy only (2 VB, 4 PVB), but 3 of these patients were referred because of evidence of activity in the para-aortic region.

It is too early to know whether lymphadenectomy will improve the prognosis for these patients with bulky metastases. However, most of these lumps were technically inoperable, and the time seems ripe for controlled trials of multi-modality treatment, amongst which surgical removal of residual bulk disease could reasonably form a part.

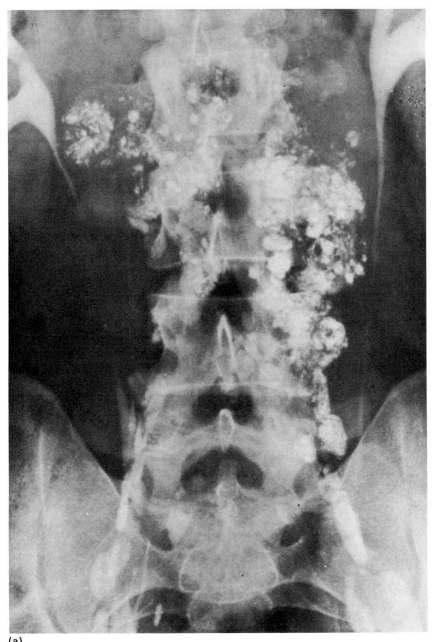

(a)
Fig. 12.1 Malignant teratoma testis. Diffuse involvement of para-aortic and paracaval lymph nodes (a) Before removal.

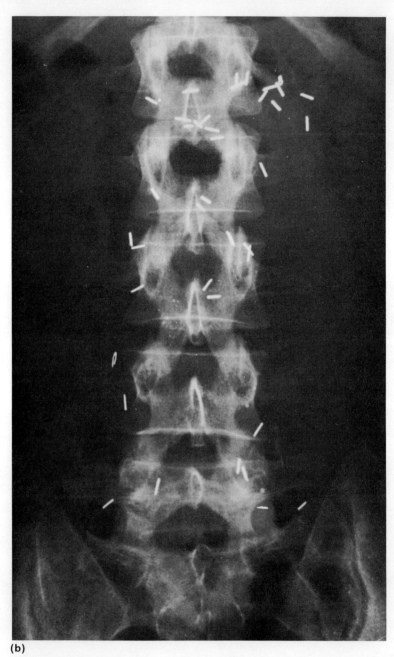

(b)

Fig. 12.1 Malignant teratoma testis. Diffuse involvement of para-aortic and paracaval lymph nodes **(b)** After removal.

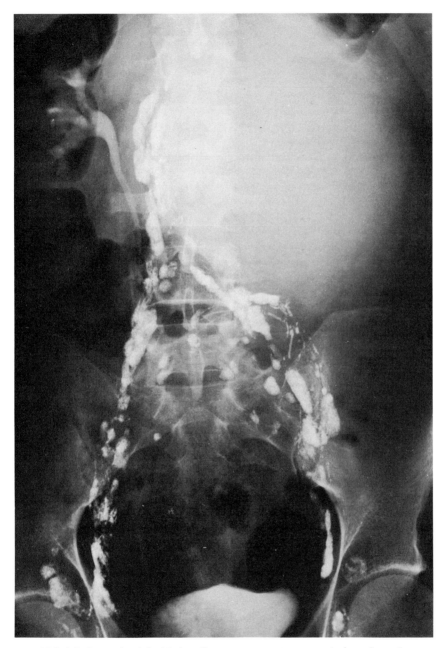

Fig. 12.2 (a) A massive left-sided malignant teratomatous mass before chemotherapy; although some function had returned to the left kidney, nephrectomy was necessary.

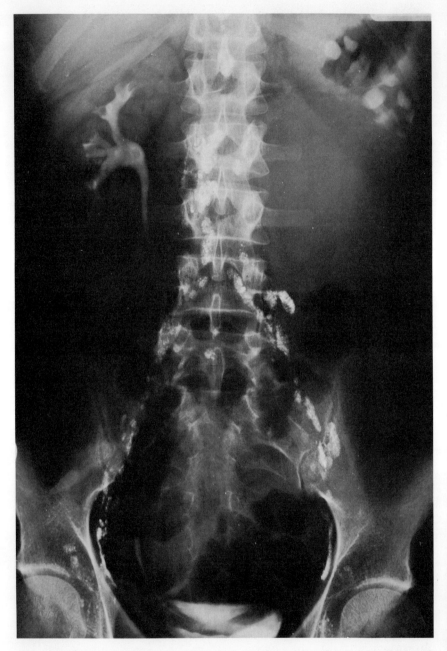

Fig. 12.2 (b) A massive left-sided malignant teratomatous mass after chemotherapy; although some function had returned to the left kidney, nephrectomy was necessary.

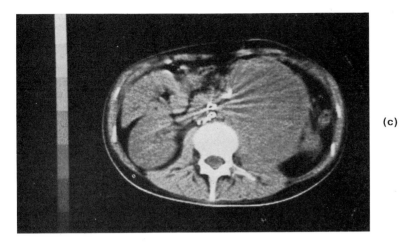

(c)

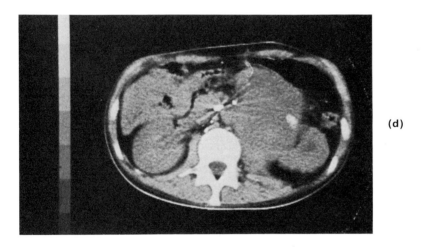

(d)

Fig. 12.2 continued. CT scans **(c)** before and **(d)** after chemotherapy; showing reduction in size of tumour mass, which lies between the left kidney and the great vessels.

Summary and conclusions

Radical lymphadenectomy is a technically difficult operation which causes considerable morbidity and produces significant interference with sexual function. Although the surgical techniques are well established, the indications for the operation are poorly defined and remain highly controversial.

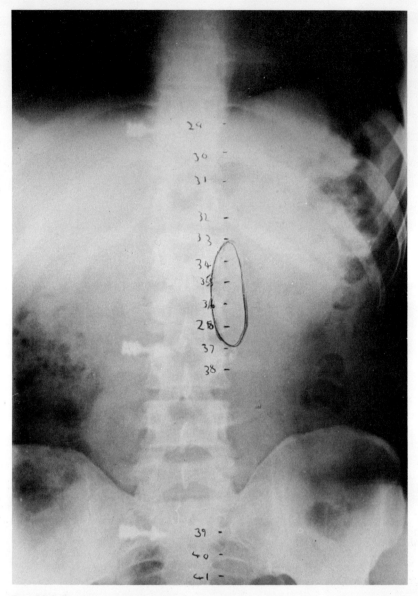

Fig. 12.3 Reconstruction of residual mass after chemotherapy and radiotherapy from a series of computerized tomographic x-ray scans.

In the author's view the procedure has no place in the routine management of early testicular teratomas, although we are exploring its use in the management of bulky lymph node metastases as part of a combined treatment policy. In these circumstances, it is essential to define the extent of the disease accurately before operation and to plan the surgical approach accordingly.

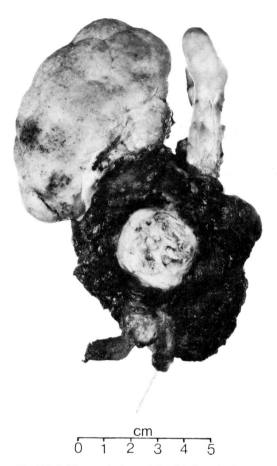

cm

0 1 2 3 4 5

Fig. 12.4 Metastasis from right-sided testicular teratoma involving the right ureter and invading vena cava. Note the finger-like projection which extended up towards the heart.

Table 12.5 Retroperitoneal node resection: pathology of primary testicular tumour related to treatment group (Royal Marsden Hospital)

Group	Total no. of patients	Pathology of testis		
		TD	MTI	MTU
Old series (1968–1976)	13	2	10	1
Chemotherapy and radiotherapy (protocol)	13*		7	5
Chemotherapy only	7		1	6
Total	33	2	18	12

* Includes one seminoma with increased markers.

Table 12.6 Retroperitoneal node resection: pathological findings in excised lymph nodes (compared with Table 12.5) (Royal Marsden Hospital)

Group	Total no. of patients	Pathology of nodes			
		NEM*	TD	MTI	MTU
Old series	13	1	4	5	3
Chemotherapy and radiotherapy (protocol)	13	4	7	1	1
Chemotherapy only	7	1	2	1	3

* No evidence of malignancy.

References

Bland-Sutton, J. (1909). *Lancet* **109**, 1406.
Bracken, R. B. and Johnson, D. E. (1976). *Urology* **7**, 35.
Bradfield, J. S., Hagen, R. D. and Ytredal, D. O. (1973). *Cancer* **31**, 633.
Castro, J. R. (1969). *Cancer* **24**, 87.
Chevassu, M. (1910). *Revue de Chirurgie* **41**, 628.
Comisarow, R. H. and Grabstald, H. (1976). *Journal of Urology* **115**, 569.
Cooper, J. F., Leadbetter, W. F. and Chute, R. (1950). *Surgery, Gynecology and Obstetrics* **90**, 486.
Culp, D. A., Boatman, D. L. and Wilson, B. (1973). *Journal of Urology* **110**, 548.
Guinn, G. A. (1972). Treatment, surgical management. In *Testicular Tumours*, pp. 161–180. Ed. by D. E. Johnson. Kimpton, London.
Hendry, W. F., Barrett, A., McElwain, T. J., Wallace, D. M. and Peckham, M. J. (1980). *British Journal of Urology* **52**, 38.
Hinman, F. (1919). *Surgery, Gynecology and Obstetrics* **28**, 495.
Hinman, F., Gibson, T. E. and Kutzmann, A. A. (1923). *Surgery, Gynecology and Obstetrics* **37**, 429.
Jamieson, J. K. and Dobson, J. F. (1910). *Lancet* **1**, 493.
Johnson, D. E., Bracken, R. B., Ayala, A. G. and Samuels, M. C. (1976). *Journal of Urology* **116**, 66.
Johnson, D. E., Bracken, R. B. and Blight, E. M. (1976). *Journal of Urology* **116**, 63.
Kademian, M. and Wirtanen, G. (1977). *Urology* **9**, 218.
Kaswick, J. A., Bloomberg, S. D. and Skinner, D. G. (1976). *Journal of Urology* **115**, 70.
Leiter, D. and Brendler, H. (1967). *Journal of Urology* **98**, 375.
Lewis, L. G. (1948). *Journal of Urology* **59**, 763.
Lindsey, C. M. and Glenn, J. F. (1976). *Journal of Urology* **116**, 59.
Lowry, E. C., Beard, D. E., Hewitt, L. W. and Barner, J. L. (1946). *Journal of Urology* **55**, 373.
Maier, J. G. and Sulak, M. H. (1973). *Cancer* **32**, 1217.
Maier, J. G., van Buskirk, K. E., Sulak, M. H., Perry, R. H. and Schamber, D. T. (1969). *Journal of Urology* **101**, 356.
Mallis, N. and Patton, J. F. (1958). *Journal of Urology* **80**, 501.
Most (1898). *Virchows Archiv für pathologische Anatomie und Physiologie und für klinische Medizin* **154**, 138.
Ray, B., Hajdu, S. I. and Whitmore, W. F. (1974). *Cancer* **33**, 340.
Roberts, J. B. (1902). *Annals of Surgery* **36**, 539.
Safer, M. L., Green, J. P., Crews, Q. E. and Hill, D. R. (1975). *Cancer* **35**, 1603.
Skinner, D. G. (1976). *Journal of Urology* **115**, 65.
Skinner, D. G. and Leadbetter, W. F. (1971). *Journal of Urology* **106**, 84.
Staubitz, W. J., Early, K. S., Magoss, I. V. and Murphy, G. P. (1974). *Journal of Urology* **111**, 205.
Staubitz, W. J. Magoss, I. V., Grace, J. T. and Schenk, W. G. (1969). *Journal of Urology* **101**, 350.

Tavel, F. R., Osius, T. G., Parker, J. W., Goodfriend, R. B., McGonigle, D. J., Jassie, M. P., Simmons, E. L., Tobenkin, M. I. and Schulte, J. W. (1963). *Journal of Urology* **89**, 241.

Walsh, P. C., Kaufman, J. J., Coulson, W. F. and Goodwin, W. E. (1971). *Journal of the American Medical Association* **217**, 309.

Wettlaufer, J. N. (1976). *Journal of Urology* **116**, 593.

Whitmore, W. F. (1968). Germinal tumours of the testis. In *Proceedings of the Sixth National Cancer Conference*, p. 219. J. B. Lippincott, Philadelphia.

13

Radiotherapy in testicular teratoma

M. J. Peckham and A. Barrett

Metastases from malignant teratoma of the testis are moderately radiosensitive and can be eradicated when the tumour volume is small. Prior to the introduction of more effective chemotherapy, radiotherapy and surgery were the only two treatment methods available. In this section it is proposed to review the results of radiotherapy in relation to clinical stage and to consider the potential future role of radiotherapy in combination with chemotherapy and surgery.

The response of testicular teratoma metastases to radiation

Subclinical metastases

For many years and following orchidectomy, the clinical Stage I patient has been managed by irradiation of the ipsilateral pelvic nodes and the para-aortic lymph node area extending to the lower dorsal region. The overall results in this group are good (*vide infra*), but it is pertinent to consider whether this is a

Table 13.1 Histologically proven metastases from testicular teratoma in negative-lymphogram patients

References	No. of patients with negative lymphograms	Positive histology
Fein and Taber (1969)	30	10
Wallace and Jing (1970)	49	8
Hussey *et al.* (1977)	73	13
Maier and Schamber (1972)	24	6
Hultén *et al.* (1973)	16	4
Jonsson *et al.* (1973)	10	2
Safer *et al.* (1975)	21	3
Durant and Barrat (1977)	14	6
Kademian and Wirtanen (1977)	16	4
Lasser *et al.*, (1977)	11	4
Cook *et al.* (1965)	12	4
Seitzman and Halaby (1964)	12	6
Storm *et al.* (1977)	28	10
	316	80 (25%)

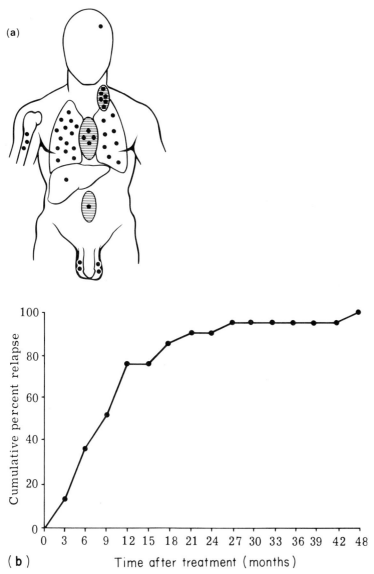

Fig. 13.1 (a) Sites of relapse in Stage I and IIA testicular teratoma patients treated by orchidectomy and nodal irradiation. (b) Time to relapse in thirty-two patients treated for Stage I and IIA testicular teratoma (Royal Marsden Hospital, 1962–1975).

reflection of the absence or low frequency of metastases in retroperitoneal nodes of the lymphogram-negative patient, or whether the high disease-free survival rate can be attributed to the eradication of small volume deposits of tumour. Table 13.1 summarizes details on 316 patients with negative lymphograms who subsequently had histological examination of the nodes. Approximately 25 per cent of patients had pathologic evidence of tumour despite the negative lymphogram. In an analysis of the sites of relapse following irradiation for early-stage disease, we have reported previously that relapse in the irradiated abdominal nodes is a rare event (Fig. 13.1a; Peckham *et al.*, 1977), and it may be concluded therefore that subclinical deposits of tumour are eradicated by nodal irradiation. Further evidence bearing on this aspect has come from the analysis of alphafetoprotein and human chorionic gonadotrophin levels in relation to orchidectomy and irradiation in the clinical Stage I patient (*vide infra*). Such a study is complicated by the need for sequential marker measurements following orchidectomy (with, if possible, a pre-orchidectomy sample) since clearance of marker produced by the primary tumour may be incomplete by the time irradiation is commenced. Thus, a single sample may not reflect marker production by subclinical metastases. The prognostic significance of marker production *per se* and of elevated titres due to metastases rather than persistence of marker from the primary tumour, need to be distinguished and results of a preliminary analysis are presented in Chapter 4 and below. Persistent elevation of marker after radiation therapy is, of course, a clear indication of the presence of residual tumour.

Clinically detectable tumour metastases

Lymph node metastases

The incidence of histologically negative nodes in lymphogram-positive patients undergoing surgery is low and, even allowing for the variability in criteria for lymphographic interpretation, it is clear that the large majority of patients with clinical Stage II disease may be assumed to have nodal metastases. Approximately 50 per cent of patients in Stage II are cured by orchidectomy and radiation therapy (*vide infra*). In a retrospective analysis we drew attention to the dependence of therapeutic response on metastatic volume (Tyrrell and Peckham, 1976; Fig. 13.2a and b). In this study, patients with abdominal node metastases less than 2 cm in maximum diameter showed a low local recurrence rate and an overall cure rate of 80 per cent; whereas, in patients with more bulky tumour deposits, only 35 per cent survived and local recurrence was associated invariably with treatment failure. These observations, made on a small number of patients, indicate that the small-volume clinically apparent tumour deposit can be eradicated, but that radiation therapy alone is inadequate treatment for bulkier disease. Maier and Mittemeyer (1977) reported a three-year disease-free survival of 9 of 11 Stage II patients following radiation therapy, and noted that the smaller-volume metastases tended to fall into this group. Further indirect evidence of the response of nodal deposits to radiation may be adduced from the results of those centres employing pre-operative irradiation before node dissection. Thus, Klein and Maier (1977), comparing experience at the Walter Reed and M. D. Anderson Hospitals, reported that the incidence of positive nodes was reduced in patients receiving 2500–3000 rad before surgery. These observations are summarized in Table 13.2.

Pulmonary metastases

There is little documented evidence defining the response of lung metastases to radiation. In general terms, clinically apparent metastases receiving lung tolerance doses of the order of 2000 rad regress and regrow with a volume

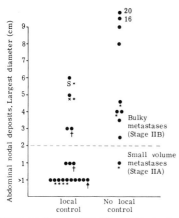

† Subsequent dissection (fully differentiated teratoma) not
   considered as relapses
‡ Also had and responded to actinomycin D
x Very high dose. 5600 rad in split course
S Deposits thought to be seminomatous
∗ Combined tumours
two cases excluded because of inadequate follow up of
   abdominal nodes

(a)

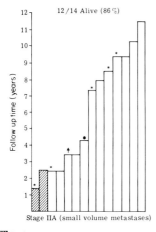

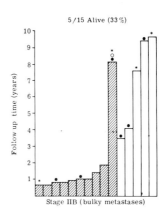

Stage IIA (small volume metastases)

▨ Died
∗ Combined tumour with seminoma
† Lung metastases at 3 months (off actinomycin D 2 years)
● Subsequent dissection

Stage IIB (bulky metastases)

▨ Died
∗ Combined tumour with seminoma
● Subsequent dissection
o Recurred at 3 years

(b)

Fig. 13.2 (a) The response to irradiation of retroperitoneal nodal metastases from testicular
teratoma according to size of metastasis. (b) **Left:** survival of patients with small-volume
(2 cm or less in diameter) retroperitoneal node metastases from testicular teratoma treated
with postorchidectomy irradiation. **Right:** survival of patients with bulky (>2 cm in diameter) retroperitoneal node metastases from testicular teratoma treated with postorchidectomy irradiation.

Table 13.2 Results of node dissection ± pre-operative irradiation (from Klein and Maier, 1977)

Clinical stage	Pre-operative radiation therapy	Incidence of histologically positive nodes at dissection	
		M. D. Anderson	Walter Reed
I	−	18/106 (17%)	6/24 (25%)
	+	0/5 (0%)	1/30 (3%)
II	−	20/22 (91%)	32/35 (91%)
	+	15/28 (54%)	11/21 (52%)

growth delay of two to three months. Van der Werf Messing (1976) has reported a 40 per cent cure rate for a small group of highly selected patients with a limited number of metastases who received 3000 rad to the lungs and boost doses to identifiable deposits. Since solitary pulmonary metastases are associated commonly with subclinical deposits in the lungs, this observation adds some support to the observations made for Stage I disease that small aggregates of tumour appear responsive to moderate doses of radiation.

The relationship between dose and response

No firm dose–response data are available for teratoma testis. As shown in Fig. 13.3, in the Royal Marsden Hospital series no obvious relationship between nominal standard dose (NSD) and local control could be identified. The observations cited above from Klein and Maier suggest that small aggregates of tumour may be eradicated by moderately low radiation doses.

Radiotherapeutic management prior to 1976

Before the routine use of the vinblastine–bleomycin and later the cis-platinum, vinblastine, bleomycin schedules (see Chapter 14), radiotherapy was employed as follows (Einhorn and Williams, 1978).

Stage I. Irradiation of the para-aortic and ipsilateral pelvic lymph node chain.

Stage II. In addition to infradiaphragmatic lymph node irradiation, supra-diaphragmatic irradiation was employed, treating the mediastinum and both supraclavicular areas.

Stage III. Infra- and supradiaphragmatic irradiation was employed.

Stage IV. In selected patients, whole lung irradiation was considered, par-ticularly when disease control at other sites had apparently been achieved and lung disease was minimal.

Treatment technique

A 6 or 8 MeV linear accelerator enables adequate doses to be delivered to the para-aortic and pelvic nodes and, because of the small focal spot, provides a

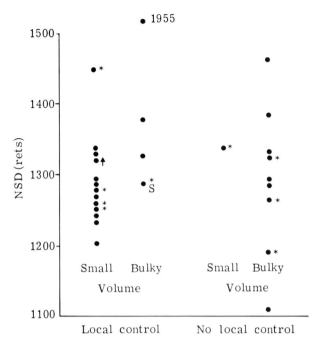

* Combined tumours
↑ Also had and responded to actinomycin D
S Deposits probably seminoma

Fig. 13.3 Response to irradiation of retroperitoneal node metastases from testicular teratoma according to NSD.

well-defined beam with sharp cut-off at the edges of the field. The latter factor
is important since it helps to minimize unnecessary renal irradiation, while
allowing adequate coverage of lymph nodes at the renal hilum.

Because of the large field sizes needed, an increase in the focal skin distance
(FSD) is necessary. Using an FSD of 142 cm, a maximum field length of 42 cm
is achieved. The patient is treated in the prone and supine positions. Anterior
and posterior planning films are taken on a simulator at 142 cm FSD. The
patient lies straight for both treatment positions, with the arms at the sides,
toes together and heels apart. Two tattoo marks are made on the skin for each
field, in order that the perspex template can be aligned correctly (*vide infra*).
A ring of wire is placed over each tattoo and a ruler with 1-cm radiopaque
marks is placed on the skin. From this the dimensions of the field can be
calculated.

The lymphogram and intravenous urogram which are carried out routinely
as part of the staging procedure provide information about the position of
nodes and kidneys for localization on the planning films. In some cases, it is
preferable to perform a pyelogram by injecting contrast at the time of treatment
planning. This ensures that the position of the nodes at the renal hilum can be
localized accurately, since the renal pelvis can be visualized.

Using the planning films, a template of perspex is made in the mould room. This is interposed between the treatment head and the patient. The treatment field is outlined on the template in wire and, when the skin tattoos are aligned accurately with the corresponding markers on the template, the shadow cast by the template wire defines the field on the skin surface and avoids the use of skin marks.

Once the template has been made, a check radiograph is taken on the simulator to check its accuracy. As a final check, a film is taken on the accelerator at the time of the first prone and first supine treatment (Fig. 13.4).

Abdominal node irradiation

Parallel opposed, anterior and posterior fields are employed. The upper border of the field is the lower border of D10 and the lower border the midobturator foramen. In the para-aortic area, the field extends laterally to cover nodes at the renal hila, i.e. usually between 8 cm and 9.5 cm wide at the skin, depending on the position of the kidneys and the size of the patient. The pelvic field extends from the medial border of the obturator foramen to 2 cm beyond the pelvic brim.

The point of inflexion between the para-aortic and pelvic area is at the lower border of L5 on the medial side and approximately at the transverse process of L4 on the lateral side. This ensures adequate inclusion of the common iliac nodes in the angle between L5 and the sacrum.

The remaining testis is protected from scattered radiation by the placement of 1-cm thick cups.

Scrotal irradiation and modification of the lymph node irradiation field

If there was prior scrotal interference surgically, i.e. transcrotal needle biopsy or scrotal orchidectomy, or in those patients where there was tumour invasion of the scrotum or possible altered lymphatic drainage following surgery for testicular maldescent or herniorrhaphy, it has been our policy to irradiate the ipsilateral scrotal sac and to extend the pelvic field to include the inguinal lymph nodes.

Orthovoltage x-rays (250 kV) have been employed to treat the scrotal sac using a direct field and preparing a lead cut-out to shield the penis and contralateral testis. The position of the shield is maintained by means of a flexible plastic support fitted in the mould room at the time the lead cut-out is prepared.

Irradiation treatment of contralateral pelvic nodes

In the large majority of patients only the ipsilateral pelvic nodes have been irradiated. However, in those rare instances where the patient presents with synchronous bilateral testicular tumours or in those patients where the lower para-aortic nodes are involved with consequent risk of retrograde lymphatic extension, the contralateral pelvic lymph node chain has been irradiated using an 'inverted Y' technique.

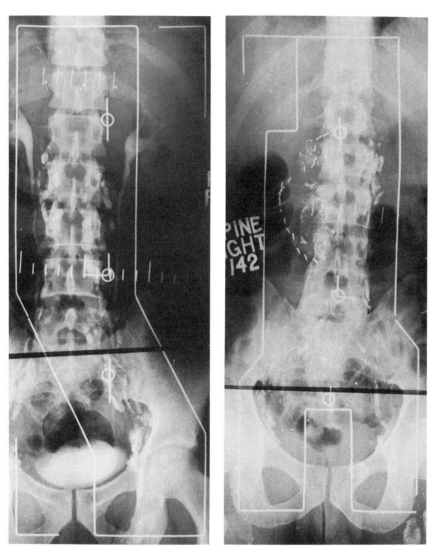

Fig. 13.4 (a) Simulator films showing radiation field to treat the para-aortic and pelvic lymph nodes. **Left:** showing field in relation to kidneys; **right:** Stage II seminoma showing treatment field in relation to tumour defined at laparotomy. *Note.* Both pelvic lymph node areas are included because of the presence of low para-aortic disease.

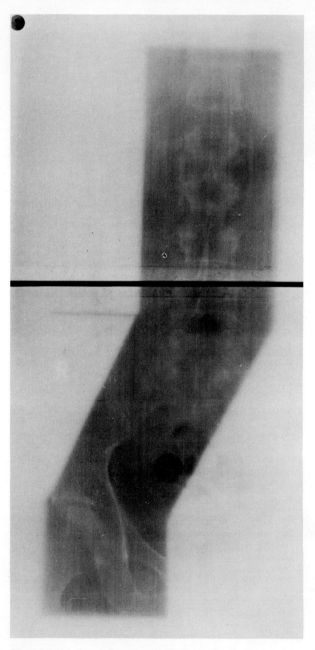

Fig. 13.4 (b) Check film taken with the patient in the treatment position on a 6 MeV linear accelerator.

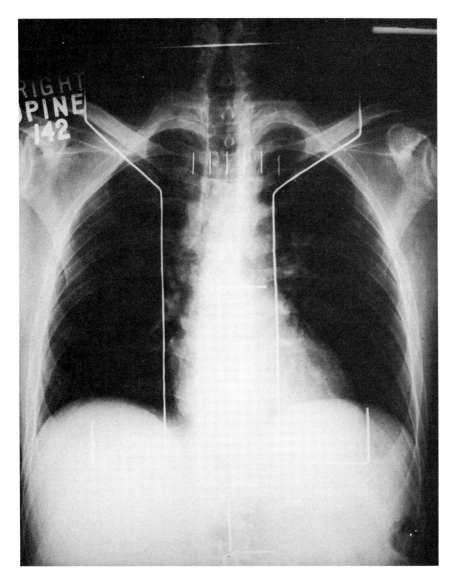

Fig. 13.4 (c) Planning film showing supradiaphragmatic field.

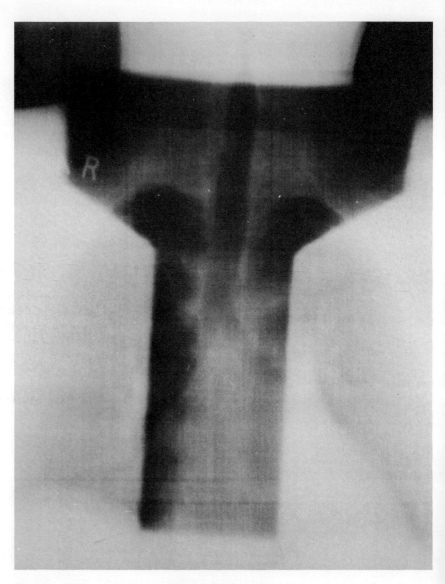

Fig. 13.4 (d) Check film of supradiaphragmatic field.

Boost radiation doses to involved nodes

In patients with involved para-aortic nodes, a boost dose may be delivered using smaller fields. In some patients, the reduced field irradiation has been given through anterior and posterior fields, but in others a three-field technique employing lateral wedged fields and an anterior field can be used satisfactorily (*vide infra*).

Treatment of the mediastinum and supraclavicular nodes

In Stage II and III patients, a four-week interval is allowed after abdominal radiation before initiating supradiaphragmatic irradiation. It is essential to calculate the gap to be left at the skin surface between the upper border of the abdominal field and the lower border of the supradiaphragmatic field individually for each patient.

The upper border of the supradiaphragmatic field is high enough to include adequately both supraclavicular fossae. The upper border of the abdominal field is tattooed at the end of treatment to ensure correct placement of the calculated gaps. The gap is calculated from the isodose curves at the field size employed, from anatomical data derived from lateral simulator films. The posterior fields are approximated with a gap calculated to avoid spinal cord overlap, so that the fields abut at the level of the lymph node chain. The anterior gap is calculated so that the fields abut at the level of the nodes.

The lateral borders of the field are placed so that the supraclavicular fossae are covered adequately. The mediastinal field extends at least 1 cm beyond recognized mediastinal lymph nodes, and the inferior border of the supraclavicular component of the field extends along the lower border of the clavicles with the larynx protected throughout treatment.

The spinal cord is shielded posteriorly at 15 Gy (midplane dose) in seminoma and at 20 Gy in teratoma patients.

The fields employed are illustrated in Fig. 13.4.

Radiation dose

In patients with Stage I disease a midplane dose of 40 Gy in 20 fractions over four weeks has been employed. A similar dose was given to the supradiaphragmatic node areas. In patients with positive abdominal nodes (Stages II and III), boost doses of 5–10 Gy are given, depending upon the volume of tissue irradiated.

Results of treatment at the Royal Marsden Hospital prior to 1976

Smithers *et al.* (1971) have reported the results of earlier experience at the Royal Marsden Hospital. The survival results obtained in patients receiving radiotherapy between 1931 and 1966 are summarized in Table 13.3.

The improvement in survival figures is difficult to interpret, since changes in staging methods occurred during this period. However, the findings of lymphography introduced in 1961 would not have modified the decision to treat the patient with radiation and it is therefore probable that better survival

Table 13.3 Results of radiotherapy for testicular teratoma (Royal Marsden Hospital, 1931–1966). (Data from Smithers *et al.* 1971)

Years	Radiation facility	Total no. of patients treated	Percentage survival	
			3 years	5 years
1931–1949	200–400 kV x-rays	32	47	47
1950–1961	2 MeV x-rays	52	59	59
1961–1966	6 MeV x-rays	16	75	—

figures were obtained by using more penetrating radiation beams to treat deeply seated nodes.

Van der Werf Messing (1976) has reported treatment results obtained in 203 patients with non-seminomatous tumours managed between 1950 and 1974. A cure rate of 90 per cent was reported for Stage I patients and 45 per cent for patients with clinical node involvement. Similar results were reported by Hussey *et al.* (1977), with three-year disease-free survival rates of 78.2 per cent for Stage I, 46.7 per cent for Stage IIA and 17.6 per cent for Stage IIB. Maier and Mittemeyer (1977) reported the results of a randomized prospective study carried out between 1968 and 1973 and comparing radiotherapy with pre- and postoperative irradiation and radical node dissection. These results are summarized in Table 13.4 and show radiotherapy to be as effective as the combined approach. In this study it should be noted that radiotherapy included supradiaphragmatic nodes.

Table 13.4 Teratoma testis: three-year disease-free survival rates in the Walter Reed trial (Maier and Mittemeyer, 1977)

Treatment	Stage I Total no. of patients	Stage II Total no. of patients
Radiotherapy	29 (86%)	11 (82%)
Node dissection and pre- and postoperative radiotherapy	30 (97%)	21 (81%)

Between 1962 (when lymphography was introduced and the linear accelerator became available) and 1977, 363 men with malignant teratomas have been treated by the testicular tumour unit at the Royal Marsden Hospital. The results of this group are analysed in two series. Between 1962 and the end of 1975 ineffective chemotherapy was employed. Since 1976 vinblastine–bleomycin without, and more recently with, cis-platinum has been employed and the results of combined modality treatment are discussed in Chapter 15 (Peckham *et al.*, 1979).

Stage I (Table 13.5)

Between 1962 and the end of 1975, 108 Stage I patients were treated by orchidectomy and radiotherapy, as described above. Of this group, 89 (82.4 per cent) remain alive and disease free.

Table 13.5 Survival of Stage I testicular teratoma patients treated by orchidectomy and radiotherapy prior to the introduction of effective chemotherapy (Royal Marsden Hospital, 1962–1975)

Histology	No. of patients	No. of patients free of disease
MTI	57	52 (91%)
MTU	48	34 (71%)
MTT	3	3 (100%)
Total	108	89 (82%)

Influence of histology

As shown in Fig. 13.5 and Table 13.5, the survival rate was significantly worse for MTU patients than MTI. There were only three MTT patients and all these have survived.

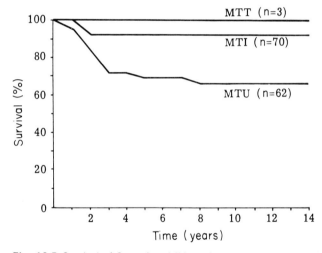

Fig. 13.5 Survival of Stage I and IIA testicular teratoma, according to histology (1962–1975).

Pattern of relapse

As shown in Fig. 13.1a, only one example of retroperitoneal relapse was encountered and the predominant sites of initial relapse were in the lungs and supradiaphragmatic nodes. The majority of relapses occurred within the first year after treatment (see Fig. 13.1b).

Analysis of prognostic factors in Stage I testicular teratomas

As discussed in Chapter 15, treatment of Stage I patients by irradiation after orchidectomy, deferring chemotherapy until early relapse is documented in the 20 per cent of patients who develop pulmonary metastases, has proved successful with 41 out of 43 (95 per cent) patients managed between December 1976 and April 1979 alive and free from disease. In spite of these excellent results, it cannot be assumed that such an approach is optimal therapy, particularly since it appears likely that an appreciable proportion of Stage I patients are cured by orchidectomy alone. The increasing precision of clinical staging manœuvres, including the judicial use of serum markers and CT scanning, allows more detailed patient evaluation. Furthermore, since chemo-therapy is effective for small-volume disease, deferral of any form of therapy in selected patients undergoing orchidectomy only is rendered a practicable possibility. The objective of such a study would be to define prognostic factors as accurately as possible so that a rational approach to future management could be established. The following sections discuss the evidence bearing upon the constitution of the clinical Stage I group.

False negative lymphography

Table 13.1 represents a collected series from the literature in which lympho-graphic interpretation has been compared with the histology of resected lymph nodes. Approximately 25 per cent of lymphogram-negative patients have occult retroperitoneal lymph node metastases and, since retroperitoneal relapse following radiotherapy has been uncommon in our experience, there is a high probability that small-volume metastases are eradicated with radiotherapy.

CT scanning

As discussed in Chapters 7 and 9, prior to radiotherapy and following orchi-dectomy, 4 out of 21 (19 per cent) clinical 'Stage I' patients were shown to have small pulmonary metastases which were not detected by conventional pulmonary radiography.

Tumour markers in Stage I

We have studied 59 patients treated between 1973 and 1978 in order to better understand the role of serum markers as prognostic indicators in patients treated by elective lymph node irradiation (Raghavan et al., 1980). The patients were divided into two groups.

Group A. These patients have elevated serum markers (AFP and/or HCG) which following orchidectomy, either remained elevated or fell more slowly than was compatible with rapid plasma clearance due to production by the primary tumour alone.

Group B. These patients either had persistently negative markers or marker elevation prior to orchidectomy which cleared rapidly (half-time for AFP five days and for HCG twenty-four hours) following removal of the primary tumour and before institution of radiation therapy.

Table 13.6 summarizes the results of the study. As shown, more than half of Group A patients relapsed with extralymphatic metastases. The disease-free survival curves for the two groups are shown in Fig. 13.6.

Involvement of the spermatic cord

As discussed in Chapter 7, the pathological staging classification employed by the British Testicular Tumour Panel correlated both with the histology of the primary tumour and with prognosis. These data, however, referred to patients inadequately staged by current standards.

Table 13.6 Relapse rate according to serum-marker status following radiotherapy for clinical Stage I teratoma testis (Royal Marsden Hospital, 1973–1978)

Group	Total no. of patients	No. of patients relapsed
A	11	7 (64%)
B	48	7 (15%)

Difference significant p<0.01.

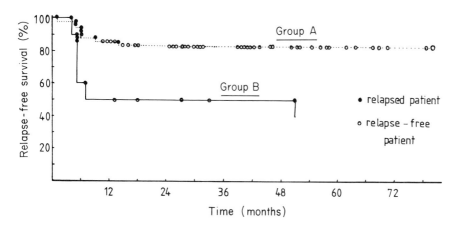

Fig. 13.6 Disease-free survival of Stage I patients treated by orchidectomy and radiotherapy. Group A, serum markers negative or, if positive, fall rapidly to normal after orchidectomy. Group B, serum markers remaining elevated or falling slowly after orchidectomy.

Unfortunately, in the past it was rarely possible to obtain adequate pathological material for detailed pathological staging of the primary tumour, although such a study is now in progress.

In the study referred to above it was possible to examine the spermatic cord in 49 patients. The data are summarized in Table 13.7 and show that the prognosis of patients with involvement of the cord (P_2, P_3) is significantly worse than the prognosis for those without cord invasion (P_1) (P<0.01).

Table 13.7 Relapse rate, in relation to invasion by tumour, of the spermatic cord in clinical Stage I teratoma testis treated by irradiation after orchidectomy (Royal Marsden Hospital, 1973–1978)

Cord histology	Total no. of patients	No. of patients relapsed
Negative	39	7 (18%)
Positive	10	6 (60%)

Difference significant p<0.01.

Tissue markers
As part of the study described above, histological sections from the primary tumour were stained by the immunoperoxidase technique for the presence of HCG (see Chapter 3). Human chorionic gonadotrophin-positive cells were identified in 27 tumours but were not seen in 21. There was no difference in relapse rate between these two groups.

Vascular invasion in the primary tumour
This has not been evaluated so far in our own series, although evidence of both vascular and lymphatic invasion will be sought in the prospective no-treatment study discussed below. Sandeman (1979) has reported that patients with T2 tumours (vascular invasion in testis or cord) fared considerably worse than patients with T1 tumours (no cord or vessel involvement) both for MTI and MTU.

Histology of the primary tumour and pathological stage
As noted in Chapter 7, MTU primary tumours have a higher probability of being associated with involvement of the spermatic cord than MTI. Thus in the analysis referred to above, 11/16 MTU primaries were P_2 or P_3 compared with 5/33 MTI.

Conclusions
As a result of the experience quoted above and the observation that between 10 and 20 per cent of patients who have histologically negative nodes at radical node dissection subsequently relapse, usually with pulmonary metastases, it is possible to attempt a tentative analysis of the constitution of clinical Stage I disease. This is shown schematically in Fig. 13.7.

No-treatment study
In Group B patients where the relapse rate following radiotherapy is low and where CT scanning may be expected to remove a further small number of high-risk patients, it is probable that 60–80 per cent of patients are cured by orchidectomy alone and require neither radiotherapy nor chemotherapy. In this group a no-treatment study has been initiated to define the cure rate with orchidectomy and to understand prognostic factors. The site of relapse will be monitored closely and, if the retroperitoneum is the initial site at which metastases are detected, this will provide a rational basis in the future for radiotherapy. To date there are scanty data on well-staged patients undergoing orchidectomy alone. Table 13.8 summarizes our preliminary experience in a group of 12 patients. So far we have not observed relapse in 5 patients with MTI primary tumours, but, interestingly, all 3 MTU patients have relapsed in the retroperitoneum. If an unacceptably high proportion of patients do relapse and require chemotherapy, it will be necessary to re-adopt the previous policy of radiotherapy, particularly since we have shown that a policy of radiotherapy and deferred chemotherapy can be highly successful (see Chapter 15).

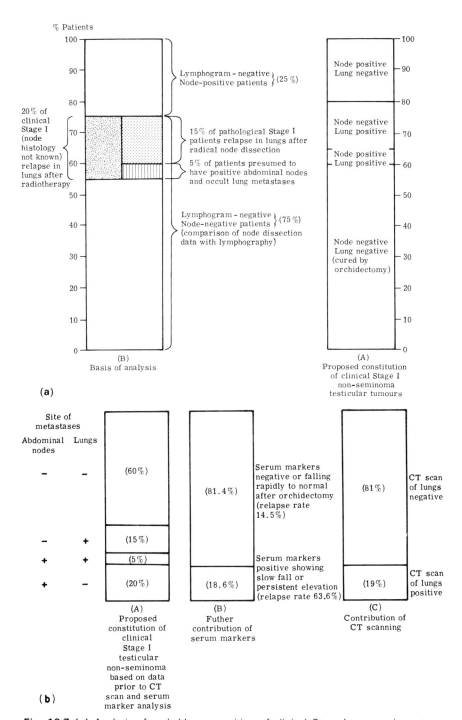

Fig. 13.7 (a) Analysis of probable composition of clinical Stage I non-seminomatous germ-cell tumours of the testis prior to introduction of CT scanning and routine application of serum markers. **(b)** Contribution of CT scanning and serum markers to the investigation of clinical Stage I non-seminomatous germ-cell tumours of the testis.

Table 13.8 Clinical Stage I germ-cell tumours of the testis: watch policy after orchidectomy

Patient	Histology	Initial markers		Primary tumour extent	Relapse Site	Time (months)	Marker elevation		Total follow up (months)
		AFP	HCG				AFP	HCG	
1	MTI								6
2	MTI		29	Rete+					10
3	MTI								15
4	MTI	119	340						8
5	MTI		349						3
6	MTU			Lymphatics+	Abdomen	5	18		7
7	MTU			Lymphatics+	Abdomen	5		12	10
8	MTU			Lymphatics+ vascular	Abdomen	2	22		4
9	MTD*								39
10	MTI								6
11	Seminoma	310							7
12	Seminoma*			Vascular+					12

* Not treated because of horseshoe kidney.

Patients with documented metastatic disease treated prior to 1976
As shown in Table 13.9 and Fig. 13.8, with the exception of patients with IIA (small-volume abdominal node metastases), patients with teratoma treated prior to December 1975 fared poorly with only 22 out of 152 (14.4 per cent) remaining alive.

Table 13.9 Results of treatment of patients with metastatic testicular teratoma prior to the use of effective chemotherapy (Royal Marsden Hospital, 1962–1975)

Stage	Total no. of patients	No. of patients disease-free
IIA	21	17 (81%)
IIB, IIC	24	6 (25%)
III	16	5 (31%)
IV	112	11 (10%)

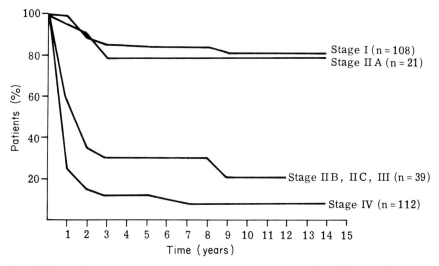

Fig. 13.8 Results of treatment of testicular teratoma by Stage. (Royal Marsden Hospital, 1962–1975.)

Stage IIA

As described above and shown in Fig. 13.2, in a retrospective analysis of the Royal Marsden Hospital series it was demonstrated that abdominal node metastases < 2 cm in maximum diameter could be controlled satisfactorily with radiation therapy. Hitherto, our policy in this group has been to treat as for Stage I, adding a supplementary dose of 5–10 Gy using small fields to treat the involved node(s). Previously, it was policy to treat the mediastinum and neck but this has been abandoned since the probability of supradiaphragmatic node involvement is low (Table 13.10). Futhermore, when supradiaphragmatic node involvement is present, the probability of extranodal extension is

Table 13.10 Occult supraclavicular node metastases in teratoma patients with abdominal node metastases (Stage II)

References	No. of patients sampled	Histology positive
Buck et al. (1972)	23	3
Donohue et al. (1977)	14	3
	37	6 (16%)

high, rendering localized therapy inappropriate. In addition, irradiation of a large volume of bone marrow compromises subsequent chemotherapy should this become necessary. In practice, the Stage IIA category is extremely uncommon and, as described below, because of the difficulty of delivering chemotherapy if infra- and supradiaphragmatic radiotherapy have been given, it is now our policy to employ two cycles of chemotherapy before irradiation. The rationale of this approach is based on the finding by Williams et al. (1980) that two cycles of PVB were effective as an adjuvant to surgery in node-positive patients.

Stages IIB, IIC and III

In this group of patients, results with radiotherapy alone are poor (*vide infra*) and treatment should be initiated with chemotherapy. This is discussed in more detail in Chapter 15.

Future proposals for patients with metastatic disease

Systemic treatment for 'Stage I' disease

As shown above, patients with persistent elevation of serum markers after orchidectomy show an unacceptably high relapse rate despite lymph node irradiation, which clearly indicates that extralymphatic dissemination has occurred (see Fig. 13.6). This group, therefore, requires chemotherapy as initial and probably their only treatment.

Stage IIA

Despite the good results obtained with radiotherapy, 20 per cent of patients relapse. Furthermore, the results quoted above were obtained employing a policy in which supradiaphragmatic nodes were always irradiated. The effectiveness of the PVB regime in dealing with small-volume abdominal disease, together with the risk of chemotherapy toxicity after infra- and supradiaphragmatic irradiation, has led us to propose the use of four cycles of chemotherapy followed by radiotherapy limited to the initially involved lymph nodes.

Stages IIB, IIC, III and IV L_1 L_2

In these groups of patients, initial sites of bulky lymph node disease are irradiated following chemotherapy. Details of this approach are given in Chapter 15. It is essential that careful planning is carried out, particularly in view of the prior exposure to intensive chemotherapy. Recently, this has been facilitated by the incorporation of CT scanning into treatment planning.

Computerized axial tomographic scanning and radiotherapy planning

As discussed in more detail in Chapter 15, radiotherapy is being employed to treat sites of lymph node disease in selected patients treated initially with chemotherapy. The accurate localization of retroperitoneal and mediastinal lymph node metastases by CT scanning, and the information provided on the disposition of normal structures, as well as the tumour, on a cross-sectional display of the body, provide a valuable contribution to accurate radiotherapy planning. The role of CT is discussed in detail in Chapter 9, but it is pertinent at this point to discuss its contribution to planning. Computed tomography scans are performed with several objectives. These include staging, monitoring of response to therapy, radiotherapy planning and surgical planning (Fig. 13.9).

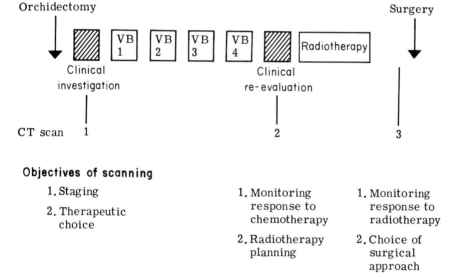

Fig. 13.9 CT scanning and sequential chemotherapy–radiotherapy for teratoma testis. This illustrates the four roles of CT scanning: staging, monitoring, response to treatment, radiation therapy planning and selection of surgical approach.

A system has been developed recently whereby CT scan information can be transferred into a dedicated digital computer and used as a basis for therapy planning (Hobday *et al.*, 1979). The relevant CT section is selected and transferred into the planning computer. The section is displayed on the planning viewing screen and information on tumour outline and position of normal structures passed into the computer by the clinician using a touch-sensitive light pencil. Using this method, the target volume is delineated as well as critical structures such as kidneys, spinal cord and lungs. An accurate patient contour is obtained also. The operator interacts with the computer to derive a satisfactory field arrangement which is permanently recorded, either as a plan superimposed on a grey-scale CT scan or as an isodose distribution on the patient outline with those structures marked with the light pencil included. The computer programme includes correction for inhomogeneous radiation absorption. This is particularly relevant if lung tissue is included in the treatment field.

The sequence of steps in deriving a CT plan to irradiate residual tumour in the retroperitoneum is illustrated in Fig. 13.10. Further details on the critical evaluation of CT scanning as a basis for therapy planning have been published elsewhere (Hobday et al., 1979).

Toxicity of nodal irradiation

The toxicity of well-planned abdominal node irradiation is low compared with the reported side effects and small mortality of radical node dissection (Table 13.11).

Acute toxicity

Acute morbidity varies from one individual to another, but is rarely severe enough to interrupt therapy. A degree of anorexia and nausea is common, vomiting should rarely pose a problem with adequate symptomatic treatment. Looseness of the motions may occur and require treatment. These symptoms subside promptly following cessation of therapy.

Long-term sequelae

The long-term morbidity has been minimal in our series. In the few cases of peptic ulcer the tumour dose employed has generally exceeded 4000 rad in four weeks and there has often been a history of prior dyspepsia.

Fertility after unilateral orchidectomy and radiation therapy

An important advantage of radiotherapy over radical node dissection is the preservation of normal sexual function. Furthermore, fertility is preserved in a proportion of patients, provided efforts are made to avoid irradiating the remaining testis. The human testis is extremely sensitive to radiation. The effect of single doses of between 8 and 600 rad were studied in detail by Rowley et al. (1974). The prompt reduction in sperm count following irradiation is accompanied by a sharp rise in urinary gonadotrophin levels. This coincided with denuding of the germinal epithelium and persisted until histological recovery occurred. With repopulation of the germinal epithelium, the total gonadotrophin levels returned to normal. Urinary LH levels did not change, but FSH levels paralleled total gonadotrophins. Rises in plasma FSH levels were dose related and significant increases occurred between 75 and 600 rad. Plasma LH behaved similarly. Plasma testosterone levels were unchanged. Spermatogonia showed morphological and quantitation changes at all dose

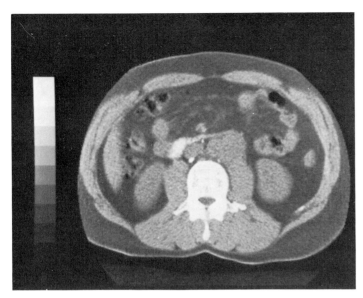

(a)

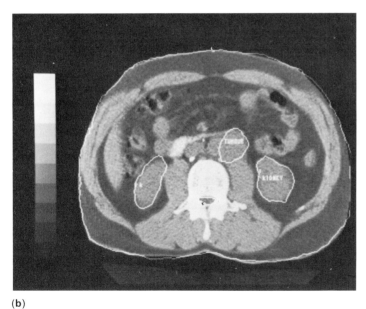

(b)

Fig. 13.10 (a) Computerized axial tomographic x ray scanning and radiation therapy planning. (b) CT scanning showing mass of involved nodes in the retroperitoneum.

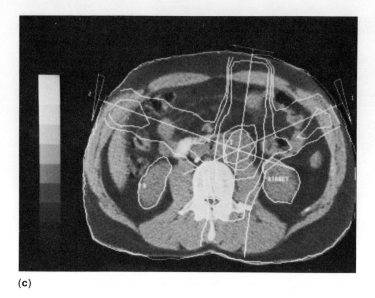

(c)

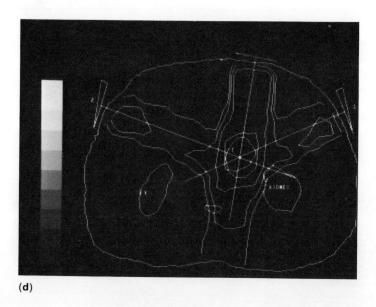

(d)

Fig. 13.10 (c) Therapy plan with isodose distribution superimposed on a grey scale CT scan. **(d)** Therapy plan on patient outline.

Table 13.11 Relative merits and disadvantages of radical node dissection and nodal irradiation in early testicular cancer

	Radical node dissection (%)	Radiotherapy (%)
Performance as a curative procedure (percentage cure rate)		
Negative nodes*	83†	82‡
Positive nodes	49	51
Complications	11§	<2
Mortality	1	0
Interference with sexual function	Retrograde ejaculation	None, fertility often preserved
Compromising effect on subsequent chemotherapy	None expected	*Immediate* chemotherapy— risk of gut toxicity; subsequent chemotherapy not compromised by abdominal node irradiation
Clinical v. pathological staging	Pathological staging data provided; major operative procedure required to obtain it	25% false negative lymphogram rate; irrelevant since radiation therapy and deferred chemotherapy give a high disease-free survival

* i.e. histology −ve or +ve for radical node dissection; lymphography −ve or +ve for radiotherapy.
† Data from Chapter 12.
‡ Data from Chapter 13 (note most +ve lymphogram patients now receive chemotherapy initially—the figure of 51% refers to radiotherapy alone).
§ Data from Williams (1977).

levels (except 8 rad, where no samples were taken). Approximately seventy days were necessary for the expression of azoospermia at all dose levels above 80 rad. Moderate oligospermia was observed with 20 rad. Histological recovery was seen at about six to eight months, and the first sperm or sperm-number increase in seminal fluid at six months following 20 rad and twenty-four months after 600 rad.

It is well documented clinically that, following orchidectomy and abdominal node irradiation, fertility may be preserved, although temporary oligospermia is generally observed. Sandeman (1966) reported a total of eighteen testicular tumour patients fathering children following radiotherapy. In this study, sequential sperm counts were carried out and showed, in most men, oligospermia with recovery between one and two years.

Amelar *et al.* (1971) reported recovery of sperm count in 4 men, with fathering of children subsequently in 3. Van der Werf Messing (1976) reported that 31 men in her series of patients fathered children after successful radiation therapy. Orecklin *et al.* (1973) described 28 patients who attempted to father children following treatment of a testicular tumour. Of these, 18 (64 per cent) were successful, 16 of whom had received prior irradiation. Smithers *et al.* (1973), reporting on the Royal Marsden Hospital series, described 34 irradiated patients who fathered 52 children. Thermoluminescent dosimetry has shown that employing testicular shielding and with the shaply defined beam

of the linear accelerator, the testicular radiation dose is of the order of 0.5–
0.7 Gy. If inappropriate surgery, past history or tumour extent demand scrotal
and inguinal node irradiation, a higher testicular dose is inevitable and the
chances of preserving fertility correspondingly reduced. In a study of six
patients who received scrotal irradiation and where radiation doses to the
remaining testis ranged from 135–201 rad, azoospermia was demonstrated in
all cases (Thomas *et al.*, 1977). In contrast, in a prospective study of three
patients who did not receive scrotal radiotherapy and in whom treatment was
confined to the para-aortic and ipsilateral pelvic lymph nodes, recovery of
spermatogenesis was demonstrated. In these patients the testicular radiation
doses were 31, 33 and 52 rad. The proportion of men with pretreatment sperm
counts within the normal range who preserve fertility is unknown, although
studies are in progress to shed light on this point.

References

Amelar, R. D., Dubin, L. and Hotchkiss, R. S. (1971). *Journal of Urology* **106**, 714.

Buck, A. S., Schamber, C. T., Maier, J. G. and Lewis, E. L. (1972). *Journal of Urology* **107**, 619.

Cook, F. E., Lawrence, D. D., Smith, J. R. and Gritti, E. J. (1965). *Radiology* **84**, 420.

Donohue, R. E., Pfister, R. R., Weigel, J. W. and Stonington, O. G. (1977). *Urology* **9**, 546.

Durant, J-C. and Barrat, F. (1977). *Annales d'urologie, Vol. 11* **1**, 25.

Einhorn, L. H. and Williams, S. D. (1978). *Cancer Treatment Reports* **62** (9), 1351.

Fein, R. L. and Taber, D. O. (1969). *Cancer* **24**, 248.

Hobday, P., Hodson, N. J., Husband, J., Parker, R. P. and Macdonald, J. S. (1979). *Radiology* **133**, 477.

Hultén, L., Kindblom, L-G., Lindhagen, J., Rosencrantz, M., Seeman, T. and Wahlqvist, L. (1973). *Acta. Chirurgica Scandinavica* **139**, 746.

Hussey, D. H., Luk, K. H. and Johnson, D. E. (1977). *Radiology* **123**, 175.

Jonsson, K., Ingemansson, S. and Ling, L. (1973). *British Journal of Urology* **45**, 548.

Kademian, M. and Wirtanen, G. (1977). *Urology* **9(2)**, 218.

Klein, K. A. and Maier, J. G. (1977). *International Journal of Radiation Oncology Biology Physics* **2**, 1229.

Lasser, Ph., Michel, G., Lacour, J., Catalogne, G. de and Thony, H. (1977). *Annales d'urologie, Vol. 11* **1**, 21.

Maier, J. G. and Mittemeyer, B. (1977). *Cancer* **39**, 981.

Maier, J. G. and Schamber, D. T. (1972). *American Journal of Roentgenology* **114**, 482.

Orecklin, J. R., Kangman, J. J. and Thompson, R. W. (1973). *Journal of Urology* **109**, 293.

Peckham, M. O., Hendry, W. F., McElwain, T. J. and Calman, F. M. B. (1977). The multimodality management of testicular teratomas. In *Adjuvant Therapy of Cancer*, p. 305. Ed. by S. E. Salmon and S. E. Jones. North Holland Publishing Company, Amsterdam, Oxford and New York.

Peckham, M. J., Barrett, A., McElwain, T. J. and Hendry, W. H. (1979). *Lancet* **ii**, 267.

Raghavan, D., Gibbs, J., Costa, Nogueira., Kohn, J., Orr, A.H., Barrett, A. and Peckham, M. J. (1980). *British Journal of Cancer* **41**, Suppl. IV, 191.

Rowley, M. J., Leach, D. R., Warner, G. A. and Heller, C. G. (1974). *Radiation Research* **59**, 665.

Safer, M. L., Green, J. P., Crews, Q. E. Jr. and Hill, D. R. (1975). *Cancer* **35**, 1603.

Sandeman, T. F. (1966). *British Journal of Radiology* **39**, 901.

Sandeman, T. F. (1979). *Australian Radiology* **23**, 136.

Seitzman, D. M. and Halaby, F. A. (1964). *Journal of Urology* **91**, 301.

Smithers, D. W., Wallace, D. M. and Austin, D. E. (1973). *British Medical Journal* **4**, 77.

Smithers, D. W., Wallace, I. N. K. and Wallace, D. M. (1971). *British Journal of Urology* **43**, 83.

Storm, P. B., Kern, A., Loening, S. A., Brown, R. C. and Culp, D. A. (1977). *Journal of Urology* **118**, 1000.

Thomas, P. R. M., Mansfield, M. D., Hendry, W. F. and Peckham, M. J. (1977). *British Journal of Surgery* **64**, 352.

Tyrrell, C. J. and Peckham, M. J. (1976). *British Journal of Urology* **48**, 363.

Van der Werf Messing, B. (1976). *International Journal of Radiation Oncology. Biology Physics* **1**, 235.

Wallace, S. and Jing, B. S. (1970). *American Medical Association* **213**, 94.

Williams, C. (1977). *Cancer Treatment Reviews* **4**, 275.

Williams, S. D., Einhorn, L. H. and Donohoe, J. P. (1980). *Proceedings of the American Association for Cancer Research (AACR) and American Society of Clinical Oncology (ASCO)* **21**, 421.

14

Chemotherapy of testicular teratoma

C. A. Juttner and T. J. McElwain

Introduction

Of a group of 275 patients with malignant testicular teratoma treated at the Royal Marsden Hospital between 1962 and 1975, only 48 per cent remain alive (Peckham *et al.*, 1977). At presentation, 56 per cent of the total had disease limited to the testicle (Stage I) or with spread to infradiaphragmatic lymph nodes only (Stage II) and the majority of long-term survivors come from these groups. Only about 15 per cent of men with supradiaphragmatic nodal spread (Stage III) or extranodal disease (Stage IV) remain alive and disease-free.

The majority of patients who die of their disease have extensive tumour at diagnosis, relapse with generalized disease, or have Stage II disease with bulky para-aortic retroperitoneal nodal involvement. Tyrrell and Peckham (1976) have shown that only one-third of patients in Stage II, with abdominal nodal metastases larger than 2 cm in diameter, are controlled by radical nodal radiotherapy. Although a small proportion of this latter group may be salvaged by laparotomy and lymphadenectomy, it is clear that many of them, as well as the patients with Stage III and IV disease, would be helped and possibly cured by effective chemotherapy, either alone or as part of a planned multimodality management approach.

Hitherto, the major problem in the chemotherapy of testicular teratoma was not a lack of drugs to which the tumour responded, but rather the low complete remission rates achieved.

Smithers (1972) reviewed the published experience with chemotherapy for metastatic testicular teratoma and found 65 cases of adequately documented complete remission. Of these, 25 lasted more than two years and 11 more than five years. Partial response rates were very much higher than remission rates and the majority of partial responses were short lived. Only six drugs produced complete remission when used alone—mithramycin, actinomycin D, methotrexate, vinblastine, nitrofurazone and hydroxyurea. Chlorambucil, vincristine and cyclophosphamide were found commonly in combinations producing complete remissions, whereas 5-fluorouracil melphalan and nitrogen mustard were occasionally part of successful combinations. Thus, the tumours were sensitive to drugs from all major functional groups—antimetabolites, alkylating agents, vinca alkaloids and antitumour antibiotics.

The first use of combination chemotherapy in testicular teratoma was reported by Li *et al.* in 1960. This was one of the earliest studies using drugs with differing toxicities in combination and the principle has been developed extensively since then.

Single-agent chemotherapy

Smithers (1972) found 31 cases of complete remission after chemotherapy with single drugs. Seventeen followed mithramycin therapy, 5 actinomycin-D, 4 vinblastine, 2 methotrexate, 2 nitrofurazone and 1 hydroxyurea. Complete remissions have been described subsequently with cyclophosphamide (Buckner *et al.*, 1974), ifosphamide (Hoefer-Janker *et al.*, 1975), cis-diammino-dichloroplatinum (Higby *et al.*, 1974a and 1974b) and bleomycin (EORTC, 1970).

The most effective drug when used as a single agent has probably been mithramycin. Many workers have described good regressions and a significant number of complete remissions (Kennedy, 1970), but there was often an unacceptable morbidity and, in one series, a drug-associated mortality of 25 per cent—3 out of 12 patients (Brown and Kennedy, 1965). Laboratory investigations revealed a marked dissociation between the rate of recovery of mithramycin-induced inhibition of RNA synthesis in mouse glioma and normal mouse liver. Since the normal tissue recovered in twenty-four hours whereas tumour recovery was incomplete at forty-eight hours, Kennedy postulated that the drug could be given on alternate days with reduced toxicity but no loss of cytotoxic effect (Kennedy, 1970). He reported a series of 23 patients treated on an alternate-day schedule and found a similar response rate (10 responses, 5 complete) compared with an earlier series of 21 patients treated with daily mithramycin (10 responses, 6 complete). The clinical and biochemical toxicity was less in the alternate-day group and there was no mortality due to therapy in this group. Nevertheless, mithramycin remains a toxic drug and probably should not be used in first line treatment, either alone or in combinations, particularly since other drugs with more manageable and predictable toxicities are now known to be effective.

Bleomycin as a single agent has produced response rates of 33 to 42 per cent (Samuels, 1971; Carter and Wasserman, 1975) and at least three complete responses have been reported (EORTC, 1970; Blum *et al.*, 1973).

Adriamycin produces responses in up to 70 per cent of patients treated (Bonadonna, 1971; Monfardini *et al.*, 1972). O'Bryan reported responses in 3 of 6 patients with teratocarcinoma (MTI) (O'Bryan *et al.*, 1973). This is of interest since MTI tends to respond less well to most single agents and combinations than does the more common histology of MTU (embryonal carcinoma).

There is little published information on response rates to cis-dichlorodiamminoplatinum (cis-DDP) used alone in teratomas, but Higby (1974b) reported responses in 9 of 11 patients with testicular tumours treated in a Phase I study and complete remissions have been seen in 4 of 22 patients treated with cis-DDP as a single agent at the Royal Marsden Hospital, and in 7 of 16 patients treated at Roswell Park Memorial Institute (Gottlieb and Drewinko, 1975).

Buckner and his co-workers used cyclophosphamide in a dose of 60–120 mg/kg (Buckner *et al.*, 1974). There were 8 responses in 9 patients, of which 2 were complete remissions. One of the complete remitters remained disease-free at twenty-four months, but all other responses were of short duration.

Ifosphamide in high dosage has been used by Hoefer-Janker et al. (1975) and Schnitker et al. (1976). Hoefer-Janker claimed 23 complete remissions in 39 patients with non-seminomatous testicular tumours. Schnitker described 9 complete remissions in 23 patients. It is not clear whether ifosphamide was used as a single agent in all these patients. Schmoll et al. (1978) described a complete remission rate of 65 per cent (15 of 23 patients) using ifosphamide in combination with vinblastine and bleomycin.

In 1970, Samuels and Howe described their first experience with vinblastine in high dosage. Eleven of 21 patients responded and in 4 of these the responses were complete. One of the complete responders remained disease free at forty-two months. The addition of melphalan appeared to confer no benefit.

Newlands and Bagshawe (1977) have reported 4 responders in 5 patients with drug-resistant malignant teratoma treated with the epipodophyllin derivative VP 16-213. Cavalli et al. (1977) had 4 responses in 7 patients with advanced malignant teratoma and we have treated 7 patients with end-stage disease, producing 3 responses. In a more recent study, 26 patients (25 with malignant teratoma and 1 with seminoma) were treated with VP 16 and, of 24 assessable for tumour response, 3 (12.5 per cent) achieved complete remission (Table 14.1) (Fitzharris et al., 1979).

Table 14.1 Response of advanced testicular teratoma to VP 16–213. (From Fitzharris et al., 1979.)

Total no. of patients	No response	No assessable disease	Improvement	Complete response	Duration of complete response (weeks)
24	12	4	5	3 (12.5%)	40+ 52+ 32+

Combination chemotherapy

The present improvement in the results of chemotherapy for testicular teratoma has followed the work of Li, Whitmore, Golbey and Grabstaldt from the Memorial Hospital, New York (1960). They reported a series of 23 patients treated with chlorambucil, actinomycin-D and methotrexate. Twelve of these showed an objective response, of which 7 were complete or nearly complete. One patient was free of disease at eighteen months and 2 at nine months, but the rest had relapsed by four months.

In 1969, Ansfield et al., described experience with the same regime. Two-thirds of the patients with measurable disease had at least a 50 per cent response, but relapse occurred usually within three months. Four patients had complete remissions, which were maintained. The longest was over seven years in a patient with a trophoblastic teratoma.

The accumulated Memorial Hospital experience was reviewed by Mackenzie in 1966. Twenty-three of 154 patients were rendered completely free of detectable disease. Only five regimes of the many tried were successful in producing complete remissions. The regime of Li *et al.* was used in 90 patients. In 72 it was the first chemotherapy given and complete remissions occurred in 10 cases. (In 2 of these an elevated urinary chorionic gonadotrophin was the only evidence of metastatic disease.) No responses were seen in the 18 patients who had received previous chemotherapy, and only 2 showed a partial response.

Actinomycin-D and chlorambucil without methotrexate produced complete responses in 5 of 31 patients. Again, previously treated patients showed only partial response. Four of 11 patients having actinomycin-D alone, administered in a variety of ways, had complete responses. Chlorambucil alone produced occasional complete remissions, but only in patients with pure seminoma. One patient had an elevated urinary chorionic gonadotrophin return to normal after treatment with 6-mercaptopurine and 6-diazo levonorleucine. There was no other evidence of tumour in this patient.

Mackenzie concluded that the most effective regime was actinomycin-D used alone in a dose of 1.0 mg daily for five days.

McElwain and Peckham have reported their experience (1974) with vinblastine, actinomycin-D and methotrexate. These drugs were combined because each produced complete remissions when used alone. Forty-four patients were treated, with an overall response rate of 57 per cent. The response rate was higher for MTU (67 per cent) than for MTI (27 per cent). Complete remissions were seen more commonly in lung metastases (7 out of 42 patients, 17 per cent) than in abdominal nodal disease (1 of 32 patients, 3 per cent). There were no complete responses in patients with liver metastases. Seven of the 8 complete remissions were in patients with MTU. This difference in response according to histology has been described by several other workers and it has been found that MTU (embryonal carcinoma) is consistently more responsive than MTI (teratocarcinoma). Few series have more than a small number of cases of MTT (choriocarcinoma) and response rates are generally low here, although complete responses do occasionally occur.

Peckham and McElwain (1975) have reported results using DTIC and adriamycin. Only 1 of 5 patients with MTU responded, while 8 of 13 with MTI showed a significant response.

Vinblastine–bleomycin combinations

In 1971, Samuels and his co-workers (personal communication) described their first use of the combination of vinblastine and bleomycin. Eight patients were treated and all eight responded. Samuels further developed this combination (Samuels, Holoye and Johnson, 1975; Samuels, Johnson and Holoye, 1975; Samuels *et al.*, 1976) and reported the results with two different combinations of vinblastine and bleomycin. In the VB_1 regime vinblastine 0.4 mg/kg is given in two divided fractions intravenously on days 1 and 2, with bleomycin 30 mg intramuscularly twice weekly (Samuels, Holoye and Johnson, 1975). Courses are repeated at four to six week intervals, depending on toxicity. In the VB_3 regime vinblastine is given in the same dosage on days 1 and 2, followed by bleomycin 30 mg/day for five days by continuous intravenous infusion. Both regimes are extremely toxic and patients need to be in hospital. Samuels also used bleoCOMF, a combination of bleomycin, cyclophosphamide, vincristine, methotrexate and 5-fluorouracil.

In MTU, complete response rates were 7 of 26 patients (27 per cent) with VB$_1$ and 21 of 36 patients (58 per cent) with VB$_3$. In MTI, the rates were 10 of 24 patients (42 per cent) with VB$_1$ and 7 of 21 patients (33 per cent) with VB$_3$. Because MTI is known to respond less well to chemotherapy, patients with MTI were treated with bleoCOMF as well as VB$_1$. Of the 10 complete responders with MTI to VB$_1$/bleoCOMF, only 1 relapsed. Nine remained free of disease at between 153 and 276 weeks from diagnosis. It is of interest that 6 of these long-term remitters had minimal disease, with gynaecomastia plus or minus an elevated HCG being the only evidence of disease in 2.

Of 7 complete responders with MTU to VB$_1$/bleoCOMF, 3 have relapsed. Two of the 4 long-term remitters had small-volume disease.

There were 9 patients with MTT treated with vinblastine–bleomycin regimes. There were only 2 complete remissions. Only 1 of these remained alive and disease-free. Thus, this histological subtype is as unresponsive to these more effective regimes as it is to other forms of chemotherapy.

The results of Wittes et al. (1976) and Monfardini et al. (1976) are less good than those of Samuels. Both these former series involved the use of vinblastine and bleomycin with the addition of actinomycin-D in one case and mithramycin in the other. Doses of vinblastine and bleomycin were lower than Samuels used and responses were also lower. Wittes reported a 34 per cent response rate with 15 per cent complete response, and Monfardini reported 3 responses in 11 patients treated. It is possible that actinomycin and mithramycin may interfere with the action of vinblastine and bleomycin, but it is more likely that the superiority of Samuels' regimes lies in the high doses of drugs used and the probable need to produce considerable reversible normal tissue damage in order to achieve remissions.

Royal Marsden Hospital series

Following the investigation of the VAM regime (McElwain and Peckham, 1974) and DTIC and adriamycin, and prior to the introduction of VB and later cis-platinum, vinblastine, bleomycin, high dose cyclophosphamide and high-dose cis-DDP were tested as single agents. There was also a more limited study of ifosphamide.

Staging and patient selection
Criteria for staging are described in Chapter 7. The deployment of chemotherapy in overall management is outlined in Chapter 11 and discussed in Chapter 15.

The criteria for response in chemotherapy studies
Complete remission (CR)
Complete disappearance of all clinical radiological and biochemical evidence of disease, including the return to normal of elevated levels of both alphafetoprotein and beta-HCG.

Partial response (PR)
A decrease of 50 per cent or more in the sum of the products of maximum perpendicular diameters of all measurable lesions, with no evidence of progres-

sion of any lesion and without the appearance of any new lesion. The response must last for at least four weeks.

No response (NR)
Any response less than a partial response or any progression of disease.

Cyclophosphamide

Following the report by Buckner *et al.* (1974), a study was performed in which 25 patients were treated with high-dose cyclophosphamide on one to five occasions. Twenty-three of these patients had received no previous chemotherapy. Twenty-one had 5 gm as an intravenous bolus on one to three occasions. Four patients had smaller doses because of previous nephrectomy, obstructive uropathy or small body size.

All patients received intravenous hydration with 6–8 litres of fluid per twenty-four hours, starting two hours before cyclophosphamide and continuing for twenty-four hours after the drug was given. This prevented haemorrhagic cystitis in most courses of treatment. Nausea and vomiting were intense but short lived. Alopecia was universal and granulocytopenia was more marked than thrombocytopenia. The nadir of the white cell count occurred in the second week after cyclophosphamide. No patient developed clinical or bacteriological evidence of infection.

Five patients were not fully assessable. Three, who responded, had radiotherapy to their metastases starting within one to five days of cyclophosphamide. One patient with pulmonary metastases had simultaneous bilateral primary tumours, one MTU, one pure seminoma. His pulmonary metastases responded, but they may have been pure seminoma. There is no record of response in one patient. There are 20 assessable patients, whose responses are shown in Table 14.2.

Table 14.2 Malignant teratoma (Royal Marsden Hospital, 1975–1976). Cyclophosphamide chemotherapy

Histology	No. of patients	CR		PR		Overall response	
MTU	14	1	(7%)	2	(14%)	3	(21%)
MTI	4	0		0		0	
MTT	1	0		0		0	
Other (mediastinal)	1	0		0		0	
Total	20	1	(5%)	2	(10%)	3	(15%)

All responders had MTU and came from the group of 13 patients with pulmonary metastases, thus confirming the increased chemosensitivity of this histological subtype and this metastatic pattern.

Although the overall response rate was very low, a much greater number of patients, about 50 per cent, showed an early response with significant reduction in the size of metastases at two weeks, but with regrowth already evident as haematological recovery occurred during the third week after cyclophosphamide. It is difficult to explain the disparity between these results and those described by Buckner, particularly since he used the same criteria for partial response. He used somewhat higher doses, up to 120 mg/kg, whereas no patient exceeded 40 mg/kg in our study; with the exception of the 3 responders and the 1 patient with bilateral simultaneous primaries, it was found that repeated doses as soon as haematological toxicity allowed did not prevent the rapid early regrowth phenomenon so commonly seen. Buckner described the same phenomenon in at least one of his patients.

Table 14.3 Malignant teratoma Royal Marsden Hospital, 1976–1977). cis-DDP chemotherapy

Histology	No. of patients	CR		PR		Overall response	
MTU ± seminoma	14	4	(29%)	4	(29%)	8	(57%)
MTI ± seminoma	4	0		2		2	(50%)
MTT ± seminoma	2	0		0		0	
Mediastinal teratoma	1	0		0		0	
Orchioblastoma	1	1		0		1	
MTD/yolk-sac	0	0		0		0	
Total	23	5	(22%)	6	(26%)	11	(48%)

The conclusion was that cyclophosphamide, at least in the dosage used, had little place as a single agent in the management of testicular teratomas.

Cis-dichlorodiamminoplatinum
The reports by Higby *et al.* (1974a; 1974b) of the effect of Cis-DDP in testicular tumours, and the more recent reports (Cvitkovic, Spaulding *et al.*, 1977; Hayes *et al.*, 1977) demonstrating that nephrotoxicity could be largely prevented by forced diuresis led to a study of the drug as a single agent in doses of 50–130 mg/ m^2 by intravenous infusion over twenty to thirty minutes. Mannitol was used with normal saline, 6 litres per twenty-four hours, and intravenous frusemide as required to ensure a high urine flow. Infusions were repeated at three-week intervals, depending on haematological and biochemical toxicity. Nephrotoxicity was monitored carefully using EDTA clearances.

Twenty-five patients received one to four infusions of Cis-DDP. Twenty-three can be fully assessed. One patient received radiotherapy starting five days after cis-DDP, another had cis-DDP after multiple lung metastases had remitted on vinblastine and bleomycin. Both were disease-free sixty-four and forty-six weeks from the end of all therapy. Three of the assessable patients received low doses (50 mg/m²) of cis-DDP. Two showed no response. The other, who had haemoptysis without evidence of a lesion, responded. The haemoptysis ceased for forty-one weeks and then recurred in association with visible pulmonary metastases. This is assessed as a complete response.

The remaining 20 patients received cis-DDP in doses of 100 to 130 mg/m². Results are presented in Table 14.3.

Although there were 5 complete remissions, all these patients had small-volume disease. Two had lung metastases less than 1 cm in diameter, 1 (already mentioned) had haemoptysis without a visible lesion and 2 had elevated alphafetoprotein as the only evidence of disease. Three of the 5 relapsed within three to 10 months. Two remain disease-free after other treatment. Only 5 patients had not received previous chemotherapy. Two had partial response, 1 cannot be assessed and 2 showed no response.

Table 14.4 shows responses according to the site of metastases. Although the numbers are small, results support the previously described finding (Peckham and McElwain, 1975) that pulmonary metastases appear to be more responsive to chemotherapy than abdominal metastases.

Table 14.4 Response of testicular teratoma metastases to cis-DDP, by site

Site	No. of patients	CR	PR	Overall response
Lung	18	3 (17%)	6 (33%)	9 (50%)
Abdomen	9	—	1 (11%)	1 (11%)

Toxicity was not a problem with cis-DDP. There was a transient fall in haemoglobin by 1–2 gm per cent which always recovered by three weeks. White cell count did not fall below 3000, or platelets below 100 000, except in a small group of patients who had had extensive prior chemotherapy and/or radiotherapy. Four patients admitted to tinnitus, which has been described as a side effect by Gottlieb and Drewinko (1975), although audiograms were not performed. Figure 14.1 shows serial EDTA clearances in a patient having two infusions of cis-DDP.

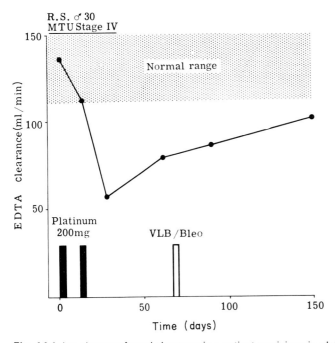

Fig. 14.1 Impairment of renal clearance in a patient receiving cis-platinum chemotherapy.

We conclude that cis-DDP has a useful place in the chemotherapy of tera-tomas. Its value in combination with other more effective agents having qualitatively different toxicities is discussed below.

Ifosphamide

Because of reports of complete remission induced by ifosphamide (Hoefer-Janker *et al.*, 1975; Schnitker *et al.*, 1976), 5 patients were treated with this drug alone in high dosage. Ifosphamide is claimed to be less myelotoxic than cyclophosphamide but more toxic to urothelium. Patients received $4 \, gm/m^2$ by rapid i.v. infusion, daily for five days. Haematuria could largely be prev-ented by intravenous hydration, 12 litres per twenty-four hours, and cathet-erization to keep the bladder empty. All patients had refractory end-stage disease. One patient had a transient partial response of lung metastases, lasting for six weeks. None of the others responded, and one died soon after chemo-therapy with septicaemia and progressive renal failure. Autopsy showed ex-tensive haemorrhage into both renal pelves. Haematological toxicity was pro-found and usually recovery did not begin until eighteen to twenty days from the end of the course. All patients experienced severe psychological depression in the recovery phase.

Vinblastine-bleomycin

The success of Samuels' (Samuels, Holoye and Johnson, 1975; Samuels, John-son and Holoye, 1975; Samuels *et al.*, 1976) vinblastine–bleomycin regimes led to a study of their effect beginning in late 1975. A small group of patients was treated with vinblastine $9 \, mg/m^2$ on days 1 and 2, followed by bleomycin 30 mg intramuscularly twice weekly for five weeks. One patient with extensive lung metastases has been in remission for 126 weeks and off all treatment for 99 weeks. The increased complete remission rate described with the VB_3 regime led to the adoption of a slight modification of this regime in early 1976. Vinblastine $9 \, mg/m^2$ was given by intravenous injection on days 1 and 2 and bleomycin, 30 mg per day by continuous infusion over twenty-four hours, was started after the first injection of vinblastine and continued for five days, to a total dose of 150 mg per course. Courses were repeated at four to five week intervals, depending on haematological toxicity.

Initially, no patients received more than two courses of vinblastine and bleomycin because the overall treatment plan included whole lung irradiation as a later treatment option. However, this policy was modified subsequently, the majority of patients receiving four courses and selected patients up to a maximum of six courses of vinblastine and bleomycin.

Fifty-seven patients received from one to six courses of vinblastine–contin-uous bleomycin (VB_3) to December 1977. Three patients cannot presently be assessed because of lack of follow-up information. Three patients had VB_3 as an adjuvant when in remission. One has relapsed and died. Two remain disease-free sixty and eighty-five weeks from the end of all treatment. Fifty-one patients are currently assessable for response. Seven of the partial responders have been rendered disease-free by subsequent radiotherapy and/or surgery.

Table 14.5 sets out the response rates overall and subdivided according to histology.

The majority of responses occurred in patients with undifferentiated tera-

Table 14.5 Malignant teratoma (Royal Marsden Hospital, 1976–1977). Vinblastine/continuous bleomycin chemotherapy

Histology	No. of patients	CR		PR		Overall response	
MTU ± seminoma	31	15	(48%)	12	(39%)	27	(87%)
MTI ± seminoma	10	1	(10%)	2	(20%)	3	(30%)
MTT ± seminoma	6	1	(17%)	1	(17%)	2	(34%)
Other teratomas (mediastinal, retroperitoneal, differentiated)	4	0		3	(75%)	3	(75%)
Total	51	17	(33%)	18	(35%)	35	(69%)

toma. The response rates in intermediate and trophoblastic teratoma were low, although patient numbers were small.

Responses were analysed according to the site of metastases. Table 14.6 shows complete and partial response rates for pulmonary, abdominal nodal, supraclavicular and mediastinal nodal and hepatic metastases. Numbers are small in the last two groups, but there is a definite difference in complete response rate between pulmonary metastases and abdominal nodal metastases. Much of this probably can be explained by the large number of patients with bulky abdominal metastases.

Table 14.6 Malignant teratoma (Royal Marsden Hospital, 1976–1977). VB$_3$ chemotherapy. Response of metastases according to site

Site	No. of patients	CR		PR		Overall response	
Lung	41	21	(51%)	10	(24%)	31	(76%)
Abdominal nodes	27	6	(22%)	11	(41%)	17	(63%)
Supraclavicular and mediastinal nodes	8	3	(38%)	5	(63%)	8	(100%)
Liver	5	1	(20%)	2	(40%)	3	(60%)

Analysis of this group of patients made it clear that both the site and the volume of metastases were important predictors of response. Tyrrell and Peckham (1976) have shown this to be true for abdominal disease treated by radiotherapy alone and Samuels et al. (1976) have described similar findings with chemotherapy. The results of his accumulated chemotherapy experience have led Samuels to alter his approach to staging (Samuels et al., 1976). Similarly, the differing responses according to bulk and site have led to a change in the detailed staging system used at The Royal Marsden Hospital and to our overall approach to advanced malignant teratoma.

Tables 14.7 and 14.8 show VB response according to subclass of abdominal and pulmonary metastases, using the staging criteria described in Chapter 7.

It is seen that the likelihood of both complete remission and partial response decreases with increasing bulk of abdominal node and pulmonary metastases.

So far as the lung metastases subclassification is concerned, the system used

Table 14.7 Malignant teratoma (Royal Marsden Hospital, 1976–1977). VB_3. Response according to bulk of abdominal nodal disease

Subclass	No. of patients	CR		PR		CR+PR	
A	3	3	(100%)	0		3	(100%)
B	6	2	(33%)	4	(67%)	6	(100%)
C	18	1	(6%)	7	(39%)	8	(44%)

Table 14.8 Malignant teratoma (Royal Marsden Hospital, 1976–1977). VB_3. Response according to subclass of pulmonary metastesas

Subclass	No. of patients	CR		PR		Overall response	
L_1	11	9	(82%)	0		9	(82%)
L_2	10	7	(70%)	1	(10%)	8	(80%)
L_3	20	5	(25%)	9	(45%)	14	(70%)
Total	41	21	(51%)	10	(24%)	31	(76%)

partially overlaps with Samuels' 'minimal pulmonary disease' and 'advanced pulmonary disease'. The emphasis, however, is different because of our initial approach using both chemotherapy and radiotherapy for a particular and common subgroup of early pulmonary disease. Our assessment is that the size of individual metastases is more important than their number in predicting chemotherapy remissions. We have seen several cases where two or three metastases 3–4 cm in diameter have failed to respond completely, whereas forty to fifty metastases, all less than 2 cm in diameter, have disappeared completely after one or two courses of chemotherapy. Clearly, there is a much greater total volume of tumour in the latter example, but this subclass is more susceptible to chemotherapy.

The findings summarized in Tables 14.7 and 14.8 are similar to those described by Samuels *et al.* (1976), who reported a complete response rate of 81 per cent for minimal lung disease, 57 per cent for advanced lung disease and 17 per cent for advanced abdominal disease, all with VB_3.

Mediastinal and supraclavicular metastases
Only 8 of the total group of 51 patients had disease in the mediastinal or supraclavicular nodes the response of which to chemotherapy could be assessed adequately. Five patients had mediastinal disease, of which 2 had complete remissions and 3 partial responses. All 8 had supraclavicular nodal metastases and all 8 responded, 3 completely. Samuels and his co-workers have reported (1976) that mediastinal disease is particularly resistant to chemotherapy, but probably this is related more to tumour volume than to site. We have applied the subclassification by diameter of metastases (less than 2 cm, 2 cm–5 cm and greater than 5 cm) to our group of patients and none of them had mediastinal or supraclavicular metastases greater than 5 cm diameter.

Hepatic metastases

Peckham and McElwain (1975) demonstrated the poor response rate and short survival in patients with liver metastases treated with vinblastine, actinomycin-D and methotrexate.

In this series there are only 5 patients with unequivocal liver metastases. One had no response to VB_3 and is dead. One had a complete response to six courses of VB_3 but the follow up is short. Two had almost complete responses after four courses of VB_3; one of these relapsed six months later after no further chemotherapy; the other continues on VB_3. The fifth showed clinical evidence of response but relapsed and died while still on chemotherapy.

There is not definite evidence as yet to show that VB_3 is as effective in liver metastases as it is in other sites. Assessment of disease and of response is much less exact in this site.

Previous chemotherapy

Several reports (Kardinal *et al.*, 1976; Wittes *et al.*, 1976; Einhorn and Donohue, 1977) have suggested that previous chemotherapy and/or radiotherapy prejudices the chance of responding to subsequent chemotherapy of various types. Eighteen patients from the Royal Marsden Hospital series had received previous chemotherapy. The response rates of the two groups are compared in Table 14.9.

Table 14.9 Response of advanced teratoma testis to VB_3 chemotherapy by previous treatment status

	No. of patients	CR		PR		Overall response	
Previous chemotherapy	18	3	(17%)	9	(50%)	12	(67%)
No previous chemotherapy	33	12	(36%)	11	(33%)	23	(70%)

The previously treated group were often end-stage, with refractory disease. The overall response rates are very similar although, as expected, fewer complete remissions occurred in those who had received previous chemotherapy.

The longer-term results of patients receiving VB either alone or in combination with radiotherapy and surgery are discussed in Chapter 15.

Toxicity

The vinblastine–continuous bleomycin regime is extremely toxic. There were two treatment deaths in our series, both associated with septicaemia. One, a man aged 56 years with MTU who relapsed with minimal lung disease following radiotherapy for Stage II disease, died soon after his second course. The other was a young man with extensive pulmonary disease and small-volume abdominal disease who had had no previous treatment. He died during the neutropenic phase, following his first course of VB_3, with septicaemia and necrotizing enterocolitis with bowel perforation. Autopsy confirmed complete remission in both. Since then, all patients have been treated with oral non-absorbable antibiotics as used in acute leukaemia (Storring *et al.*, 1977) and no further deaths have occurred. Infectious complications remain the major danger of treatment and may require therapy with granulocyte transfusions as well as appropriate systemic antibiotics. Neutropenia reaches its nadir, usually below 600 WBC/mm³, on days 8 to 10 with recovery evident by day 14 (Fig. 14.2). Thrombocytopenia occurs on days 2 to 4, often below 30 000/mm³, with recovery proceeding through the period of leukopenia. Haemorrhage has occurred in only one patient, with duodenal invasion by massive abdominal disease. He had a haematemesis while responding well during his first course of VB₃. Subsequent courses were not associated with bleeding.

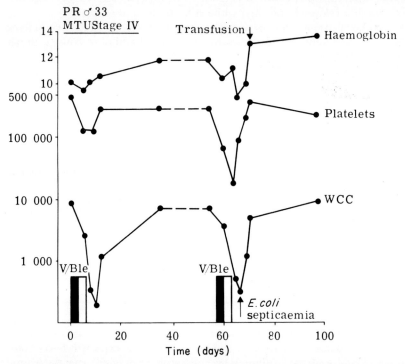

Fig. 14.2 Blood count changes following chemotherapy with vinblastine and bleomycin.

Less significant but almost universal side effects are alopecia, stomatitis and constipation; the latter two require vigorous local treatment. The haemoglobin falls by 1 to 3 gm per cent with each course, but recovers between courses and transfusion is rarely required. Bleomycin skin rashes and pigmentation are common and bleomycin also produces febrile reactions and symptoms rather like severe influenza. No bleomycin pneumonitis has been seen, other than in patients who have had previous lung irradiation. Patients usually lose from 5 to 10 kg in weight with each course, but most recover to near their pretreatment weight between courses.

All aspects of toxicity tend to become more severe with continuing treatment. One patient had chemotherapy terminated after the fifth course with severe neuropathy, gastrointestinal upset and inability to regain weight.

The toxicity is such that this regime should be used only by those experienced in the management of neutropenic patients, in a hospital with adequate facilities.

Cis-platinum, vinblastine and bleomycin combination (PVB)
Cis-DDP is an interesting drug to combine with vinblastine and bleomycin. Its toxicity is qualitatively different from both vinblastine and bleomycin and there is experimental evidence that it may have a specific effect on tissues arising from the urogenital anlage, in that it produces testicular atrophy in monkeys (Higby et al., 1974a).

Einhorn and Donohue (1977) have reported results in 50 patients treated with cis-DDP, vinblastine and bleomycin, with continuation therapy consisting of vinblastine and BCG for two years. Three patients were considered non-evaluable because of massive disease with early death within two weeks of beginning chemotherapy. Of the remaining 47 patients, 74 per cent attained complete remission. The other 12 patients all had partial remissions and 5 of these became disease-free following subsequent surgery.

In a recent progress report on this initial series (Einhorn, 1979), 32 (68 per cent) patients remain alive and 28 (60 per cent) remain alive and disease-free.

In a subsequent study, a further 79 patients were randomized in a three-arm study employing PVB with different doses of vinblastine and PVB plus adriamycin. Overall, 53 patients (67 per cent) achieved complete remission and an additional 10 patients (13 per cent) were rendered disease-free by subsequent surgery. Of this total of 63 patients achieving complete remission, only 7 (11 per cent) have relapsed. No differences were observed between the three arms of the study. Thus, overall in this later study, 70 per cent of patients remain disease-free and it is clear that the PVB combination constitutes a major advance in the management of advanced teratoma testis. In these two series reported by Einhorn and his colleagues, all but one relapse occurred within a year of initiating treatment.

As with other combination chemotherapy regimes in testicular teratoma, better results were seen in MTU (84 per cent CR) than in MTI (55 per cent CR) or choriocarcinoma (60 per cent CR).

A regime (VAB III) which included bleomycin, vinblastine, cis-DDP, actinomycin-D, cyclophosphamide and chlorambucil has been investigated by Golbey and his colleagues (Golbey et al., 1979). In a group of 92 patients a complete remission rate of 62 per cent was reported, 27 per cent of whom subsequently relapsed. Cvitkovic, Cheng et al. (1977) described a further combination (VAB IV) in which the same drugs were employed in a modified sequencing. As with the VAB III regime, maintenance chemotherapy with vinblastine, actinomycin D and chlorambucil was employed. Of 55 evaluable patients, 29 (53 per cent) achieved complete remission. Thus it does not appear at the present time that these more complex regimes offer more advantages than the PVB regime developed by Einhorn.

The influence of tumour bulk on PVB response
As with the VB regime, small-volume disease is associated with a higher complete response rate to PVB than bulky disease, particularly in the abdomen (Einhorn and Donohue, 1977). There was a 90 per cent complete remission rate in patients with small-volume lung disease, 88 per cent in minimal

abdominal and pulmonary disease compared with 56 per cent in advanced abdominal disease and 67 per cent in advanced lung disease. The influence of tumour volume on chemotherapy response is discussed further in Chapter 15.

Toxicity of PVB
The major toxicity of the PVB regime is neutropenia. Of the initial series of 47 patients reported by Einhorn, 18 (38 per cent) required hospitalization for presumed sepsis. Of these 47 patients, 7 (15 per cent) had documented septicaemia and 1 patient died. The major myelosuppressive drug in the PVB regime is vinblastine, and randomization in the subsequent prospective study has demonstrated that a lower dose (0.3 mg/kg) gives equally good results as the initial higher dose of drug (0.4 mg/kg). Other side effects of vinblastine include myalgia and constipation. Cis-platinum is a nephrotoxic drug and renal clearance studies are essential before each course of treatment. In most patients impairment of renal function is not a clinical problem if adequate saline hydration is employed with each cis-platinum administration. Bleomycin, as noted below, is associated with skin changes and potentially with pulmonary fibrosis, although in this age group the latter complication is uncommon.

Chemotherapy: conclusions

Remission rates and response rates have improved considerably since the early single-agent studies and the first combination chemotherapy of Li. Although several recent regimes (Kardinal et al., 1976; Klepp et al., 1977) have produced complete remission rates of around 30 per cent, it is only the VB and PVB regimes that have been associated with complete remission rates significantly higher than this. The results reported by Einhorn are particularly encouraging and the complete response rate of 70 per cent is comparable with the results achieved with quadruple chemotherapy in Hodgkin's disease. Patients who remain in complete remission for two years after stopping chemotherapy appear to have a high probability of cure, but the present intensive regimes may be associated with later relapses and careful long-term follow up is essential. It is clear that assessment of many reported studies is complicated by the absence of precise details of site and size of metastases.

The current major problems are the extreme toxicity of present chemotherapeutic regimes and difficulty in controlling bulky disease in the lung and abdomen. The use of other drugs, such as VP16-213, particularly in combination with vinblastine, bleomycin and cis-DDP, seems likely to lead to even higher remission rates and may produce more responses in the more refractory subgroups.

References

Ansfield, F. J., Korbitz, B. C., Davis, H. L. and Ramirez, G. (1969). *Cancer* **24**, 442.
Blum, R. H., Carter, S. K. and Agre, K. (1973). *Cancer* **31**, 903.
Bonadonna, G. (1971). *Acta Chirurgica Belgica* **70**, 393.
Brown, J. H. and Kennedy, B. J. (1965). *New England Journal of Medicine* **272**, 111.
Buckner, C. D., Clift, R. A., Fefer, A., Funk, D. D., Glucksber, H., Newman, P. E., Paulsen, A., Storb, R. and Thomas, E. D. (1974). *Cancer Chemotherapy Reports* **1(58)**, 709.

Carter, S. K. and Wasserman, T. H. (1975). *Cancer* **36**, 729.

Cavalli, F., Sonntag, R. W. and Brunner, K. W. (1977). *Lancet* **ii**, 326.

Cvitkovic, E., Cheng, E., Whitmore, W. F. and Golbey, R. B. (1977). *Proceedings of the American Society of Clinical Oncology* **18**, 324.

Cvitkovic, E., Spaulding, J., Bethune, V., Martin, J. and Whitmore, W. F. (1977). *Cancer* **39**, 1357.

Einhorn, L. H. (1979). *Cancer Treatment Reports* **63**, 1659.

Einhorn, L. H. and Donohue, J. (1977). *Annals of Internal Medicine* **87**, 293.

EORTC (1970). *British Medical Journal* **2**, 643.

Fitzharris, B. M., Kaye, S. B., Saverymuttu, S., Newlands, E. S., Barrett, A., Peckham, M. J. and McElwain, T. J. (1979). *European Journal of Cancer* **16**,1193.

Golbey, R. B., Reynolds, T. F. and Vugrin, D. (1979). *Seminars in Oncology* **6**, 82.

Gottlieb, J. A. and Drewinko, B. (1975). *Cancer Chemotherapy Reports* **59**, 621.

Hayes, D. M., Cvitkovic, E., Golbey, R. B., Scheiner, E., Helson, L. and Krakoff, I. H. (1977). *Cancer* **39**, 1372.

Higby, D. J., Wallace, H. J., Albert, D. J. and Holland, J. F. (1974a). *The Journal of Urology* **112**, 100.

Higby, D. J., Wallace, H. J., Albert, D. J. and Holland, J. F. (1974b). *Cancer* **33**, 1219.

Hoefer-Janker, H., Scheef, W., Günther, W. and Hüls, W. (1975). *Medizinische Welt (Stuttgart)* **26**, 972.

Kardinal, C. G., Jacobs, E. M., Bull, F., Bateman, J. R. and Pajak, T. (1976). *Cancer Treatment Reports* **60**, 953.

Kennedy, B. J. (1970). *Cancer* **26**, 755.

Klepp, O., Klepp, R., Host, H., Asbjornsen, G., Talle, K. and Stenwig, A. E. (1977). *Cancer* **40**, 638.

Li, M. C., Whitmore, W. F., Golbey, R. and Grabstaldt, H. (1960). *Journal of the American Medical Association* **174**, 145.

McElwain, T. J. and Peckham, M. J. (1974). *Proceedings of the Royal Society of Medicine II* **67**, 297.

Mackenzie, A. R. (1966). *Cancer* **19**, 1369.

Monfardini, S., Bajetta, E., Musumeci, R. and Bonadonna, G (1972). *The Journal of Urology* **108**, 293.

Monfardini, S., Fossati, V., Pizzocaro, G. and Bonadonna, G. (1976). *Tumori* **62**, 435.

Newlands, E. S. and Bagshawe, K. D. (1977). *Lancet* **ii**, 87.

O'Bryan, R. M., Luce, J. K., Talley, R. W., Gottlieb, J. A., Baker, L. H. and Bonadonna, G. (1973). *Cancer* **32**, 1.

Peckham, M. J., Hendry, W., McElwain, T. J. and Calman, F. M. B. (1977). In *Adjuvant Therapy of Cancer*, p. 305. Ed. by S. E. Salmon and S. E. Jones. Elsevier/North Holland Biomedical Press, Amsterdam.

Peckham, M. J. and McElwain, T. J. (1975). In *Clinics in Endocrinology and Metabolism*, Vol. 4, No. 3, p. 665. W. B. Saunders, London.

Samuels, M. L. (1971). *The Cancer Bulletin* **25**, 26.

Samuels, M. L., Holoye, P. Y. and Johnson, D. E. (1975). *Cancer* **36**, 318.

Samuels, M. L. and Howe, C. D. (1970). *Cancer* **25**, 1009.

Samuels, M. L., Johnson, D. E. and Holoye, P. Y. (1975). *Cancer Chemotherapy Reports* **1(59)**, 563.

Samuels, M. L., Lanzotti, V. J., Holoye, P. Y., Boyle, L. E., Smith, T. L. and Johnson, D. E. (1976). *Cancer Treatment Reviews* **3**, 185.

Schmoll, H. J., Rhomberg, W. and Diehl, V. (1978). In *Current Chemotherapy. Proceedings of the Tenth International Congress on Chemotherapy*, p. 1089. Ed. by W. Siegenthaler and R. Luthy. American Society for Microbiology, Washington DC.

Schnitker, J., Brock, N., Burkert, H. and Fichtner, E. (1976). *Arzneimittel-Forschung* **26**, 1783.

Smithers, D. W. (1972). *British Journal of Urology* **44**, 217.

Storring, R. A., Jameson, B., McElwain, T. J., Wiltshaw, E. W., Spiers, A. S. D. and Gaya, H. (1977). *Lancet* **ii**, 837.

Tyrrell, C. J. and Peckham, M. J. (1976). *British Journal of Urology* **48**, 363.

Wittes, R. W., Yagoda, A., Silvay, O., Magill, G. B., Whitmore, W., Krakoff, I. H. and Golbey, R. B. (1976). *Cancer* **37**, 637.

15

Non-seminomas: current treatment results and future prospects

M. J. Peckham

Malignant teratomas of the testis constitute a unique group of tumours. Their responsiveness to chemotherapy and their curability were predictable from earlier experience which demonstrated that a small proportion of patients with advanced disease could be cured with low-dose single-agent chemotherapy. Thus, teratomas cannot be regarded as a model system for the common solid malignancies. It is of interest to review the details of patients who achieved cures with single agents such as actinomycin-D. Figure 15.1 shows the chest radiograph and volume growth and regression curves of several large metas-

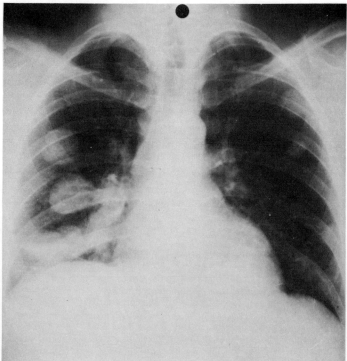

Fig. 15.1 Patient with Stage IV testicular teratoma (MTU) treated in 1967 with actinomy-cin-D. The patient remains alive and disease-free thirteen years later. **(a)** Chest film showing bulky metastases.

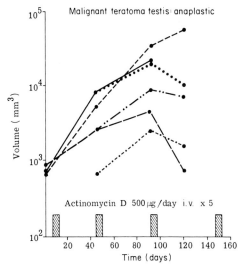

Actinomycin D 500 µg/day i.v. x 5

Fig. 15.1 continued **(b)** Tumour growth curves. Note the slow pattern of response with continual growth of metastases for more than two months after the initiation of chemotherapy.

tases in a patient cured by intermittent low-dose intravenous actinomycin-D. Two aspects are noteworthy. Firstly, the patient would have been substaged by the current classification as IV L_3 which, even with modern combination therapy, constitutes a poor risk group, and secondly, tumour growth continued under therapy with slow regression occurring after two months. In this patient, treated thirteen years ago, one retrocardiac opacity remains on the chest radiograph. It may be speculated that in addition to drug-induced killing of clonogenic cells, differentiation of the proliferating cell pool accounted at least in part for the observed pattern of response and tumour inactivation.

Current chemotherapy results

The best chemotherapy results reported to date have been those obtained using the cis-platinum, bleomycin, vinblastine (PVB) combination (see Chapter 14). Results using this combination, which has been under investigation by

Table 15.1 Results of PVB chemotherapy for malignant teratoma testis (Einhorn, 1979)

	Total pts.	Evaluable	Complete remission	Rendered disease-free with surgery	Relapses in CR group	Continuing CR
Group I (1974–1976)	50	47*	33 (70%)	5 (11%)	8/38 (21%)	30/47 (64%)
Group II (1976–1979)	79	79	53 (67%)	10 (13%)	7/63 (11%)	55/79† (70%)

* Three died soon after referral and have been excluded.
† One patient died from pulmonary embolus.

Einhorn and his colleagues since 1974, have been updated recently (Einhorn, 1979) and are summarized in Table 15.1. In the initial study, for which adequate follow up is available, 64 per cent of patients are surviving disease-free.

Einhorn and his colleagues have tested two dose levels of vinblastine and the value of adding adriamycin to the PVB regime. As shown in Table 15.2, no significant differences were seen between the three arms of the study. Patients all received maintenance vinblastine for two years (0.3 g/kg every four four weeks). Experience with a combination of cyclophosphamide, vinblastine, actinomycin-D, bleomycin, chlorambucil, adriamycin and cis-platinum (VAB IV protocol) has been reported by Golbey *et al.* (1979) and is summarized in Table 15.3. The complete response rate appears inferior to that reported by Einhorn, but the details of substage distribution and the proportion of patients with large-volume metastatic disease were not detailed adequately to allow an assessment of comparability of the two series to be made.

Table 15.2 Results of randomized trial in the chemotherapy of teratoma testis, 1976–1979 (Einhorn, 1979)

Groups	Regime	Vinblastine dose (mg/kg)	Total no. of patients	CR		Remaining in CR	
I	PVB	0.3	27	16	(59%)	17	(63%)
II	PVB	0.4	26	18	(69%)	18	(69%)
III	PVB + adriamycin	—	26	19	(73%)	20	(77%)

Table 15.3 Chemotherapy of testicular teratoma with VAB IV protocol (Golbey *et al.*, 1979)

Total no. of patients	CR with chemotherapy alone		Complete remission with surgery		Continuing complete remission	
55	29	(52.7%)	11	(20%)	33	(60%)

The influence of tumour volume in chemotherapy response

It is clear that the size of tumour metastases exerts an important influence on the probability of control with chemotherapy. Table 15.4 summarizes data on the vinblastine–bleomycin and PVB regimes showing that, whereas the com-

Table 15.4 Influence of tumour volume on chemotherapy response in testicular teratoma

References	Small volume			Large volume		
	Total	CR	Percentage	Total	CR	Percentage
Samuels *et al.* (1976)	26	23	88.5	63	24	38.1
Juttner and McElwain (See Chapter 14)	24	19	79.2	44	8	18.2
Total (VB)	50	42	(84)	107	32	(29.9)
Einhorn and Donahue (1977)	22	20	91	25	15	(60)
Stoter *et al.* (1979)	3	3	100	36	20	(55.6)
Total (PVB)	25	23	92	61	35	(57.4)

plete remission rate with small-volume tumour is high, with bulky disease the proportion of incomplete responses increases.

Results using a five-drug combination consisting of cis-platinum, actinomycin-D, vinblastine, cyclophosphamide and bleomycin (Anderson *et al.*, 1979) also have demonstrated clearly the adverse influence of tumour volume, both in terms of achievement of complete remission and the maintenance of it (Table 15.5).

Table 15.5 Influence of tumour volume on chemotherapy response using a combination of cis-platinum, actinomycin D, vinblastine, cyclophosphamide and bleomycin (Anderson *et al.*, 1979)

	Total no. of patients	CR	Relapses in CR group
'Minimal' tumour	11	9 (82%)	0/9
Remaining patients	14	2 (14%)	2/2

The Royal Marsden Hospital experience
In approaching the problem of devising a comprehensive approach to the management of patients in all stages, we were influenced by several factors, including the effect of tumour volume both on radiation response and chemotherapy response, the desirability of avoiding intensive treatment with any modality wherever possible and the possibility of developing an essentially non-surgical approach using drugs and radiation in selected patients with advanced disease.

Protocols
Between 1976 and early 1978 the protocols summarized in Fig. 15.2 were employed. Following orchidectomy, radiotherapy was the sole treatment for Stages I and IIA, chemotherapy being deferred until relapse occurred (see Chapter 13) and chemotherapy with vinblastine and bleomycin (VB) being initial treatment for Stages IIB, IIC, III and Stage IV patients (see Chapter 14; Peckham *et al.*, 1979).

Table 15.6 summarizes in more detail the striking relationship between tumour volume and drug response using the VB regime. With these data in mind it was postulated that chemotherapy would effectively control presumed subclinical extralymphatic metastases (Stages IIB, IIC, III) or demonstrable small-volume lung metastases (Stage IVL$_1$ L$_2$), whereas it was more likely to fail in bulky lymph node masses, or when there was advanced extralymphatic disease (IV L$_3$, IV H +). Furthermore, the demonstrated influence of tumour volume on radiation response (see Chapter 13) indicated that radiotherapy as prior or sole treatment for Stages IIB, IIC or III would be ineffective, but that cytoreduction by prior drug therapy might enable residual tumour foci to be eliminated by irradiation. The initial approach to, and rationale of management can be summarized as shown in Table 15.7.

In January 1978, cis-platinum was added to the treatment regime and the combination, reported by Einhorn and Donohue (1977), used either alone or in conjunction with radiotherapy and/or surgery as outlined above (Fig. 15.3).

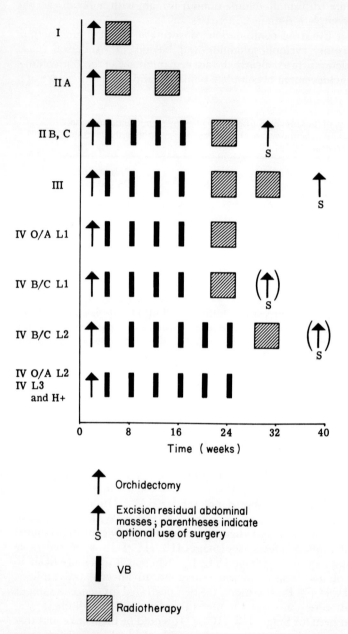

Fig. 15.2 Protocols for management of teratoma testis Stages I–IV (Royal Marsden Hospital, 1976–1978).

Table 15.6 Results of treatment of testicular teratoma with vinblastine-bleomycin according to tumour volume

References	Stage	Complete remission rate	
Samuels *et al.* (1976)	III B_2 (minimal lung)	9/11	(82%)
	III B_3 (advanced lung)	12/21	(57%)
	III B_4 (advanced abdomen)	3/17	(18%)
Royal Marsden Hospital	Abdominal nodes		
series	A	3/3	(100%)
	B	2/6	(33%)
	C	1/18	(6%)
	Lung metastases		
	L_1	9/11	(82%)
	L_2	7/10	(70%)
	L_3	5/20	(25%)

Table 15.7 Non-seminomas—summary of treatment protocols (Royal Marsden Hospital, 1976–1979)

Category	Stages	Treatment
Early stage disease	I, IIA	Lymph-node irradiation Chemotherapy for relapse
Advanced stage Group I	IIB, IIC, III, IVL_1L_2	Chemotherapy to (i) eliminate small extralymphatic metastases; (ii) reduce the volume of lymph-node masses, followed by radiotherapy to eliminate residual tumour in lymph nodes Surgery for residual masses
Advanced stage Group II	IVL_3, H +	Chemotherapy alone

Results of treatment (1976–1979)

The results described below relate to 98 previously untreated patients with non-seminomatous testicular tumours referred to the Royal Marsden between December 1976 and April 1979 (Data analysis, April 1980; Peckham *et al.*,

Table 15.8 Outcome of treatment in 98 patients with previously untreated teratoma testis (Royal Marsden Hospital, 1976–1979)

Stage	Total no. of patients	Relapsed	Disease-free		Alive with disease	Dead of disease	Dead of intercurrent disease or treatment
I	39	8	37	(95%)	—	—	2
IIA	4	1	4	(100%)	—	—	—
IIB–III	17	1	13	(76.5%)	2	1	1
IVO A L_1 L_2	9	—	9	(100%)	—	—	—
IVB C L_1 L_2	10	—	6	(60%)	2	1	1
IVO A L_3	8	—	5	(62.5%)	—	3	—
IVB C L_3	5	—	1	} (9%)	2	2	—
IV H+	6	—			—	6	—
Total	98	10	75	(76.5%)	6	13	4

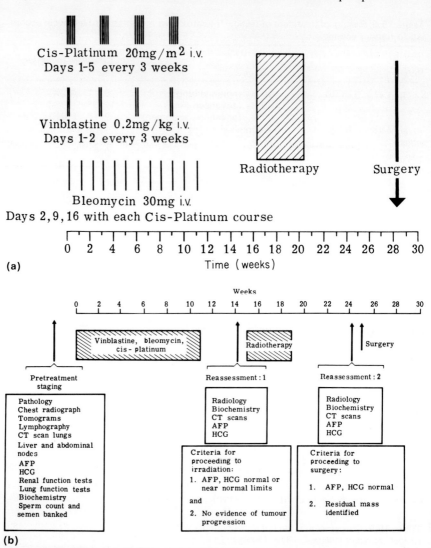

Fig. 15.3 (a) Royal Marsden Hospital protocols for combined management of selected patients with advanced teratoma testis (1979–1980*). **(b)** Protocol for patient assessment during combined therapy of advanced testicular teratoma.
    *Vinblastine replaced by VP16-213 in 1980.

1981). As shown in Table 15.8, 83 per cent of men in this group are alive and 77 per cent are alive without any evidence of disease. The results for men referred with relapse following radiation therapy will be considered separately.

Stage I

As shown in Table 15.8, there were 39 patients with clinical Stage I disease, all of whom received abdominal node irradiation after orchidectomy. Of these, 8 (20.5 per cent) relapsed and received chemotherapy. Six are alive and disease-free, 1 man died of uncontrolled gastrointestinal haemorrhage and a second death occurred in a man of 67 years from a cerebrovascular accident fifteen months after therapy. Thus, 37 patients (95 per cent) are alive and disease-free. As shown in Table 15.9, 74 per cent (29 out of 39) of Stage I patients had an MTI primary tumour. The relapse rates for MTI and MTU were comparable (20.6 per cent and 22.2 per cent respectively). The survival curve for Stage I and IIA patients is shown in Fig. 15.4.

Table 15.9 Early stage malignant teratoma testis receiving orchidectomy, lymph node irradiation and chemotherapy for relapse. Outcome by histology. (Royal Marsden Hospital, 1976–1979)

Stage	Histology	Total no. of patients	Relapses	Currently disease-free		Death from tumour	Death from intercurrent disease
I	MTD	1	—	1		—	—
I	MTI	29	6	28		—	1
I	MTU	9	2	8		—	1
IIA	MTI	2	1	2		—	—
IIA	MTU	2	—	2		—	—
Total		43	9	41	(95.3%)	—	2

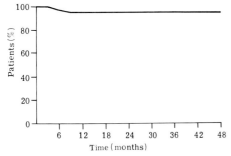

Fig. 15.4 Stage I and IIA non-seminomatous germ-cell tumours of the testis: disease-free survival of 43 patients. (Royal Marsden Hospital, 1976–1979.)

Stage IIA
This is an uncommon stage presentation and during the three-year period under consideration only 4 patients were treated. These had infra- and supra-diaphragmatic irradiation, as described in Chapter 13. As shown in Tables 15.8 and 15.9, all 4 are alive and disease-free. One patient who relapsed has been treated successfully with chemotherapy. Thus, of the Stage I and IIA group, 41 out of 43 (95.3 per cent) men are alive and disease-free.

Stages IIB, IIC and III
As shown in Table 15.8, 13 out of 17 (76.5 per cent) patients in this category remain alive and disease-free, despite initially bulky lymph node disease, hitherto carrying a poor prognosis (see Chapter 13).

Stage IV O A L_1 L_2
Patients in this category had small-volume lung disease associated either with

no evidence of retroperitoneal node involvement or, if present, metastases were <2 cm in diameter. All 9 men in this group are alive and disease-free.

Stage IV B C L, L₂
The association of bulky abdominal disease with small-volume pulmonary disease was encountered in 10 patients, 6 of whom are alive and free from tumour.

Stage IV O A L₃
Eight patients had large multiple lung metastases associated with small-volume abdominal disease or a negative lymphogram and, of these, 5 (62.5 per cent) are disease-free.

Stage IV B C L₃ and Stage IV H+
The association of bulky abdominal lymph node disease and bulky multiple pulmonary metastases was seen in 5 men, and liver involvement in 6. These two categories are associated with a poor prognosis with only 1 out of 11 (9 per cent) patients remaining disease-free.

The latter group of patients, for convenience, has been designated Advanced Stage Group II (ASG II) and Stages IIB, IIC, III and Stage IV O–C L₁ L₂, collectively as Advanced Stage Group I (ASG I). Patients in the ASG I

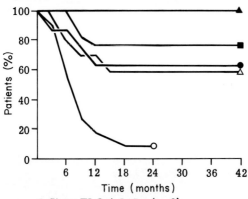

▲ Stage IV O,A,L₁L₂ (n = 9)

■ Stage IIB,IIC,III (n = 17)

● Stage IV O,A,L₃ (n = 8)

△ Stage IV B,C,L₁L₂ (n = 10)

○ Stage IV B,C,L₃ and stage IV H+ (n = 11)

Fig. 15.5 Previously untreated advanced non-seminomatous germ-cell tumours of the testis: disease-free survival by stage. (The Royal Marsden Hospital, 1976–1979.) The following differences are significant:

IV O A L₁L₂ > IV B C L₁L₂ (p < 0.05)
IV O A L₁L₂ > IV B C L₃H+ (p < 0.05)
II, III   > IV B C L₃H+ (p < 0.001)
IV B C L₁L₂ > IV B C L₃H+ (p = 0.05)
IV O A L₃ > IV B C L₃H+ (p = 0.005).

category are eligible for the sequential chemotherapy–radiotherapy–surgery protocol (see above and Chapter 13), whereas patients in the ASG II group are managed with chemotherapy alone.

Within the advanced stage categories the importance of substage based on tumour volume needs to be emphasized. The disease-free survival curves for the subgroups described above are shown in Fig. 15.5 and demonstrate that disease-free rates ranging from 100 per cent to < 10 per cent can be obtained within the Stage IV category. The implications for the comparison of results from different centres are obvious and, unless there is a clear statement of the extent and size of metastatic disease, direct comparisons are impossible to interpret in a meaningful way.

Previously irradiated patients

In addition to the 98 previously untreated patients, 33 men were treated with chemotherapy for disease relapsing after prior irradiation (Table 15.10). Of

Table 15.10 Chemotherapy for patients with testicular non-seminoma relapsing after radiation therapy. Outcome of treatment by stage. (Royal Marsden Hospital, 1976–1979)

Stage*	Total no. of patients	Disease-free		Alive with disease	Death from tumour	Death from intercurrent disease
IIB CIII	9	4	(44%)	2	2	1
IVO A L_1L_2	11	7	(64%)	3	—	1
IV B C L_1L_2	5	2	(40%)	2	1	—
IV O A L_3	5	2	(40%)	1	1	1
IV B C L_3 H+	3	0		—	2	1
Total	33	15	(45.5%)	8 (24.2%)	6 (18.2%)	4 (12.1%)

* Represents stage at time of initiation of chemotherapy.

these, 23 are alive (69.7 per cent) and 15 (45.5 per cent) are disease-free. The relationship between substage and disease-free rate is observed also in this group, with the best results obtained in patients with small-volume lung and abdominal disease (7 out of 11 disease-free). The disease-free survival curve for the whole series of advanced-stage patients and previously irradiated and unirradiated groups are shown in Fig. 15.6. The difference between the two latter groups is not significant. In Fig. 15.7, the influence of prior irradiation is examined in relation to advanced stage grouping. In the ASG I (see above) patients the results obtained in previously unirradiated patients were considerably better than those observed in men relapsing after radiotherapy. The difference did not quite reach significance (p = 0.07). One possible explanation for this difference could relate to the difficulty of delivering adequate chemotherapy following radiotherapy. In practice, this has not been our experience. An alternative explanation is the contribution from radiotherapy following chemotherapy which could be employed only in those patients who had not been exposed previously to abdominal lymph node irradiation. No differences were observed in the ASG II patients in relation to prior treatment status.

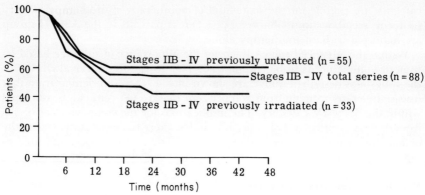

Fig. 15.6 Advanced non-seminomatous germ-cell tumours of the testis: disease-free survival. (Royal Marsden Hospital, 1976–1979).

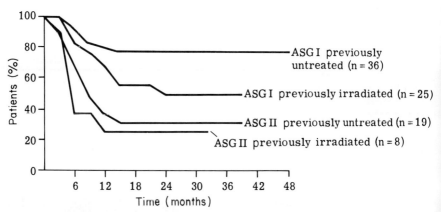

Fig. 15.7 Advanced non-seminomatous germ-cell tumours of the testis: disease-free survival by prior treatment status. (Royal Marsden Hospital, 1976–1979.)

Radiotherapy following chemotherapy

In the ASG I previously untreated patients, 26 men received elective irradiation to sites of initial disease (Table 15.11). Of these, 23 (88.4 per cent) are alive, 21 (80.8 per cent) without evidence of tumour. Patients who are alive have been followed from twelve to forty-five months (median twenty-six months). Of those patients who did not receive irradiation after chemotherapy, either because they were referred after prior radiotherapy or because they were treated with chemotherapy ±surgery only, 19 out of 35 (54.3 per cent) are currently free from evidence of disease.

The tolerance to radiotherapy after chemotherapy has been satisfactory and the two late complications encountered relate to the use in the early phase of the study of high doses of radiation given in an attempt to control residual bulky tumour. One patient is disease-free at forty months, having had surgery for an infarcted segment of bowel at thirty-two months, and a second has

Table 15.11 Radiotherapy to sites of initial disease after intensive chemotherapy for advanced testicular teratoma (Royal Marsden Hospital, 1976–1979)

	Elective radiotherapy after chemotherapy	No radiotherapy after chemotherapy	
		Previously untreated patients	Previously irradiated patients
Total no. of patients	26	10	25
NED	21	6	13
Percentage	80.8	60	52
Total	21/26 (80.8%)	19/35 (54.3%)	

Range 12–45 months (median 32 months).

developed partial cord damage but is stable and disease-free at forty-seven months.

Surgery after chemotherapy ± radiotherapy

As discussed in Chapter 12, retroperitoneal node resection is carried out in selected patients who have evidence of residual masses after chemotherapy and radiotherapy, or who have persistent large-volume abdominal disease after chemotherapy. The value of surgery has not been established clearly. In particular, it is not clear whether the resection of residual viable tumour contributes to patient cure directly, or whether its value is diagnostic, indicating the necessity for further chemotherapy. Present evidence indicates that if surgery is carried out in patients with elevated serum markers, or histological evidence of residual malignancy, there is a high risk of relapse and further chemotherapy is indicated. Furthermore, the significance of apparently completely differentiated structures in the resected specimen does not preclude disease reactivation. Indeed, prompt and rapid tumour growth both locally and in the lungs may occur after the resection of well-differentiated teratoma.

In the present series, a total of 15 patients underwent surgical resection of residual masses in the retroperitoneum (14) or thorax (1). Eleven patients had had prior irradiation and 9 showed no evidence of residual malignancy. Of the 15 men who came to surgery, 12 (80 per cent) are disease-free compared with 16 out of 21 (76.2 per cent) ASG I patients who did not.

More recent data are summarized in Table 15.12. The proportion of patients who had residual malignancy in excised masses is lower in those receiving radiotherapy after chemotherapy than reported experience in patients proceeding directly to surgery after chemotherapy.

Influence of type of chemotherapy on treatment results

The decision to employ a three-drug combination which included cis-platinum, rather than the vinblastine–bleomycin regime, was based on the experience of

Table 15.12 Advanced testicular teratoma: histology of resected tissue after prior chemotherapy ±radiotherapy

Series	Total no. of patients	Fibrosis		Mature teratoma		Carcinoma	
Chemotherapy followed by surgery							
Einhorn (1980)	40	15		12		13	
Garnick *et al.* (1980)	15	2		8		5	
Royal Marsden Hospital	14	2		7		5	
Total	69	19	(27.5%)	27	(39.1%)	23	(33.3%)
Chemotherapy followed by radiotherapy and surgery							
Royal Marsden Hospital	13	9	(69.2%)	2	(15.4%)	2	(15.4%)

Table 15.13 Chemotherapy for advanced teratoma testis (Royal Marsden Hospital, 1976–1979)

Regime	No. of patients		No. of courses	Average
VB	47		1–6	3.6
PVB	16		1–6	3.8
PVB+VB	25	{ PVB	1–6	2.8
		{ VB	1–5	2.3

VB, vinblastine, bleomycin; P, cis-platinum.

Einhorn and his colleagues (Einhorn and Donohue, 1977; Einhorn, 1979) who
reported complete remission rates almost twice those reported for VB by
Samuels *et al.* (1976).

As shown in Table 15.13, some patients in the present series received VB,
some PVB and others in the intermediary period both VB and PVB. The total
number of courses varied, since initially only two courses of VB were given
and subsequently a minimum, whenever possible, of four. Table 15.14 shows
the outcome of treatment by stage group and chemotherapy. For each of these
subgroups, no difference in disease-free survival rate is seen between patients
treated with VB only and those having in addition cis-platinum throughout or

Table 15.14 Outcome of treatment for advanced teratoma testis by type of chemotherapy
(Royal Marsden Hospital, 1976–1979)

Stage	Chemotherapy	Total no. of patients	No. disease-free	Percentage
II III IV B C L_1 L_2	VB	20	13	65
	PVB±VB	20	12	60
IV O A L$_1$ L$_2$	VB	13	11	84.6
	PVB±VB	8	5	62.5
IV L_3 H+	VB	14	5	35.7
	PVB±VB	13	3	23.1

during part of their chemotherapy. Although it is not possible to draw any firm conclusion from this non-randomized comparison, it highlights the difficulty of interpreting and comparing data from different centres without detailed knowledge of stage distribution.

The influence of histology

As shown in Table 15.15, the disease-free survival rates for MTI (40 per cent) are lower than those achieved for MTU (66.7 per cent) in the advanced-stage patients. Figure 15.8 shows the survival curves for previously untreated patients according to histology. The MTU patients fared significantly better than those with an MTI primary tumour $(p < 0.05)$.

Figure 15.9 shows disease survival by advanced-stage group and histology. In ASG I there was a marked and significant advantage for the MTU patients,

Table 15.15 Results of treatment of advanced teratoma testis: influence of histology (Royal Marsden Hospital, 1976–1979)

Stage	Histology			
	MTI	MTU	MTT	YS
ASG I	10/22*	28/35	3/4	—
ASG II	2/8	6/16	0/2	0/1
Overall	12/30 (40%)	34/51 (66.7%)	3/6 (50%)	0/1

MTI, malignant teratoma intermediate; MTU, malignant teratoma undifferentiated; MTT, malignant teratoma trophoblastic; YS, yolk-sac carcinoma; ASG, advanced stage group (see text).
* Number of disease-free/total patients.

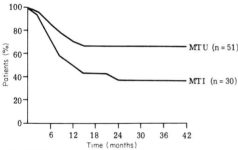

Fig. 15.8 Advanced non-seminomatous germ-cell tumours of the testis: disease-free survival by histology. (Royal Marsden Hospital, 1976–1979.)

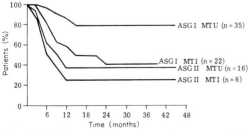

Fig. 15.9 Advanced non-seminomatous germ-cell tumours of the testis: disease-free survival by stage and histology. (Royal Marsden Hospital, 1976–1979.)

compared with the MTI group. In the ASG II patients no significant difference was observed. Although significant differences between MTU and MTI have emerged for disease-free survival, this is not yet reflected in a difference in overall survival, since the patient with MTI disease has a more protracted course, living longer with evidence of uncontrolled malignancy.

Tumour markers and outcome of treatment in advanced disease
Serum AFP and HCG levels are of prognostic significance in early-stage disease, provided that the rate of fall following orchidectomy is monitored closely (see Chapter 13). The prognostic significance of marker elevation in advanced disease remains unclear, since both the proportion of patients with

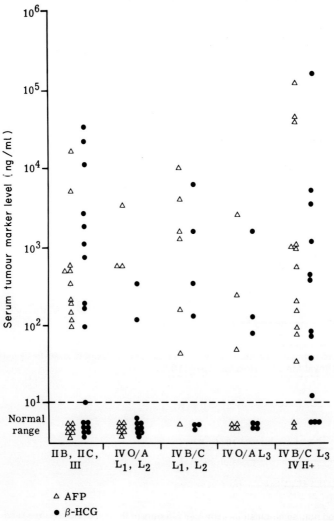

△ AFP
● β-HCG

Fig. 15.10 Serum tumour marker levels by clinical stage in advanced teratoma testis.

Table 15.16 Serum-marker status in advanced teratoma testis in relation to bulk of disease (Royal Marsden Hospital, 1976–1979)

	Both normal		Both elevated		AFP elevated only		HCG elevated only	
IV O A L_1 L_2	11	(55%)*	0		4	(20%)	5	(25%)
II III IV B C L_1 L_2	9	(22%)	17	(41%)	10	(24%)	5	(12%)
IV O A L_3	3	(23%)	4	(31%)	3	(23%)	3	(23%)
IV B C L_3 H+	2	(14%)	10	(72%)	2	(14%)	0	

* Percentage of total patients in each stage grouping.

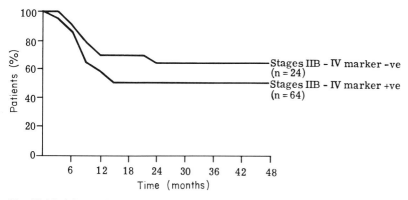

Fig. 15.11 Advanced non-seminomatous germ-cell tumours of the testis: disease-free survival by serum-marker status. (Royal Marsden Hospital, 1976–1979.)

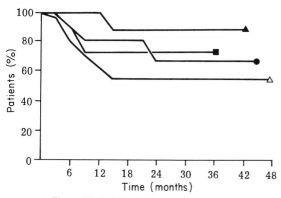

▲ Stage IV O,A,$L_1 L_2$ marker +ve (n = 9)

■ Stage IIB,IIC,III,IV B,C,$L_1 L_2$,IV O,A,L_3 marker −ve (n = 11)

● Stage IV O,A,$L_1 L_2$ marker −ve (n = 11)

△ Stage IIB,IIC,III,IVB,C,$L_1 L_2$IV O,A,L_3 marker + (n = 43)

Fig. 15.12 Advanced non-seminomatous germ-cell tumours of the testis: disease-free survival by stage grouping and serum-marker status. (Royal Marsden Hospital, 1976–1979.)

elevated marker levels and absolute marker levels are related to bulk of metastatic tumour, which is itself an extremely important determinant of prognosis (Fig. 15.10). Serum-marker status and substage category are summarized in Table 15.16. Whereas both AFP and HCG are normal in 55 per cent of Stage IV patients with minimal disease, only 14 per cent of bulky Stage IV

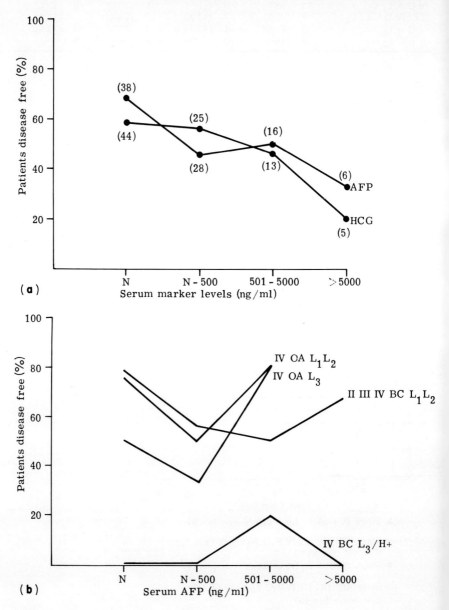

Fig. 15.13 Advanced teratoma testis. Disease-free survival rate by serum-marker levels (Royal Marsden Hospital, 1976–1979). **(a)** All stages; **(b)** by substage for alphafetoprotein.

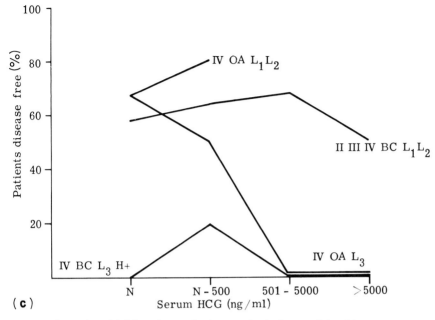

Fig. 15.13 continued **(c)** by substage for human chorionic gonadotrophin.

patients have normal marker levels. Overall, as shown in Fig. 15.11, there is a slightly better disease-free survival rate for marker-negative patients than marker-positive patients, although the difference is not significant. Indeed, if serum-marker status is examined in relation to tumour burden (Fig. 15.12), the marker-positive patients with minimal disease fared better than those with negative markers. If disease-free survival rate is examined in relation to the absolute level of serum marker, then a negative correlation is observed with a progressive fall in disease-free survial with increasing serum titre (Fig. 15.13a). However, this is expected, since the high titre group have the bulkiest disease. If marker levels are examined within substage categories, little evidence of a correlation between disease-free survival and titre is observed (Fig. 15.13b and c). This suggests that the sensitivity to therapy of AFP-producing cells, HCG-

Table 15.17 Advanced teratoma testis: initial marker status and marker pattern on relapse (Royal Marsden Hospital, 1976–1979)

					Outcome of treatment				
						Relapse			
Marker status at time of chemotherapy						Marker +		Marker −	
AFP		HCG							
+	−	+	−		NED	AFP	HCG	AFP	HCG
—	36	—	—		27	2	—	7	—
39	—	—	—		20	11	—	8	—
—	—	—	44		26	—	1	—	17
—	—	37	—		23	—	8	—	6

producing cells and cells unassociated with marker production is not markedly different and that marker levels *per se* are not prognostically significant.

Serum AFP and HCG status prior to treatment and at relapse

In Table 15.17, serum-marker status on relapse is examined in relation to initial pretreatment marker status in patients with advanced disease. Of 36 patients who were initially AFP negative, 2 of 9 relapses were associated with raised AFP levels. Only 1 of 18 initially HCG-negative patients who relapsed had elevated serum HCG levels. Conversely, of 19 relapses in patients with initially elevated AFP levels, 8 had normal AFP values. Of 14 relapses in HCG-positive patients, 6 were associated with normal HCG levels in the serum. These observations indicate that, while a raised marker level is of practical value in monitoring patients, regrowth of tumour may occur in the absence of a reappearance of either AFP or HCG in the serum. Conversely, it is essential to monitor serum-marker levels in patients who were initially marker negative, since subsequent appearance of AFP or HCG may occur.

Toxicity of treatment of advanced disease

As shown in Table 15.18, there were 5 deaths in the advanced stage series of 88 patients. One was postoperative and the other 4 related to chemotherapy.

Table 15.18 Advanced teratoma testis: deaths from treatment or intercurrent disease (Royal Marsden Hospital, 1976–1979)

Stage	Chemotherapy (no. of courses) VB	PVB	Time following start of chemotherapy to death (months)	Cause of death
Unirradiated				
II	1	3	8	Postoperative
IV A L$_3$	1	—	1	Chemotherapy
Previously irradiated				
IV O L$_1$	2	—	2	Chemotherapy
IV O L$_3$	2	4	5	Chemotherapy
IV H+	—	1	1	Chemotherapy

Total deaths from chemotherapy	4/88 (4.5%)
Total deaths from previously untreated group	1/55 (1.8%)
Total deaths from previously irradiated group	3/33 (9.1%)

The overall drug-related mortality was 4.5 per cent and was higher in the previously irradiated patients—3 out of 33 (9 per cent)—than in previously untreated patients—1 out of 55 (1.8 per cent). Of the 3 deaths in patients referred with disease relapsing after irradiation, 2 occurred in men who had had supra- and infradiaphragmatic irradiation.

The implications of treatment for fertility

Whereas it is established that a proportion of men who receive irradiation alone preserve fertility and father normal children, the outlook for men who receive chemotherapy is less clear. Initially, it was assumed that intensive chemotherapy of the VB or PVB type would inevitably produce sterility.

However, we have a small number of young men who have re-established active spermatogenesis and fathered children. On the assumption, however, that many will be sterilized, and if an initial sperm count is satisfactory, it is our policy to offer the possibility of semen banking.

Conclusions from the Royal Marsden experience

In clinical Stage I testicular non-seminoma, cure rates approaching 100 per cent are achievable by a non-invasive policy of retroperitoneal lymph node irradiation followed by chemotherapy for relapse. The hazard of chemotherapy is reduced considerably if doses of more than 40 Gray in four weeks are avoided and supradiaphragmatic irradiation not employed. Furthermore, if relapse occurs after a short interval following irradiation, the substitution of vinblastine by VP16-213 is probably as efficacious and considerably less toxic. Advances in staging methodology and our understanding of tumour markers mean that a group of patients with a high risk and a group with a low risk of occult metastases can be identified. In the former group, chemotherapy is the treatment of choice and, in the latter, a watch policy starting after orchidectomy should provide valuable data on prognostic factors and a firm basis for future management. If the retroperitoneum is the initial site of disease in those who relapse, this will provide a rationale for radiotherapy or surgery. So far as radical node dissection is concerned, the results are remarkably comparable to those achieved by radiotherapy and it is possible that this major procedure could in due course be abandoned in favour of a non-invasive management policy, as employed in our practice.

Adjuvant chemotherapy, or chemotherapy deferred until documented relapse, is equally effective in surgically managed patients. Thus, Williams et al. (1980) have reported on 57 pathological Stage I patients, 4 of whom relapsed and received PVB and all of whom are alive and disease-free. All 7 pathological Stage II patients receiving two cycles of PVB after surgery are disease-free. Of 24 Stage II patients treated with surgery alone, 7 relapsed, 6 of whom are disease-free, the remaining 1 dying of unrelated causes.

The use of two cycles as an adjuvant in Stage II disease is of interest since such an approach may be of value in the management of clinical Stage IIA disease followed by radiotherapy limited to identifiable abnormal retroperitoneal nodes. Certainly in the latter group, avoidance of supradiaphragmatic irradiation is important.

If the experience from Indiana, employing surgery and deferred chemotherapy, is compared to our experience and if pathological Stage I and II disease is equated with clinical Stage I, IIA and IIB, the results are remarkably similar. Thus 80 out of 81 (98.8 per cent) are disease-free in the former group, compared with 44 out of 46 (95.7 per cent) in the latter series. The former series were managed by radical node dissection and deferred chemotherapy and the Marsden patients by radiotherapy and deferred chemotherapy (I, IIA) or chemotherapy followed by radiotherapy (IIB).

So far as advanced disease is concerned, the improvement in prognosis is gratifying and striking. The role of radiotherapy after chemotherapy has been little explored. Sonntag et al. (1979) have reported the preliminary results of a study in which, following induction with vinblastine, bleomycin, adriamycin and cis-platinum, complete remission patients either received irradiation to initial sites of disease or maintenance chemotherapy with CCNU, methotrexate and vinblastine for two years. No unexpected toxicity was encountered in the radiotherapy arm. Six patients received whole lung irradiation after bleomycin and this was apparently well tolerated. At the time of reporting, 5 out of 20 patients in the chemotherapy arm had relapsed, compared with 2 out of 15 in the irradiated group. Although our experience does not conclusively demonstrate that elective irradiation following chemotherapy is of value, the improved survival of patients receiving radiotherapy and the low percentage of positive histology in resected masses are suggestive. A policy of sequential chemotherapy–radiotherapy is a practicable approach which needs testing in a prospective clinical trial. A reduction in the proportion of patients who have residual malignancy after chemotherapy is of obvious importance and, once the patient has been explored, our experience has been that radiotherapy is inadvisable since there may be considerable morbidity.

The significance of tumour volume needs to be stressed, particularly when comparing experience gained at different centres. Even with the advances in treatment, the results in patients with bulky abdominal and lung disease remain poor and require alternative chemotherapeutic approaches.

Final observations

The stage distribution of non-seminomatous germ-cell tumours indicates that between 50 and 60 per cent have clinical Stage I disease at presentation, and hence the management of the early-stage patient is of considerable importance. Advanced presentations may occur in patients with a short history, but are associated frequently with a delay in diagnosis, delay in referral or initially inappropriate therapy. It is essential that these young men with potentially curable tumours are referred to specialist centres. Current chemotherapy, although effective, remains toxic and associated with considerable morbidity. With the increasing precision of non-invasive staging procedures it should be possible to tailor therapy to individual needs, and the avoidance of therapy, be it surgery, radiation or chemotherapy, is an important consideration. It seems appropriate to move away from surgery and radiation as initial forms of treatment and the continuation of radical node dissection as a staging procedure is difficult to justify. The selective use of radiation as an adjunct to chemotherapy is worthy of exploration, but its role requires evaluation in a randomized clinical trial. The success of currently employed chemotherapeutic regimes should not (bearing in mind their toxicity) prevent the active exploration of newer approaches to therapy. These unusual tumours are sensitive to a wide spectrum of cytotoxic drugs and, in addition, show striking evidence of differentiation occurring spontaneously and possibly in relation to treatment. The possible manipulation and promotion of this feature of teratoma biology perhaps offers a longer-term therapeutic prospect.

References

Anderson, T., Javadpour, N., Schilsky, R., Barlock, A. and Young, R. C. (1979). *Cancer Treatment Reports* **63**, 1687.

Einhorn, L. H. (1979). *Cancer Treatment Reports* **63**, 1659.

Einhorn, L. H. (1980). *Proceedings of the American Association for Cancer Research (AACR) and American Society of Clinical Oncology (ASCO)* **21**, 159.

Einhorn, L. H. and Donohue, J. P. (1977). *Annals of Internal Medicine* **87**, 293.

Garnick, M. B., Canellos, G. P. and Richie, J. P. (1980). *Proceedings of the American Association for Cancer Research (AACR) and American Society of Clinical Oncology (ASCO)* **21**, 422.

Golbey, R. B., Reynolds, T. F. and Vugrin, D. (1979). *Seminars in Oncology* **VI**, 82.

Peckham, M. J., Barrett, A., McElwain, T. J. and Hendry, W. F. (1979). *Lancet* **ii**, 267.

Peckham, M. J., Barrett, A., McElwain, T. J., Hendry, W. F. and Raghavan, D. (1981). *British Journal of Urology* **53**, 162.

Samuels, M. L., Lanzotti, V. J., Holoye, P. Y., Boyle, L. E., Smith, T. L. and Johnson, D. E. (1976). *Cancer Treatment Reviews* **3**, 185.

Sonntag, R. W., Senn, H. J. and Cavalli, F. (1979). *Cancer Treatment Reports* **63**, 1669.

Stoter, G., Vendrik, C. P. J., Struyvenberg, A., Brouwers, Th. M., Sleijfer, D. Th., Schraffordt Koops, H., Van Oosterom, A. T. and Pinedo, H. M. (1979). *Lancet* **i**, 941.

Williams, S. D., Einhorn, L. H. and Donohue, J. P. (1980). *Proceedings of the American Association for Cancer Research (AACR) and American Society of Clinical Oncology (ASCO)* **21**, 421.

16

Testicular tumours of childhood
A. Barrett and M. J. Peckham

Introduction
Primary testicular tumours are rare in infancy and childhood, accounting for
only 0.5 per cent to 1 per cent of all solid tumours. They represent 2 per cent
to 5 per cent of all testicular tumours and are the seventh most common
malignant neoplasm of childhood. The majority are diagnosed before the age
of 2. Approximately 25 per cent may be present at birth. There is no increased
tendency for tumours to develop in the undescended testis in infants and
children as there is in adults (except in seminomas), in spite of the fact that up
to 14 per cent of male children under the age of 1 have unilateral or bilateral
cryptorchidism. Several individual cases, however, have been reported. For
most of the childhood testicular tumours, age at presentation and duration of
symptoms before diagnosis are the most important prognostic factors. Survival
is best in children under the age of 5 and poorest in the group with onset of
disease at puberty. The longer the primary lesion remains untreated, the more
likely are metastases to occur. Histological features of malignancy, such as
frequent mitoses and blood vessel invasion, seem to be of less prognostic
significance.

Presentation
The signs and symptoms of testicular tumours in children are similar to those
found in the adult. The most common finding is a painless scrotal swelling
discovered by the child's mother. Sometimes a history of trauma is elicited but
probably only draws attention to a pre-existing mass. Usually pain is associated
only with metastatic disease and is a poor prognostic sign. The skin over the
scrotum is involved very rarely and usually oedema or inflammation are seen
only secondary to trauma or infection. Early diagnosis depends on maintaining
a high degree of suspicion when presented with a scrotal swelling in a child.
Differential diagnoses to be considered include torsion of the testis, orchitis or
epididymitis.

  The incidence of a co-existing hydrocele varies in reported series from 10
per cent to 46 per cent.

Diagnosis
The diagnosis should be confirmed by exploration through an inguinal excision, with clamping of the cord before manipulation of the tumour as for any
240

adult testicular lesion. Needle biopsy should be avoided. Further investigation should include lymphangiography and intravenous pyelography, chest x-ray, and whole lung tomography if indicated, and estimation of the blood for alphafetoprotein and human chorionic gonadotrophin.

Because of the rarity of these tumours, only individual case reports or small series of patients are available for study and sometimes differences in histological classification have made comparisons difficult and uniform treatment policy impossible. In the British Testicular Tumour Panel (BTTP) series of 1859 tumours, there have been 51 cases of testicular and paratesticular tumours in children under the age of 15. The distribution of these is shown in Fig. 16.1.

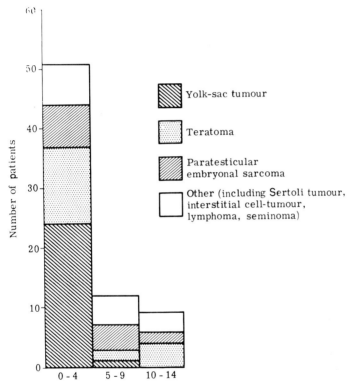

Fig. 16.1 Testicular tumours of children. Distribution by histological subtype. (Data from Pugh, 1976.)

Intrascrotal tumours can be divided conveniently into those arising from the testis itself and those having their origin in paratesticular tissues. They may also be designated histogenetically as of germ-cell or non-germ-cell origin, the former being more common (Table 16.1). The frequency of individual subtypes from a recent review by Brosman (1979) is shown in Table 16.2.

Table 16.1 Classification of childhood testicular tumours

Testicular
(i) Primary
    Germ cell   Teratoma
                             Yolk-sac tumour
                             Seminoma
    Non-germ-cell   Sertoli (androblastoma)
                             Interstitial cell
(ii) Secondary
    Leukaemia
    Lymphoma
    Solid tumour metastases (especially neuroblastoma)

Paratesticular
    Rhabdomyosarcoma
    Other soft tissue sarcomas

Table 16.2 Testicular tumours in prepubertal children. (From literature review by Brosman, 1979)

General category	Type	Total no. of patients
Germ-cell tumours		424
	Yolk-sac carcinoma	366
	Teratoma	58
Non-germ-cell tumours		132
	Sertoli cell tumour	22
	Leydig cell tumour	52
	Connective tissue tumour	58

Teratoma

Teratomas and yolk-sac tumours are the two most common testicular tumours in childhood. Unlike their adult counterparts, teratomas are most frequently benign. As well as arising in the scrotum, they may occur also in any site through which there has been germ cell migration, such as the pineal body, mediastinum, retroperitoneum or the sacrum.

Because the majority of teratomas in the paediatric age group are differentiated, the prognosis is better than in adults and orchidectomy alone is usually curative. They may be mistaken clinically for a hydrocele. They are almost always unilateral, although a bilateral case has been reported. They are usually well circumscribed, partly solid, partly cystic tumours confined to the body of the testis and containing a wide range of mature tissues—some, like cartilage, easily recognizable macroscopically. Histologically they are composed of miscellaneous types of epithelium mixed with mesodermal tissues, all fully differentiated and mature. They occur almost exclusively in children.

Of 28 testicular teratomas in boys under the age of 15 years seen by the British Testicular Tumour Panel, 21 were of the fully differentiated type (TD) and behaved as completely benign tumours.

Malignant teratoma intermediate (MTI) does occur rarely in childhood. Six cases were seen by the British Testicular Tumour Panel and were classified as such because of areas of poor differentiation. However, lack of differentiation may reflect immaturity of the tissues rather than malignancy and may make histological interpretation and classification difficult at times. Of these 6 cases, 2 who received postoperative radiotherapy died within one year; the rest are alive without recurrence. Malignant teratoma undifferentiated (MTU) and malignant teratoma trophoblastic (MTT) are extremely rare in childhood. Mixed tumours containing yolk-sac elements do occur, but mixed seminomas and teratomas are not seen in this age group. Because of their rarity, the treatment and prognosis of malignant teratoma in children have not been defined clearly in any of the published series. Abell and Holtz (1963) recorded 10 cases treated by orchidectomy alone. Seven died within one year of diagnosis; 2 additional patients had lymph node dissections and were long-term survivors. Johnson *et al.* (1970) reported 5 cases: 2 treated by orchidectomy alone developed metastases within sixteen months, 2 had bilateral lymphadenectomy and 1 had unilateral node dissection with chemotherapy, and are all surviving up to six years later.

Staubitz *et al.* (1965) treated 4 cases with node dissection and reported a three to five year survival in all.

Radiotherapy has been used infrequently and should be avoided if possible because of the problem of interference with epiphyseal growth, which will occur with doses above 2300 rad. Damage to the kidneys can be avoided usually by careful treatment planning. In these rare tumours, if metastases are present, the treatment approach advocated for adult teratoma employing a similar chemotherapeutic approach is indicated.

Seminoma

This is an extremely rare tumour in childhood and its existence as a true entity is even doubted by some authorities. Four cases are found in the British Testicular Tumour Panel series and approximately 25 cases under the age of 15 years have been reported up to May 1977 (Viprakasit *et al.*, 1977). The age range was $2\frac{1}{2}$ to 15 years, with an average of 9.7. Seminoma in children may be associated with maldescent of the testes, like their adult counterparts. There is little evidence to suggest that these tumours behave differently from those seen in adults, and the majority were cured by orchidectomy alone or with the addition of low-dose abdominal irradiation.

Yolk-sac carcinoma

The majority of children with this tumour present before the age of 2 years. Yolk-sac tumours have been described over the years by many different names, including orchioblastoma, juvenile embryonal carcinoma, adenocarcinoma of the infant testis and endodermal sinus tumour. In the last decade it has become clear that this tumour is identical histologically with the ovarian tumour considered by Teilum (1971) to arise from the yolk sac. This is a distinctive type of adenocarcinoma arising in the testis of infants or very young children, which may be regarded as originating in germ cells with differentiation towards extra-embryonic (yolk-sac) structures. Increasing familiarity with the tumour as a distinct entity has led to more frequent diagnosis. Woodtli and Hedinger

(1974) collected 92 cases and 53 cases were notified to the British Testicular Tumour Panel between 1958 and 1973.

Yolk-sac tumours present as rapidly growing, painless testicular swellings and macroscopically as unencapsulated masses, usually replacing the testis, yellow or white in colour, sometimes with cystic areas or areas of haemorrhage. Histologically the appearances are of an adenocarcinoma with papillary or tubular structures and solid and cystic areas. They are usually mucus secreting. The cells have clear cytoplasm and characteristic perivascular collections of cells of epithelial type may be seen. There are prominent 'mantles' of cells around blood vessels, but they may be difficult to find. These tumours are usually unassociated with seminoma or teratoma, but, like teratomas, they may arise in the ovary, sacrococcygeal region, mediastinum or pineal region. They tend to grow rapidly and metastasize to lymph nodes and distant sites.

In more than 50 per cent of children the history is less than three months in duration. The child presents with a firm non-tender testicular mass which may be large, exceeding 10 cm in diameter.

Staging

Yolk-sac tumours may be confined to the testis, as shown by the fact that a proportion of children are cured by orchidectomy alone. Thus, as shown in Table 16.3, in a recent survey of the literature Brosman (1979) has reported that 60 per cent of 194 children were cured by orchidectomy alone. In an earlier review by Sabio *et al.* (1974), 25 out of 52 (48 per cent) children were reported cured by orchidectomy. Findings at retroperitoneal node dissection

Table 16.3 Yolk-sac carcinoma: outcome of therapy. (From literature review by Brosman, 1979)

Treatment	Total no. of patients	Disease-free at two years	Percentage
Orchidectomy	194	117	60
Orchidectomy/chemotherapy	10	10	100
Orchidectomy/radiotherapy	64	55	86
Orchidectomy/node dissection			
negative nodes	94	78	83
positive nodes	4	3	(75)
Total	366	263	72

Table 16.4 Results of radical retroperitoneal node dissection in yolk-sac carcinoma of the testis in childhood

References	Total no. of patients undergoing surgery	No. with positive nodes
Young *et al.* (1970)	8	0
Gangai (1968)*	10	0
Drago *et al.* (1978)*	39	6
Hopkins *et al.* (1978)	11	0
Bracken *et al.* (1978)	12	0
Total	80	6 (7.5%)

* Literature review.

Table 16.5 Early-stage presentation of yolk-sac carcinoma of the testis in childhood

References	Total no. of patients	No. with tumour clinically localized to testis
Hopkins et al. (1978)	14	11
Sabio et al. (1974)	8	8
Johnson et al. (1970)	5	3
Young et al. (1970)	13	11
Total	40	33 (82.5%)

are consistent with this observation since, as shown in Table 16.4, only 7.5 per cent of children have had histologically positive nodes. As shown in Table 16.5, probably at least 80 per cent of children have no evidence of disease outside the testis at the time of orchidectomy. The usual clinical staging approach outlined in Chapter 7 is advocated. Serum alphafetoprotein levels are of great value in the management of yolk-sac tumours of childhood and, because of the lack of associated non-yolk-sac elements, marker levels provide an accurate method of monitoring therapeutic progress.

Treatment and prognosis

The predominance of early-stage presentations is reflected in a reasonably good overall prognosis for children with yolk-sac tumours.

Bearing in mind the appreciable cure rate with orchidectomy alone, the precision of modern clinical staging procedures and the use of alphafetoprotein as a tumour marker, children with Stage I disease should be monitored carefully without elective postorchidectomy treatment. On the other hand, Hopkins et al. (1978) concluded that, since 5 out of 9 patients managed by orchidectomy alone had died, all patients should receive further treatment. It should be noted, however, that their review included children seen as far back as 1930 and staging in many would have been inadequate by current standards. These authors argue that node dissection should be performed routinely, but it seems difficult to sustain this contention in view of the low yield of positive results. In the series reported by Hopkins et al., all patients since 1958 had received actinomycin-D and no child (of a total of 11) has died. There is no doubt that yolk-sac tumours are chemosensitive and a combination of vincristine, actinomycin-D and cyclophosphamide is advocated in State II, III and IV patients.

The role of radiotherapy is difficult to evaluate but, because of the desirability of avoiding irradiation in this age group, the combination of orchidectomy and chemotherapy would seem advantageous. Karamehmedovic et al. (1975) report 4 survivors treated this way and in reviewing the literature note 10 out of 10 survivors.

There are 3 reported cases of apparent cure of metastatic disease, all with solitary lung metastases, 1 with radiotherapy alone and the others with combination treatment.

Limited clinical experience indicates that alphafetoprotein, which is produced from the granules and PAS-positive globules in the lining cells of the endodermal sinuses, is an extremely useful marker in childhood yolk-sac tumours. Smith et al. (1977) report a case where rise in AFP preceded clinical evidence of metastases and enabled early initiation of chemotherapy and monitoring of response.

Reported responses to chemotherapy have been unpredictable and a variety of agents has been tried, including methotrexate, vincristine, cyclophosphamide, adriamycin and actinomycin-D. Use of high-dose, intermittent, combination chemotherapy seems to be more useful than single-agent therapy and good responses have been seen in two of our patients treated with combinations of vincristine, cyclophosphamide and adriamycin or actinomycin-D.

Paratesticular rhabdomyosarcoma

These are unusual testicular tumours occurring relatively more frequently in children than in adults and comprising less than 2 per cent of all intrascrotal tumours. In a report from the Intergroup Rhabdomyosarcoma Study Committee (Raney et al., 1978) of 289 children with rhabdomyosarcomas, in 20 (7 per cent) the paratesticular region was the primary site. The tumour usually presents as a painless, unilateral, intrascrotal mass, which may transilluminate if there is an associated hydrocele. The history is generally short and the growth rate of the tumour rapid. The tumours usually arise adjacent to, or slightly superior to, the testis from the intrascrotal portion of the cord or, less commonly, from the inguinal canal.

Paratesticular rhabdomyosarcomas may reach a large size. In the series quoted above, the size ranged from 3 to 15 cm diameter, with a mean of 7 cm.

The age at presentation varies widely from a few months to the late teens. In the Intergroup series the age range was 1.7 to 19 years, with an average of 9 years. The age distribution indicates a peak in early childhood under the age of 5, with a second peak in the 16 to 20 year age group.

The lymphatic drainage of the cord is the same as that of the testis and lymphatic spread is important, the abdominal nodes usually being the first site of metastases. All patients with tumours infiltrating the cord will eventually develop node metastases.

Lymphangiography, is, therefore, an important part of initial investigation and staging of the tumour.

Pathology

Macroscopically the tumour tissue may appear white or creamy with areas of haemorrhage and necrosis. There is a great variation of microscopical structure, even within a single tumour, and any of the following patterns may be seen.

1. A predominantly myxomatous tissue composed of irregular stellate and fusiform cells separated by abundant connective tissue mucin.
2. Undifferentiated spheroidal and angulated cells which may be closely packed together.
3. Small, round or ovoid cells with eosinophilic cytoplasm.
4. Undifferentiated spindle cells.
5. Long spindle-shaped cells with eosinophilic cytoplasm and longitudinal myofibrils with cross striations.

6. Large, ovoid, rounded and strap-like cells with abundant eosinophilic cytoplasm and cross striations.

Staging

The approach to clinical staging is generally similar to that described for tumours of the testis in Chapter 7. Paratesticular rhabdomyosarcomas tend to spread initially via the lymphatic system and clinically evident haematogenous spread at time of diagnosis is unusual.

The staging system generally employed is as follows.

Stage I. Primary tumour completely resected. No regional node involvement.

Stage II. Histologically demonstrable local microscopic residual tumour and/or regional node involvement.

Stage III. Gross residual tumour.

Stage IV. Distant metastases.

The stage distribution in the series reported by Raney *et al.* (1978) was Stage I 13 patients, Stage II 6, Stage III 0, and Stage IV 1 patient.

There is a high incidence of positive retroperitoneal nodes at presentation. Data from the literature are summarized in Table 16.6, showing that 43 per

Table 16.6 Paratesticular rhabdomyosarcoma in childhood: incidence of positive nodes at radical node dissection (RND)

Total no. of patients undergoing RND	Histologically positive	Percentage
54	23	42.8

Data from

Arlen *et al.* (1969)	Jaffe *et al.* (1973)
Brosman *et al.* (1974)	Johnson *et al.* (1970)
Burrington (1969)	Jungling and Culp (1975)
Cromie *et al.* (1979)	Littman *et al.* (1972)
Ghavimi *et al.* (1973)	Raney *et al.* (1978)
Gray and Biorn (1960)	Rosas-Uribe *et al.* (1970)
Hays *et al.* (1969)	Skeel *et al.* (1975)
Hoffman and Baird (1960)	Tank *et al.* (1972)
Hopkins *et al.* (1978)	Tefft *et al.* (1967)

cent of patients undergoing radical node dissection have positive nodes. There are scant data on the accuracy of lymphography but, of 6 patients with negative lymphograms coming to surgery in the Intergroup series, 1 had positive nodes. Inguinal nodes are less common and of 13 patients only 2 (15 per cent) had positive histology. In keeping with the lower frequency of clinically detectable metastases outside the lymphatic system, the incidence of vascular invasion within the primary tumour is low—3 out of 20 (15 per cent)—in the Intergroup series.

Treatment and prognosis

Survival data from historical series treated by orchidectomy alone suggest a survival rate of 19 to 50 per cent for all stages considered together, with survival being poorest in the group with onset at puberty (Littman *et al.*, 1972). The British Testicular Tumour Panel series shows a survival rate of 45 per cent at three years (Gowing, 1976). The prognosis for rhabdomyosarcomas in general has improved with the development of a multidisciplinary approach to treatment. It has been established for rhabdomyosarcomas in general that adjuvant chemotherapy improves the results of treatment. Table 16.7 summarizes the

Table 16.7 Randomized study of adjuvant chemotherapy in rhabdomyosarcoma: children's study group A (Heyn *et al.*, 1974)

Stage	Treatment	Total no. of patients	Relapses	
I	Local only	15	8 (53%)	
	*Local + chemotherapy	17	3 (17.6%)	p = 0.03
IIA	Local + chemotherapy	11	0	

* Actinomycin D and vincristine.
p = 0.002 for pooled I and IIA patients receiving chemotherapy v. control Stage I patients.

results of the Children's Study Group in a trial reported by Heyn *et al.* (1974). In this study, actinomycin-D and vincristine significantly improved the disease-free survival rate in early-stage patients. The roles of node dissection and radiotherapy are less clear. The former is associated with retrograde ejaculation and infertility, and radiotherapy may be preferable to control retroperitoneal node disease. On the other hand, it is necessary to deliver doses of the order of 40 Gray in four weeks and the timing of radiation in relation to chemotherapy needs to be considered carefully, as discussed in Chapter 15 for testicular tumours. It is clear that the introduction of chemotherapy has improved prognosis. In a review of results since 1960, Raney *et al.* (1978) reported that 44 out of 74 (59.5 per cent) children were disease-free at two years. In the Intergroup series of 20 patients, 89 per cent were disease-free at a median time of twenty-three months.

Cromie *et al.* (1979) report the results of combined modality treatment in 5 patients with paratesticular rhabdomyosarcomas. All patients underwent node dissection, which was positive in all 5 children. Three patients subsequently had radiotherapy, 4 had VAC chemotherapy and 1 had vincristine and actinomycin-D. At the time of reporting, all patients were free of tumour at 12 to 108 months.

A report from Curnes *et al.* (1977) shows that no patients with paratesticular tumours treated with orchidectomy, radical node dissection and chemotherapy have died and this series includes one patient who presented with metastatic disease.

Currently, in patients who do not have evidence of haematogenous spread, a policy of chemotherapy and radiotherapy is employed. Treatment is started with two cycles of combination chemotherapy (vincristine, actinomycin-D and cyclophosphamide). Following this, radiation therapy is delivered to the para-aortic and ipsilateral pelvic nodes (40 Gy in four weeks) with continuation of VAC chemotherapy four weeks after radiotherapy, cycles being given at three-weekly intervals for one year.

Sertoli-cell tumours

These rare tumours are histogenetically related to non-germ cells of the primary sex cords and/or the primitive mesenchyme of the gonad. They show a considerable variety of structures and may be associated with endocrine effects. They represent only a very small proportion of the total of childhood testicular tumours. Macroscopically they are well demarcated, firm, white or creamy yellow in colour and cystic areas are commonly seen. Microscopy shows tubular formations with or without a lumen lined by radially arranged cells resembling Sertoli cells. They usually present clinically with a painless enlarged testis. The hormonally inactive Sertoli-cell tumour of the testis is clinically indistinguishable from more common tumours such as that arising from the yolk-sac, but hormone-producing tumours may present with signs of virilization or feminization. Only one case has been reported to the British Testicular Tumour Panel and a review of the literature (Weitzner and Gropp, 1974) reveals only 23 cases, 16 of whom were aged less than 1; 2 children had bilateral tumours and one occurred in an undescended testis. In most cases the tumour had been present for a short time only before diagnosis, but in 3 patients the history was longer than one year. Three patients had gynaecomastia and 1 showed signs of precocious puberty with penile enlargement and increased urinary 17-keto steroid extretion. The very small number of hormonally active Sertoli-cell tumours in children precludes histopathological correlation, but two of the boys with gynaecomastia had tumours consisting almost entirely of epithelial components. Only one case is reported to have metastasized, but the patient survived after radical node dissection. All other cases were benign. However, careful follow up may be indicated if features of malignancy are seen histologically, such as large tumours, infiltration of testis or paratesticular tissue, increased mitoses, pleomorphism and poor differentiation with scanty tubule formation.

Interstitial-cell tumours

These are uncommon, characteristically benign growths formed of interstitial (Leydig cells) with or without endocrine activity. Leydig cells are scattered throughout the intertubular tissues of the testis and produce androgenic (C_{19}) steroid hormones under gonadotrophin control. They are more common in later childhood than in infancy; they present with signs of virilization and sexual precocity, but occasionally feminization may occur (Melicow et al., 1949). They may be confused clinically with the syndrome of adrenocortical hyperplasia and high 17-keto steroid levels may be found. Chorionic gonadotrophin is absent. Investigations should exclude hyperplasia by measurement of urinary oestrogens, pregnanetriol, 17-hydroxy- and 17-keto steroids and plasma cortisone levels before and after ACTH stimulation and dexamethazone suppression (Dalgaard and Hesselberg, 1957). Plasma testosterone levels and FSH and LH may be useful. Macroscopically they are well-circumscribed, rounded, and solid tumours of yellowish brown colour, and histologically a compact mass of eosinophilic cells is seen arranged in sheets or dispersed through a fibrocellular stroma. Focal calcification may be seen. Melicow *et al.* (1949) reported 10 cases of interstitial-cell tumour appearing before puberty. All were benign and none recurred following simple orchidectomy.

Leukaemic infiltrates

The incidence of leukaemic infiltration of the testis, as a complication of acute lymphoblastic leukaemia (ALL) in childhood, has increased as longer remission from bone marrow and meningeal disease has been achieved. A report from the Medical Research Council (1978) has shown that 4 out of 60 patients had testicular disease at the time of initial diagnosis, 13 were found to be involved at the time of first marrow relapse; 29 out of 60 developed clinical signs of testicular involvement during the first remission without other signs of leukaemic recurrence, and 14 cases followed bone marrow relapse. It seems possible that the reason for the worse prognosis for boys with ALL compared with girls is due to testicular infiltration, and routine biopsy of the testis and prophylactic testicular irradiation are being considered in some centres as part of the primary treatment. There is a low risk of testicular relapse during maintenance chemotherapy and ways of delivering more effective chemotherapy are also being sought. A dose of 2400 rad is commonly given to the testes to prevent or treat leukaemic infiltration.

References

Abell, M. R. and Holtz, F. (1963). *Cancer* **16**, 965.
Arlen, M., Grabstald, H. and Whitemore, W. F. Jr. (1969). *Cancer* **23**, 525.
Bracken, R. B., Johnson, D. E., Cangir, A. and Ayala, A. (1978). *Urology* **11**, 376.
Brosman, S. A., Cohen, A. and Fay, R. (1974). *Urology* **3**, 568.
Brosman, S. A. (1979). *Urology* **13**, 581.
Burrington, J. D. (1969). *Journal of Pediatric Surgery* **4**, 503.
Cromie, W. J., Raney, R. B. and Duckett, J. W. (1979). *Journal of Urology* **122**, 80.
Curnes, J. T., Pratt, C. B. and Hustu, H. O. (1977). *Journal of Urology* **118**, 662.
Dalgaard, J. B. and Hesselberg, F. (1957). *Acta Pathologica et Microbiologica Scandinavica* **41**, 219.
Drago, J. R., Nelson, R. P. and Palmer, J. M. (1978). *Urology* **12**, 499.
Gangai, M. P. (1968). *Cancer* **22**, 658.
Ghavimi, F., Exelby, P. R., D'Angio, G. J., Whitmore, W. F., Lieberman, P. H., Lewis, J. L. Jr., Mike, V. and Murphy, M. L. (1973). *Cancer* **32**, 1178.
Gowing, N. F. C. (1976). In *Pathology of the Testis*, p. 317. Ed. by R. C. B. Pugh. Blackwell, Oxford.
Gray, C. P. and Biorn, C. L. (1960). *Journal of Urology* **84**, 562.
Hays, D. M., Mirabal, V. Q., Patel, H. R., Shore, N. and Wooley, M. M. (1969). *Surgery* **65**, 845.
Heyn, R. M., Holland, R., Newton, W. A. Jr., Tefft, M., Breslow, N. and Hartmann, J. R. (1974). *Cancer* **34**, 2128.
Hoffman, W. W. and Baird, S. S. (1960). *Journal of Urology* **84**, 376.
Hopkins, T. B., Jaffe, N., Colodny, A., Cassady, J. R. and Filler, R. M. (1978). *Journal of Urology* **120**, 96.
Jaffe, N., Filler, R. M., Farber, S., Traggis, D. G., Vawter, G. F., Tefft, M. and Murray, J. E. (1973). *American Journal of Surgery* **125**, 482.
Johnson, D. E., Kuhn, C. R. and Guinn, G. A. (1970). *Journal of Urology* **104**, 940.

Jungling, M. J. and Culp, D. A. (1975). *Journal of Urology* **114**, 313.

Karamehmedovic, O., Woodtli, W. and Plüss, H. J. (1975). *Journal of Pediatric Surgery* **10**, 109.

Littman, R., Tessler, A. N. and Valensi, Q. (1972). *Journal of Urology* **108**, 290.

Medical Research Council Working Party on Leukaemia in Childhood (1978). *British Medical Journal* **1**, 334.

Melicow, M. M., Robinson, J. N. and Rainsford, L. K. (1949). *Journal of Urology* **62**, 672.

Pugh, R. C. B. (1976). In *Pathology of the Testis.* p. 139. Ed. by R. C. B. Pugh. Blackwell Scientific Publications, London.

Pugh, R. and Cameron, K. M. (1976). In *Pathology of the Testis,* p. 199. Ed. by R. C. B. Pugh. Blackwell Scientific Publications, London.

Raney, R. B., Hays, D. M., Lawrence, W., Soule, E. H., Tefft, M. and Donaldson, M. H. (1978). *Cancer* **42**, 729.

Rosas-Uribe, A., Luna, M. A. and Guinn, G. A. (1970). *American Journal of Surgery* **120**, 787.

Sabio, H., Burger, E. O., Farrow, G. M. and Kelalis, P. P. (1974). *Cancer* **34**, 2118.

Skeel, D. A., Drinker, H. R. Jr. and Witherington, R. (1975). *Journal of Urology* **113**, 279.

Smith, I. E., Eckstein, H. B., Kohn, J. and McElwain, T. J. (1977). *British Journal of Urology* **49**, 427.

Staubitz, W. J., Jewett, T. C., Magoss, I. V., Schenk, W. G. and Phalakornkule, S. (1965). *Journal of Urology* **94**, 683.

Tank, E. S., Fellmann, S. L., Wheeler, E. S., Weaver, D. K. and Lapides, J. (1972). *Journal of Urology* **107**, 324.

Tefft, M., Vawter, G. F. and Mitus, A. (1967). *Radiology* **88**, 457.

Telium, G. (1971). Special tumors of ovary and testis and related extragonadal lesions. *Comparative Pathology and Histological Identification.* Munksgaard, Copenhagen.

Viprakasit, D., Navarro, C., Guarin, U. K. and Garnes, H. A. (1977). *Urology* **9**, 568.

Weitzner, S. and Gropp, A. (1974). *American Journal of Diseases of Childhood* **128**, 541.

Woodtli, W. and Hedinger, Chr. (1974). *Virchows Archives A. Pathological Anatomy and Histology* **364**, 93.

Young, P. G., Mount, B. M., Foote, F. W. and Whitmore, W. F. (1970). *Cancer* **28**, 1065.

17

Extragonadal malignant germ-cell tumours

Derek Raghavan

In order to diagnose a primary extragonadal germ-cell tumour it is essential to exclude the possible presence of an occult primary testicular tumour presenting with disseminated disease. In 1927, Prym suggested the occurrence of spontaneous regression of a testicular primary in a patient with disseminated choriocarcinoma in whom examination of the right testis had revealed a small, fibrous nodule. Several other workers have documented cases either of spontaneous regression of primary testicular tumours or of apparent extragonadal primary tumours with foci or scarring or of occult residual tumour tissue in the gonads (Friedman and Moore, 1946; Rather *et al.*, 1954; Azzopardi *et al.*, 1961; Azzopardi and Hoffbrand, 1965; Asif and Uehling, 1968; Rudnick and O'Dell, 1971; Meares and Briggs, 1972).

Although these findings suggest that some extragonadal presentations may represent metastases, there is no doubt that true primary tumours originating outside the testis exist. Stowell *et al.* (1945) disputed the significance of testicular scars when reporting a well-documented case of primary extragenital choriocarcinoma, and it has even been suggested that the scars themselves might be a consequence of primary extragonadal growths (Lynch and Blewett, 1953). Ectopic testicular tissue has been reported in the retroperitoneum which could provide the basis for a primary retroperitoneal origin (Staemmler, 1934; Allen and Vespignani, 1938).

In more than thirty cases in which a diagnosis of extragonadal germ-cell malignant tumours has been made, the patients' testes have been examined histologically (Utz and Buscemi, 1971; Johnson *et al.*, 1973; Cox, 1975; Luna and Valenzuela-Tamariz, 1976; Raghavan and Barrett, 1980) and in only one of these was a focus of tumour demonstrated (0.7 × 0.5 × 0.3 cm) (Luna and Valenzuela-Tamariz, 1976). In addition, many cases have been reported in which repeated and careful clinical examination of the testicles has proved negative (Bagshaw *et al.*, 1969; Utz and Buscemi, 1971; Johnson *et al.*, 1973; Cox, 1975; Luna and Valenzuela-Tamariz, 1976; Raghavan and Barrett, 1980). Pineal teratomas have been identified in patients whose gonads have been examined histologically and proven negative for tumour (Borit, 1969; Yoshiki *et al.*, 1976).

Origins and histogenesis

It has been suggested (Fox and Hospers, 1936; Schlumberger, 1946) that extragonadal germ-cell tumours are the result of local dislocation of tissues during embryogenesis, with neoplasia developing in primitive rests of totipotential cells left during the blastular or morular stage. Thus, mediastinal tumours, for example, would arise from the third branchial pouch, the anlage of the thymus.

The principal alternative hypothesis is that these tumours arise from primordial germ cells rather than as aberrations of somatic development (Friedman, 1951; Dixon and Moore, 1952; Teilum, 1959; Teilum, 1971). Thus, tumours at different sites are postulated to arise from germ cells that have been misplaced during ontogeny and which, during their passage from the yolk-sac endoderm, have travelled in the midline through the retroperitoneum to the mediastinum, the pineal gland, or to the sacrococcygeal region, instead of to the gonadal ridges (Fig. 17.1). The hypothesis of misplaced germ cells, first

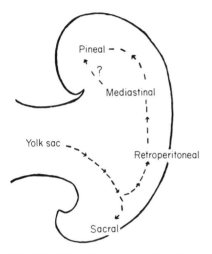

Fig. 17.1 Migration of germ cells in the genesis of extragonadal primary germ-cell tumours.

advocated by Askanazy (1907), received support from the anatomical demonstration of the pathway of germ-cell migration (Fuss, 1912; Witschi, 1948).

It has been proposed also that these tumours arise from foci of pluripotential embryonic tissue which have escaped from the influence of the primary organizer during fetal life (Willis, 1962).

Several variant hypotheses have been proposed to explain the development of germ-cell tumours at particular sites—for example, the suppressed twin/pygopagus theory (Bland-Sutton, 1922; Perlstein and Le Count, 1927) and the development from totipotent cells in Henson's node (Brindley, 1945) to explain sacrococcygeal tumours. However, most of these theories have not gained widespread support.

The marked excess of malignancy in males in most of the extragonadal sites (Donnellan and Swenson, 1968; Johnson et al., 1973; Martini et al., 1974; Schey et al., 1977) remains unexplained.

Theories regarding the biochemical and genetic bases of germ-cell malignancy and teratogenesis are beyond the scope of this review, but are discussed extensively elsewhere (Theiss et al., 1960; Linder et al., 1975; Linder, McCaw and Hecht, 1975; Riley and Sutton, 1975; Erickson and Gondos, 1976; O'Hare, 1978).

Histopathology

The histology of germ-cell tumours is similar in gonadal and extragonadal sites (Friedman, 1951; Utz and Buscemi, 1971; Schantz *et al.*, 1972; Johnson *et al.*, 1973; Luna and Valenzuela-Tamariz, 1976; Roth and Panganiban, 1976). Nevertheless, certain features appear to be characteristic of the non-gonadal tumours. Perhaps the most important difference from testicular tumours is the absence of the tunica albuginea, a tough barrier limiting local tumour spread.

Tumour histology may either be 'pure' (with only one component of seminoma or teratoma) or 'mixed' (showing the histological features of seminoma and teratoma, or of different subtypes of teratoma) and, in the case of mixed tumours, the natural history and metastatic patterns are usually those of the non-seminomatous components (*British Medical Journal*, 1969; Sickles *et al.*, 1974).

Mediastinum

One of the problems in assessing the frequency of these tumours has been the histological similarity of the mediastinal seminoma (germinoma) and the thymoma and its variants. Lattes (1962) for example, at the Penrose Cancer Conference (1960) submitted a section of 'seminoma-like tumour of the thymus' to the attending pathologists for histological assessment with the following results: 'thymoma' (93 pathologists), 'seminomatous thymoma' (23), 'teratoma' (5) and 'pseudoseminomatous thymoma' (1).

Similarly, the histological patterns now considered to represent 'teratomas' have formerly been interpreted variously as 'lymphomas', 'thymomas' and 'unclassified tumours'. It is hardly surprising that there are difficulties in interpreting early statistics regarding the incidence, pathology and behaviour of these tumours.

Pineal body

The nomenclature that has been applied to the tumours of the pineal body and surrounding regions is both confusing and controversial, with the interchangeable use of such terms as 'pinealoma', 'ectopic pinealoma', 'atypical teratoma', 'germinoma', 'embryoma', 'dysembryoma', 'teratoid tumour' and 'teratoma'.

Russell and Rubinstein (Russell, 1944; Russell and Rubinstein, 1963) described the 'atypical teratoma', consisting of sheets of moderately large, clear cells histologically identical to the seminoma (germinoma), the most common histological type of pineal tumour. Their classification of pineal tumours included 'teratomas' (described as typical and atypical), 'pinealomas' (true pineal parenchymal tumours), cysts and glial and other forms. Morphological and histochemical evidence of the similarity of atypical teratomas and seminnomas has been provided (Friedman, 1947; Beeley *et al.*, 1973) and a further similarity of these tumour types has been defined in terms of their rapid response to irradiation. Notwithstanding the confusion caused by the term 'atypical teratoma', true malignant teratomas of the pineal gland have been described (Russell, 1944; Dayan *et al.*, 1966; Bestle, 1968; Simson *et al.*, 1968; Borit, 1969; Albrechtsen *et al.*, 1972). Albrechtsen and his colleagues (1972) have broadened the classification of these tumours to include yolk sac (or endodermal sinus tumour) components, previously classified as 'pinealomas', 'teratomas', 'malignant papillomas', 'angioreticulomas' or 'unclassifiable tumours'.

The common characteristic of these 'seminomas' and 'teratomas' is their occurrence in the midline, most commonly related to the pineal body, but also in the suprasellar region or third ventricle (Albrechtsen *et al.*, 1972).

Sacrococcygeal region

Interpretation of the reported morphology of malignant tumours of the sacrococcygeum is complicated by the variable criteria employed to define malignancy. Thus, while some reports employ criteria of infiltration or metastic spread (Donnellan and Swenson, 1968), others refer to potential malignancy, by which is meant the finding of highly primitive or embryonic tissues (Conklin and Abell, 1967). Thus, the incidence of histological 'malignancy' varies from 16 per cent to 42 per cent (Conklin and Abell, 1967), depending on the criteria used.

Patient age and sex appear to be important factors in determining malignant potential. Paradoxically, tumours excised in neonates less than 1 month of age and in adults tend to be histologically and functionally benign, in comparison to those in the intervening age group (Gross *et al.*, 1951; Willcox and Mackenzie, 1961; Waldhausen *et al.*, 1963; Hickey and Martin, 1964; Donnellan and Swenson, 1968; Izant and Filston, 1975; Grosfield *et al.*, 1976). The characteristic male sex predominance of germ-cell malignancy is maintained in these tumours (Donnellan and Swenson, 1968; Schey *et al.*, 1977). One aspect of the histology of tumours in the sacrococcygeal region is the absence of germinomas (seminomas) in series reported.

Other sites

Macroscopically, extragonadal tumours in most sites are predominantly solid, with areas of necrosis, haemorrhage and cyst formation. There is often evidence of local infiltration, with lack of definition of tissue planes.

Histologically, the patterns of pure or mixed seminoma and/or teratoma may be present, with varying degrees of differentiation and variable numbers of mitoses.

Teratomas have been reported at numerous sites (including lung, face, neck, vagina, prostate, liver, stomach and thyroid) and the majority have been histologically benign. Few of the case reports stand up to critical evaluation. Thus, reports of primary malignant germ-cell tumours of the prostate (Benson *et al.*, 1978) and the liver (Misugi and Reiner, 1965; Hart, 1975) remain unsubstantiated. The well-documented histologically proven cases have been reported predominantly in infants and children, the main microscopic patterns being yolk-sac (endodermal sinus) tumour and choriocarcinoma (malignant trophoblastic teratoma).

Clinical presentation

Mediastinum

Mediastinal germ-cell tumours are uncommon. When separated from thymic tumours, they comprise 2 to 6 per cent of mediastinal tumours, and 5 to 13 per cent of mediastinal malignancies (Oberman and Libke, 1964; Joseph *et al.*, 1966; Cox, 1975), figures influenced by the criteria of reporting. They occur most commonly in patients in the second and third decades (Schantz *et al.*, 1972; Johnson *et al.*, 1973; Martini *et al.*, 1974; Sickles *et al.*, 1974; Cox, 1975). Although uncommon in children, they represent 10 to 20 per cent of childhood mediastinal tumours; about 20 per cent of them are malignant (Canty and Siemens, 1978). Although the overall sex incidence is equal, there is a clear excess of malignancy in males (Houghton, 1936; Fine *et al.*, 1962; Oberman and Libke, 1964; Wychulis *et al.*, 1971; Martini *et al.*, 1974; Cox, 1975; Canty and Siemens, 1978).

Modes of presentation are summarized in Table 17.1, 'routine examination' and 'chest pain' being the most common (British Medical Journal, leading

Table 17.1 Presentation of mediastinal germ-cell tumours

Asymptomatic/routine chest x-ray
Chest pain
Dyspnoea
Cough ± haemoptysis
Neck mass
Superior vena caval obstruction
Gynaecomastia
Non-specific/constitutional
Metastases

article, 1969; Utz and Buscemi, 1971; Besznyak *et al.*, 1973; Martini *et al.*, 1974; Sickles *et al.*, 1974; Cox, 1975; Raghavan and Barrett, 1980). Symptoms associated with these tumours are related to size, invasion of neighbouring structures and the presence of distant metastases. Because they are characteristically asymptomatic, mediastinal germ-cell tumours often present late (Fig. 17.2).

Clinical examination is directed to the assessment of (i) the size of the tumour and the severity of its local effects; (ii) the presence of metastatic disease; and (iii) the possibility that the presentation is itself a reflection of primary disease elsewhere (e.g. the gonads).

Pineal region

Tumours of the pineal region represent 0.4 to 2 per cent of all intracranial tumours (Kernohan and Sayre, 1952; Zulch, 1956; Maier and Dejong, 1967; Puschett and Goldberg, 1968). There is a marked predominance in males and most patients are younger than 25 years of age at presentation (Dayan *et al.*, 1966; Maier and Dejong, 1967; So, 1976; Sung *et al.*, 1978). In the suprasellar

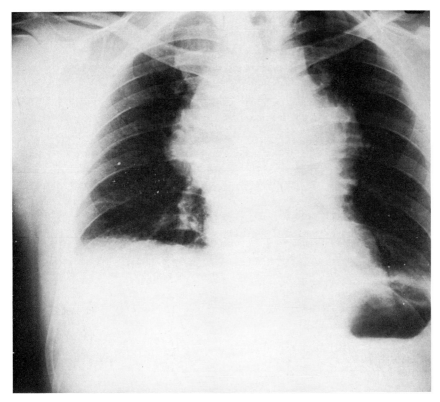

Fig. 17.2 Mediastinal germ-cell tumour of yolk-sac type presenting with superior vena caval obstruction in a 37-year-old man.

region, the sex incidence is equal (Simson *et al.*, 1968; Camins and Mount, 1974).

The clinical features are due to the presence of an expanding lesion in the pineal region, causing aqueduct obstruction with a consequent increase in intracranial pressure and hydrocephalus. Extension into the surrounding cerebral tissue may cause a variety of specific neurological syndromes (Table 17.2; Rubin and Kramer, 1965; Dayan *et al.*, 1966; Maier and Dejong, 1967; Puschett and Goldberg, 1968; Simson *et al.*, 1968; So, 1976; Spiegel *et al.*, 1976; Sung *et al.*, 1978).

Sacrococcygeal region

Although the sacrococcygeal region is one of the most common sites of teratomas, the incidence is only about 1 in 40 000 births (Ross, 1948; Dillard *et al.*, 1970). From 67 to 90 per cent of all cases occur in females (Gross *et al.*, 1951; Waldhausen *et al.*, 1963; Conklin and Abell, 1967; Donnellan and Swenson, 1968; Izant and Filston, 1975). In most reported series there is a male predominance of malignant tumours (Donnellan and Swenson, 1968; Schey *et al.*, 1977). However, Chretien *et al.* (1970) have reported 21 cases of childhood

Table 17.2 Presentation of pineal germ-cell tumours

Raised intracranial pressure
Headaches
Papilloedema
Decreased visual acuity
Visual blurring
Impaired consciousness

Involvement of occulomotor apparatus
Parinaud's syndrome
Abnormal pupillary function
Diplopia
Ptosis

Posterior extension
Cerebellar dysfunction
Impaired hearing
Loss of downward conjugate eye movement

Anterior, inferior extension (hypothalmus/midbrain)
Diabetes insipidus
Somnolence
Altered gonadal function
Pituitary insufficiency

Lateral extension
Thalamic syndrome
Pyramidal tract signs

Metastases
Cerebrum
Spinal cord

sacrococcygeal embryonal cell carcinomas, of which 17 occurred in females.

Benign sacrococcygeal germ-cell tumours occur uncommonly in adults (1 in 87 000; Miles and Stewart, 1974) and malignancy of these tumours is rare (Marcuse, 1959).

The presentation, as in other sites, is determined by local tumour bulk, its complications and the effects of distant metastases (Table 17.3).

The tumour may occur either in the midline or in the gluteal region. The American Academy of Pediatrics (Altman *et al.*, 1974) has classified sacrococ-

Table 17.3 Presentation of sacrococcygeal teratomas

Mass
Skin discolouration
Hairy naevus
Constipation
Urinary tract symptoms
Leg weakness
Pain
Peri-anal disease
Obstruction of labour
Distant metastases
Vascular or lymphatic obstruction
Local complications

cygeal tumours according to their site, type I representing an external tumour, types II and III referring to increasing intrapelvic tumour masses with associated external manifestations, and type IV being a presacral tumour with no external mass.

Urinary tract symptoms usually reflect pressure on the outflow tract and include overflow incontinence, frequency and pain.

Local complications of haemorrhage, infection and necrosis are relatively common both in benign and malignant disease. Sacrococcygeal teratomas, regardless of type, may have an associated intraspinal component (Gwinn *et al.*, 1955) and hence may show signs of spinal cord compression.

A family history of twins has been reported as an occasional association (Gross *et al.*, 1951; Hickey and Martin, 1964; Izant and Filston, 1975; Schey *et al.*, 1977). A family cluster of 26 patients in six unrelated families has been reported (Ashcraft and Holder, 1965; Hunt *et al.*, 1977) with a syndrome of presacral (type IV) teratoma and anal stenosis. Many of the family members also were noted to have vasico-ureteric reflux, skin dimples and retrorectal abscesses. In these families, the sex incidence was nearly equal and malignant potential was quite low. The pattern of inheritance was autosomal dominant.

The association of sacrococcygeal teratomas and coccygeal aplasia or agenesis has been documented also, including one report in which 9 members of a family had sacral agenesis (6 females, 3 males) and 4 of the females had presacral tumours (Laird, 1954; Kenefick, 1973).

Retroperitoneum

Retroperitoneal primary malignant germ-cell tumours may be difficult to distinguish from metastases in view of the usual pattern of spread of primary testicular tumours. The mean age at presentation of reported cases is 13 to 16 years (Palumbo *et al.*, 1949; Engel *et al.*, 1968), and 90 per cent of cases occur in the first three decades. There is no clear overall sex predominance, although more cases of malignancy have been reported in males. About 10 per cent of retroperitoneal teratomas are malignant (Engel *et al.*, 1968), as are germinomas in this area.

Presenting features of these tumours are listed in Table 17.4 (Palumbo *et al.*, 1949; Engel *et al.*, 1968; Pantoja *et al.*, 1976). Although teratomas may occur

Table 17.4 Presentation of retroperitoneal germ-cell tumours

Asymptomatic
Abdominal mass ± pain
Increasing abdominal girth
Vascular obstruction
Nausea, vomiting
Constipation
Complications
  Haemorrhage
  Infection
  Necrosis/rupture
Constitutional symptoms
Distant metastases

anywhere in the retroperitoneum, the most common site is the region of the upper pole of the kidney, especially on the left side (Engel *et al.*, 1968).

Other sites

The clinical features of malignant germ-cell tumours at unusual sites are manifestations (as above) of local tumour bulk, complications and the presence of metastases (Misugi and Reiner, 1965; Norris *et al.*, 1970; Allyn *et al.*, 1971; Ozaki *et al.*, 1971; Meares and Briggs, 1972; Bale *et al.*, 1975; Hart, 1975; Benson *et al.*, 1978; Holt *et al.*, 1978; Kimler and Muth, 1978). These tumours are extremely uncommon and will not be discussed further.

Investigation

In general, the investigative approach is similar to that employed in primary testicular malignancies (Peckham and McElwain, 1975), with an extensive initial staging approach that includes 'routine' biochemical and haematological tests, conventional X-rays, CAT and radionucleide scanning. Lymphangiography should not be carried out in patients with large mediastinal masses in the presence of symptoms and signs of respiratory embarrassment, as there is a risk of further deterioration of the ventilation/perfusion inequality due to embolism from the oily contrast medium. Gallium scanning is useful in the investigation of seminomas, but of less value in teratomas (Paterson *et al.*, 1976).

The CAT brain scanner has largely replaced invasive procedures such as pneumoencephalography, carotid arteriography and diagnostic craniotomy and biopsy (Spiegel *et al.*, 1976).

Tumour-marker substances are an essential part of the diagnostic work-up (see Chapter 4) to help to define the type of histology and in the subsequent monitoring of treatment (Peckham and McElwain, 1975; Walden *et al.*, 1977; Norgaard-Pedersen *et al.*, 1978). Even in pineal teratomas, particularly of yolk-sac and trophoblastic histological types, serum and cerebrospinal fluid alpha-fetoprotein (AFP) and human chorionic gonadotrophin (HCG) levels have a role in monitoring the response to treatment and in documenting the persistence of disease (Yoshiki *et al.*, 1976; Norgaard-Pedersen *et al.*, 1978).

The review of histology, augmented with immunocytochemical staining for AFP, HCG and other potential markers, will help to define which markers are likely to be useful parameters of clinical progress (Heyderman, 1978).

The differences in the metastatic patterns of testicular and extragonadal primaries reflect the absence of the tunica albuginea and the paucity of early symptoms, particularly in the mediastinum and retroperitoneum, with resultant delay in presentation.

Mediastinum

In the mediastinal seminomas, spread may occur to the lungs, liver, bones and regional nodes (Johnson *et al.*, 1973; Martini *et al.*, 1974; Cox, 1975; Luna and Valenzuela-Tamariz, 1976; Polansky *et al.*, 1979; Raghavan and Barrett, 1980). Other less common sites of metastasis include the brain (Martini *et al.*,

1974), spleen (Steinmetz and Hays, 1961), tonsils (Steinmetz and Hays, 1961), thyroid (Kountz *et al.*, 1963), adrenals (Steinmetz and Hays, 1961), spinal cord (El-Domeiri *et al.*, 1968) and pancreas (Raghavan and Barrett, 1980). The characteristic of this tumour when treated with irradiation is the achievement of local tumour eradication, with patients sometimes dying of distant metastases.

This is in sharp contrast to non-seminomatous germ-cell tumours, where local recurrence occurs quite frequently (Martini *et al.*, 1974) in addition to distant metastatic spread to lung, liver, brain, nodes, bones and kidneys (British Medical Journal, 1969; Johnson, *et al.*, 1973; Martini *et al.*, 1974; Sickles *et al.*, 1974; Cox, 1975).

Pineal region

Tumours of the pineal gland spread by direct extension, via the bloodstream and through the cerebrospinal fluid (Maier and Dejong, 1967). Spinal metastases are important as potential sites of treatment failure in patients who receive only local irradiation. Maier and Dejong (1967) have quoted unpublished data from the Armed Forces Institute of Pathology that 8 per cent of pineal tumours and 37 per cent of suprasellar germinomas metastasize to the cerebral or spinal subarachnoid space within six months to five years, and similar figures have been reported elsewhere (Fowler *et al.*, 1956; Dayan *et al.*, 1966; Camins and Mount, 1974). Metastasis outside the central nervous system is very rare, although Giuffre and DiLorenzo (1975) have reported a pineal choriocarcinoma that seeded to brain, lungs, liver and the left kidney in the preterminal stages.

Sacrococcygeal region

Malignant germ-cell tumours of the sacrococcygeum spread locally (involving coccyx and adjacent pelvic and abdominal viscera) and to lymph nodes (including inguinal and para-aortic), liver, bones, lung and brain. Donnellan and Swenson (1968) reported 5 out of 30 children with metastatic disease at the time of death. Chretien *et al.* (1970), in a series of 21 children with embryonal carcinoma, noted 12 with secondaries at presentation. Asymptomatic metastases are not uncommon, both at presentation and subsequently.

Treatment

The major factors that determine a management plan for these tumours are listed in Table 17.5.

Table 17.5 Factors determining management

Age of patient
Site of tumour
Histology
Volume of tumour
Sensitivity of cell type to radiotherapy and chemotherapy
Presence of metastases
Known metastatic pattern of the tumour
General physical condition of the patient

The exclusion by careful clinical examination of a gonadal primary is of particular importance when either surgery and/or local irradiation are selected as the treatment(s) of choice.

Mediastinum

Although surgery is still employed, it should not be regarded as the treatment of choice, but is essential to establish a diagnosis. Radiotherapy is the treatment of choice for mediastinal seminoma (Edland *et al.*, 1968; El-Domeiri *et al.*, 1968; Bagshaw *et al.*, 1969; Nichels and Franssila, 1972; Schantz *et al.*, 1972; Cox, 1975; Polansky *et al.*, 1979). However, if bulky lesions are present, prior chemotherapy may be employed to achieve volume reduction and facilitate irradiation. In cases of pure seminoma where neither AFP or HCG are elevated, a midplane dose of 35–40 Gray in four to four and a half weeks is adequate. To minimize normal tissue damage, a 'shrinking field' technique can be used, in which the field size is reduced as the mass regresses.

The role of chemotherapy in the treatment of seminoma is not defined clearly. Recent experience indicates that the combinations used for teratoma of the testis (vinblastine, bleomycin and cis-platinum) may be effective in advanced seminoma (see Chapter 10). However, the exquisite radiosensitivity

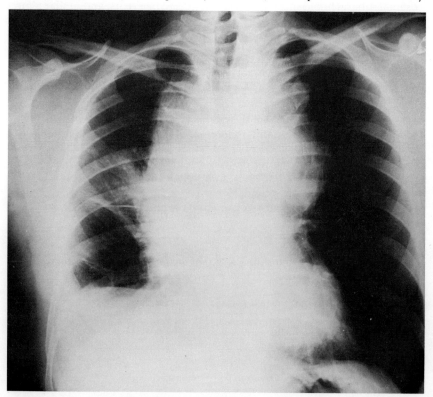

Fig. 17.3 Bulky mediastinal seminoma with extension into the right lung treated by cis-platinum, bleomycin and vinblastine. **(a)** Prior to chemotherapy.

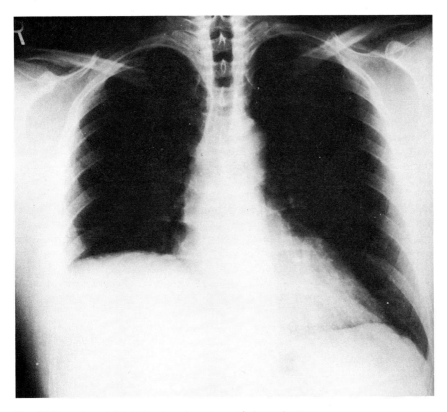

Fig. 17.3 continued **(b)** Following six courses of chemotherapy.

of seminoma should not be overlooked. In a recent report of the Royal Marsden experience of 6 patients with mediastinal seminoma (age range 13 to 43 years), 2 have died of their disease (Raghavan and Barrett, 1980). One patient had recently completed treatment and 3 were disease-free following irradiation at five, ten and eleven years.

Figure 17.3a shows the chest X-ray appearances of mediastinal seminoma before and after radiotherapy. Figure 17.3b shows regression of a bulky primary mediastinal seminoma with chemotherapy.

Optimal therapy for malignant mediastinal teratomas is controversial. Beattie (1979) reported 20 patients with non-seminomatous mediastinal germ-cell tumours, of whom only one was alive. The approach outlined in Chapter 15 is equally appropriate to the management of extra-gonadal non-seminomatous germ-cell tumours, and treatment should be initiated with chemotherapy and augmented by surgery or radiotherapy when appropriate.

Walden *et al.* (1977) have reported two apparent cures, one with surgery, radiotherapy and chemotherapy and the other with chemotherapy alone. Reynolds *et al.* (1979) has reported an experience at the Memorial Hospital,

New York, where 18 non-seminomatous tumours have been treated since 1971. Of these, 3 are alive and disease free at twelve, twenty-two and fifty-one months.

Figure 17.4 shows the chest x-ray of a patient with a primary mediastinal malignant teratoma before and after chemotherapy.

Pineal region

Germinomas and 'benign' teratomas

Early results of aggressive surgical excision of pineal tumours were disappointing because of the morbidity of the procedures and the frequency of disease recurrence (Horrax, 1949; Cole, 1971). As a result, radical operations have been abandoned in favour of more conservative shunting and biopsy procedures, followed by irradiation. The introduction of the Torkildsen shunt (Torkildsen, 1939) made it possible to treat hydrocephalus. In some centres, with the introduction of CAT scanning to aid in diagnosis, cranial irradiation is carried out without surgical intervention (Spiegel *et al.*, 1976).

Overall, treatment policies are similar in most centres, irradiation doses of 4500 to 5000 rad being delivered in four to six weeks, often preceded by one of the available shunting procedures (Rubin and Kramer, 1965; Maier and

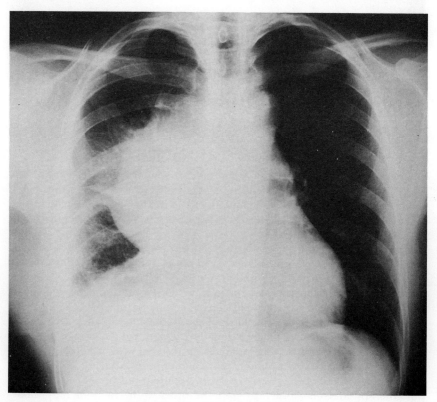

Fig. 17.4 (a) Massive mediastinal germ-cell tumour (malignant teratoma undifferentiated).

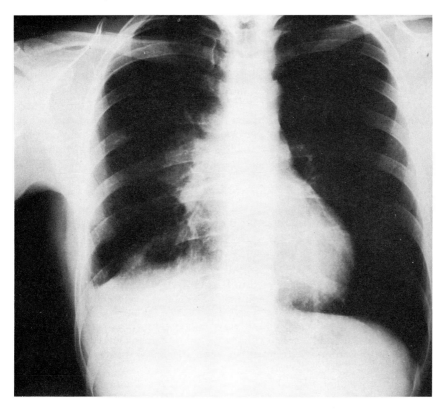

Fig. 17.4 continued **(b)** radiograph showing good partial response following chemo-therapy with cis-platinum, vinblastine and bleomycin.

Dejong, 1967; So, 1976; Sung *et al.*, 1978). Field sizes vary with estimated tumour volume (Maier and Dejong, 1967). In some centres, whole-brain irradiation is used alone, whereas in others, a lower whole-brain dose is augmented by a local tumour boost (Sung *et al.*, 1978).

The major controversy of treatment is whether or not to irradiate the spine prophylactically. As discussed above, a significant proportion of patients develop spread to the spinal cord. The usual practice in many centres is to advocate craniospinal irradiation (Cole, 1971). In addition to surgery and irradiation, hormonal treatment with pituitary replacement is essential, the symptoms and signs of hypopituitarism often persisting after the tumour has been eradicated.

An alternative to external irradiation that has been suggested is the use of interstitial radio-active gold (^{198}Au) implants, if the tumour diameter is less than 4 cm with no evidence of infiltration of surrounding structures (So, 1976).

Malignant teratomas

Malignant teratomas of this region are very uncommon, and thus experience in therapy is limited. Yolk-sac tumour, the predominant histological type reported, appears to be somewhat sensitive to radiotherapy, but results of treatment are, not surprisingly, less impressive than in germinomas.

Sacrococcygeal region

Analysis of most series reported indicates that immediate, radical, surgical excision (including the coccyx) should be the aim of treatment for childhood sacrococcygeal teratomas, regardless of the size or age of the patient at diagnosis. Surgery in the newborn, performed by experienced paediatric surgeons, is safe and allows the highest rate of complete cure. As discussed previously, delay increases the risk of the development of malignancy. The major risks to be avoided in early surgery include incomplete removal of the coccyx (with an increased risk of recurrence), postoperative shock due to inadequate blood and fluid replacement in the neonate, and unrecognized dura injury with persistent CSF leak in patients with intraspinal extension (Gross et al., 1951; Donnellan and Swenson, 1968).

The classical surgical approach of Gross et al. (1951) consists of a posterior approach with en bloc removal of the tumour and coccyx, whereas Waldhausen et al. (1963) have recommended an abdominosacral approach to ensure adequate access to the intrapelvic components of the tumours.

In adults, malignant potential is much less and the need for surgery can be balanced against the symptomatic state and general health of the patient.

In the case of recurrence, further attempts at excision may be feasible and radiotherapy is often indicated either as an adjunct to surgery or as an alternative.

The management of malignant sacrococcygeal teratomas is difficult and often unsuccessful (Donnellan and Swenson, 1968; Chretien et al., 1970). Optimum treatment probably requires the use of surgery, radiotherapy and combination chemotherapy (Donnellan and Swenson, 1968), but published experience with such cases is limited.

Retroperitoneum and other sites

The histology and bulk of the tumours in these sites largely determine the therapeutic approach. In the case of retroperitoneal seminomas, radiotherapy is the initial treatment of choice. The tumours are highly radiosensitive and the potential for cure is good.

Little experience has been gained of treating malignant retroperitoneal teratomas with current chemotherapy regimes, although Samuels et al. (1976) have reported a case treated with chemotherapy with survival in excess of two years.

Prognosis

The prognosis of seminomas (germinomas) at each site remains significantly better than of malignant teratomas, largely because of their radiosensitivity. The outlook for patients with teratomas has improved with the development of more effective chemotherapy regimens and the use of tumour markers to define more clearly the endpoints of treatment.

Seminomas

Five-year survival figures for mediastinal seminomas of approximately 75 per cent are achieved in patients treated with either radiotherapy alone or in combination with surgery and chemotherapy (Edland *et al.*, 1968; Schantz *et al.*, 1972; Polansky *et al.*, 1979). Similar figures are reported for germinomas of the pineal region (Simson *et al.*, 1968; Sung *et al.*, 1978). Although patient numbers are smaller, long-term survival is well documented for patients with retroperitoneal seminomas treated with radiotherapy, with up to 60 per cent of patients free of disease from two to twenty-four years after diagnosis. Seminomas of the mediastinum and pineal region may be associated with either late relapse or prolonged survival in the presence of active disease (Bagshaw *et al.*, 1969; Utz and Buscemi, 1971; Schantz *et al.*, 1972; Martini *et al.*, 1974).

Teratomas

Hitherto, the outlook for patients with malignant extragonadal teratomas has been less satisfactory. In all sites, mortality rates are high and life expectancy from the time of diagnosis is short (Conklin and Abell, 1967; *British Medical Journal*, 1969; Chretien *et al.*, 1970; Johnson *et al.*, 1973; Martini *et al.*, 1974; Cox, 1975; Canty and Siemens, 1978). The occasional successes reported with aggressive radiotherapy or combination chemotherapy (Wychulis *et al.*, 1971; Sickles *et al.*, 1974; Cox, 1975; Samuels *et al.*, 1976; Walden *et al.*, 1977) have not yet made a major impact on five-year survival figures or cure rates, but the encouraging results reported in the management of disseminated testicular tumours suggest that a similar pattern may emerge for malignant extragonadal teratomas.

References

Albrechtsen, R., Klee, J. G. and Moller, J. E. (1972). *Acta pathologica et microbiologica scandinavica* Section A, **80,** Suppl. 233, 32.

Allen, E. and Vespignani, P. M. (1938). *Anatomical Record* **72,** 293.

Allyn, D. L., Silverberg, S. G. and Salzberg, A. M. (1971). *Cancer* **27,** 1231.

Altman, R. P., Randolph, J. G. and Lilly, J. R. (1974). *Journal of Pediatric Surgery* **9,** 389.

Ashcraft, K. W. and Holder, T. M. (1965). *Annals of Surgery* **162,** 1091.

Asif, S. and Uehling, D. T. (1968). *Journal of Urology* **99,** 776.

Askanazy, M. (1907) *Verhandlungen der Deutschen Gesellschaft für Pathologie* **1,** 39.

Azzopardi, J. G. and Hoffbrand, A. V. (1965). *Journal of Clinical Pathology* **18,** 135.

Azzopardi, J. G., Mostofi, F. K. and Theiss, E. A. (1961). *American Journal of Pathology* **38,** 207.

Bagshaw, M. A., McLauchlin, W. T. and Earle, J. D. (1969). *American Journal of Roentgenology* **105,** 86.

Bale, P. M., Painter, D. M. and Cohen, D. (1975). *Pathology* **7,** 209.

Beattie, E. J. Jr. (1979). *Seminars in Oncology* **6,** 109.

Beeley, J. M., Daly, J. J., Timperley, W. R. and Warner, J. (1973). *Journal of Neurology (Neurosurgery) and Psychiatry* **36,** 864.

Benson, R. C., Segura, J. W. and Carney, J. A. (1978). *Cancer* **41,** 1395.

Bestle, J. (1968). *Acta pathologica et microbiologica scandinavica* **74,** 214.

Besznyak, I., Sebesteny, M. and Kuchar, F. (1973). *Journal of Thoracic and Cardiovascular Surgery* **65,** 930.

Bland-Sutton, Sir J. (1922). *Tumours Innocent and Malignant*. Paul B. Hoeber, New York.

Borit, A. (1969). *Journal of Pathology* **97,** 165.

Brindley, G. V. (1945). *Annals of Surgery* **121,** 721.

British Medical Journal (1969). Leading article *ii*, 135.

Camins, M. B. and Mount, L. A. (1974). *Brain* **97**, 447.
Canty, T. G. and Siemens, R. (1978). *Cancer* **41**, 1623.
Chretien, P. B., Milam, J. D., Foote, F. W. and Miller, T. R. (1970). *Cancer* **26**, 522.
Cole, H. (1971). *Clinical Radiology* **22**, 110.
Conklin, J. and Abell, M. R. (1967). *Cancer* **20**, 2105.
Cox, J. D. (1975). *Cancer* **36**, 1162.
Dayan, A. D., Marshall, A. H. E., Miller A. A., Pick, F. J. and Rankin, N. E. (1966). *Journal of Pathology and Bacteriology* **92**, 1.
Dillard, B. M., Mayer, J. H., McAlister, W. H., McGavrin, M. and Strominger, D. B. (1970). *Journal of Pediatric Surgery* **5**, 53.
Dixon, F. J. and Moore, R. A. (1952). *Armed Forces Institute of Pathology Fascicle* **32**, 48.
Donnellan, W. A. and Swenson, O. (1968) *Surgery* **64**, 834.
Edland, R. W., Levine, S., Serfos, L. S. and Flair, R. C. (1968). *American Journal of Roentgenology* **103**, 25.
El-Domeiri, A. A., Hutter, R. V. P., Pool, J. L. and Foote, F. W. Jr. (1968). *Annals of Thoracic Surgery* **6**, 513.
Engel, R. M., Elkins, R. C. and Fletcher, B. D. (1968). *Cancer* **22**, 1068.
Erickson, R. P. and Gondos, B. (1976). *Lancet* **i**, 407.
Fine, G., Smith, R. W. Jr. and Pachter, M. R. (1962). *American Journal of Medicine* **32**, 776.
Fowler, F. D., Alexander, E. Jr. and Davis, C. H. (1956). *Journal of Neurosurgery* **13**, 271.
Fox, J. and Hospers, C. A. (1936). *American Journal of Cancer* **28**, 273.
Friedman, N. B. (1947) *Cancer Research* **7**, 363.
Friedman, N. B. (1951). *Cancer* **4**, 265.
Friedman, N. B. and Moore, R. A. (1946). *Military Surgery* **99**, 573.
Fuss, A. (1912). *American Journal of Surgery* **132**, 378.
Giuffre, R. and DiLorenzo, N. (1975). *Journal of Neurosurgery* **42**, 602.
Grosfield, J. L., Ballantine, T. V. N., Lowe, D. and Baehner, R. L. (1976). *Surgery* **80**, 297.
Gross, R. E., Clatworthy, H. W. Jr. and Meeker, I. A. Jr. (1951). *Surgery, Gynecology and Obstetrics* **92**, 341.
Gwinn, J. L., Dockerty, M. B. and Kennedy, R. L. (1955). *Pediatrics* **16**, 239.
Hart, W. R. (1975). *Cancer* **35**, 1453.
Heyderman, E. (1978). *Scandinavian Journal of Immunology* **8** Suppl. 8, 119.
Hickey, R. C. and Martin, R. G. (1964). *Annals of the New York Academy of Science* **114**, 951.
Holt, S., Deverall, P. B. and Boddy, J. E. (1978). *Journal of Pathology* **126**, 85.
Horrax, G. (1949). *Radiology* **52**, 186.
Houghton, J. D. (1936). *American Journal of Pathology* **12**, 349.
Hunt, P. T., Davidson, K. C., Ashcraft, K. W. and Holder, T. M. (1977). *Radiology* **122**, 187.
Izant, R. J. and Filston, H. C. (1975). *American Journal of Surgery* **130**, 617.
Johnson, D. E., Laneri, J. P., Mountain, C. F. and Luna, M. (1973). *Surgery* **73**, 85.
Joseph, W. L., Murray, J. F. and Mulder, D. G. (1966). *Diseases of the Chest* **50**, 150.
Kenefick, J. S. (1973). *British Journal of Surgery* **60**, 271.
Kernohan, J. W. and Sayre, G. P. (1952). *Atlas of Tumour Pathology*. National Research Council, Washington.
Kimler, S. C. and Muth, W. F. (1978). *Cancer* **42**, 311.
Kountz, S. L., Connolly, J. E., and Cohn, R. (1963). *Journal of Thoracic and Cardiovascular Surgery* **45**, 289.
Laird, D. R. (1954). *American Journal of Surgery* **88**, 793.
Lattes, R. (1962). *Cancer* **15**, 1224.
Linder, D., Hecht, F., McCaw, B. K. and Campbell, J. R. (1975). *Nature* **254**, 597.
Linder, D., McCaw, B. K. and Hecht, F. (1975). *New England Journal of Medicine* **292**, 63.
Luna, M. A. and Valenzuela-Tamariz, J. (1976). *American Journal of Clinical Pathology* **65**, 450.
Lynch, M. J. G. and Blewett, G. L. (1953). *Thorax* **8**, 157.
Maier, J. G. and Dejong, D. (1967). *American Journal of Roentgenology* **99**, 826.
Marcuse, P. M. (1959). *Cancer* **12**, 889.
Martini, N., Golbey, R. B., Hajdu, S. I., Whitmore, W. F. and Beattie, E. J. Jr. (1974). *Cancer* **33**, 763.

Meares, E. M. Jr. and Briggs, E. M. (1972). *Cancer* **30**, 300.

Miles, R. M. and Stewart, G. S. (1974). *Annals of Surgery* **179**, 676.

Misugi, K. and Reiner, C. B. (1965). *Archives of Pathology* **80**, 409.

Nickels, J. and Franssila, K. (1972). *Acta pathologica et microbiologica scandinavica A* **80**, 260.

Norgaard-Pedersen, B., Lindholm, J., Albrechtsen, R., Arends Diemer, N. H. and Riishede, J. (1978). *Cancer* **41**, 2315.

Norris, H. J., Bagley, G. P. and Taylor, H. B. (1970). *Archives of Pathology* **90**, 473.

Oberman, H. A. and Libke, J. H. (1964). *Cancer* **17**, 498.

O'Hare, M. J. (1978). *Investigative Cell Pathology* **1**, 39.

Ozaki, H., Ito, I., Sano, R., Hirota, T. and Shimosato, Y. (1971). *Japanese Journal of Clinical Oncology* **1**, 83.

Palumbo, L. T., Cross, K. R., Smith, A. N. and Baronas, A. A. (1949). *Surgery* **26**, 149.

Pantoja, E., Llobet, R. and Gonzalez-Flores, B. (1976). *Journal of Urology* **115**, 520.

Paterson, A. H. G., Peckham, M. J. and McCready, V. R. (1976). *British Medical Journal* i, 1118.

Peckham, M. J. and McElwain, T. J. (1975). *Clinical Endocrinology and Metabolism* **4**, 665.

Perlstein, M. A. and Le Count, E. R. (1927). *Archives of Pathology* **3**, 171.

Polansky, S. M., Barwick, K. W. and Ravin, C. E. (1979). *American Journal of Roentgenology* **132**, 17.

Prym, P. (1927). *Virchows Archiv für pathologische Anatomie und Physiologie* **265**, 239.

Puschett, J. B. and Goldberg, M. (1968). *Annals of Internal Medicine* **69**, 203.

Raghavan, D. and Barrett, A. (1980). *Cancer* **46**, 1187.

Rather, L. J., Gardiner, W. R. and Frerichs, J. B. (1954). *Stanford Medical Bulletin* **12**, 12.

Reynolds, T. F., Yagoda, A., Vugrin, D. and Golbey, R. (1979). *Seminars in Oncology* **6**, 113.

Riley, P. A. and Sutton, P. M. (1975). *The Lancet* i, 1360.

Ross, S. T. (1948). *American Journal of Surgery* **76**, 687.

Roth, L. M. and Panganiban, W. G. (1976). *Cancer* **37**, 812.

Rubin, P. and Kramer, S. (1965). *Radiology* **85**, 512.

Rudnick, P. and O'Dell, W. D. (1971). *New England Journal of Medicine* **284**, 405.

Russell, D. S. (1944). *Journal of Pathology and Bacteriology* **56**, 145.

Russell, D. S. and Rubinstein, L. J. (1963). *Pathology of Tumours of the Nervous System* Edward Arnold, London.

Samuels, M. L., Lanzotti, V. J., Holoye, P. Y., Boyle, L. E., Smith, T. L. and Johnson, D. E. (1976). *Cancer Treatment Review* **3**, 185.

Schantz, R., Sewall, W. and Castleman, B. (1972). *Cancer* **30**, 1189.

Schey, W. L., Shkolnik, A. and White, H. (1977). *Radiology* **125**, 189.

Schlumberger, H. G. (1946). *Archives of Pathology* **41**, 398.

Sickles, E. A., Belliveau, R. E. and Wiernik, P. H. (1974). *Cancer* **33**, 1196.

Simson, L. R., Lampe, I. and Abell, M. R. (1968). *Cancer* **22**, 533.

So, S. C. (1976). *Australian and New Zealand Journal of Surgery* **46**, 75.

Spiegel, A. M., DiChiro, G., Gorden, P., Ommaya, A. K., Kolins, J. and Pomeroy, T. C. (1976). *Annals of Internal Medicine* **85**, 290.

Staemmler, M. (1934). *Verhandlungen der Deutschen Gesellschaft für Pathologie* **27**, 190.

Steinmetz, W. H. and Hays, R. A. (1961). *American Journal of Roentgenology* **86**, 669.

Stowell, R. E., Sachs, E. and Russell, W. O. (1945). *American Journal of Pathology* **21**, 787.

Sung, D. I., Harisadis, L. and Chang, C. H. (1978). *Radiology* **128**, 745.

Teilum, G. (1959). *Cancer* **12**, 1092.

Teilum, G. (1971). *Special Tumors of Ovary and Testis. Comparative Pathology and Histological Identification*. J. B. Lippincott Co., Philadelphia.

Theiss, E. A., Ashley, D. J. B. and Mostofi, F. K. (1960). *Cancer* **13**, 323.

Torkildsen, A. (1939). *Acta chirurgica scandinavica* **82**, 117.

Utz, D. C. and Buscemi, M. F. (1971). *Journal of Urology* **105**, 271.

Walden, P. A. M., Woods, R. L., Fox, B. and Bagshawe, K. D. (1977). *Thorax* **32**, 752.

Waldhausen, A., Kilman, J. W., Vellios, F. and Battersby, J. S. (1963). *Surgery* **54**, 933.

Willcox, G. L. and Mackenzie, W. C. (1961). *Archives of Surgery* **83**, 11.

Willis, R. A. (1962). *Borderland of Embryology and Pathology*, 2nd ed. Butterworth, Washington.

Witschi, E. (1948). *Contributions to Embryology. Publication of the Carnegie Institution* **209**, 67.

Wychulis, A. R., Payne, W. S. P., Claggett, O. T. and Woolner, L. B. (1971). *Journal of Thoracic and Cardiovascular Surgery* **62**, 379.

Yoshiki, T., Itoh, T., Shirai, T., Noro, T., Tomino, Y., Hamajima, I. and Takeda, T. (1976). *Cancer* **37**, 2343.

Zulch, H. J. (1956). *Biologie und Pathologie der Hirngeschwulste. Handbuch der Neurochirurgie Band III*. Springer-Verlag, Berlin.

18

Malignant lymphoma and uncommon testicular tumours

M. J. Peckham

Uncommon testicular tumours

Of a total of 2941 tumours of the testis and paratesticular structures recorded by the British Testicular Tumour Panel (Pugh and Cameron, 1976), germ-cell tumours totalled 2320 (78.9 per cent). The remaininng 20 per cent was composed of a wide range of different tumour types, several of which will be discussed in this chapter. These include the following.

1. Malignant lymphoma   185/2941 patients (6.3 per cent).
2. Sertoli-cell tumour   32/2941 patients (1 per cent).
3. Interstitial (Leydig)-cell tumour   43/2941 patients (1.5 per cent).
4. Mesothelioma   10/2941 patients (0.3 per cent).

In addition, mention will be made of tumours associated with testicular feminization and dysgenetic gonads. Soft tissue sarcomas are discussed in Chapter 16.

Testicular lymphoma

Malignant lymphoma may present in and be confined to the testis, or testicular involvement may be part of a generalized disease process. Overall, lymphomas comprise 7 per cent of testicular neoplasms and are seen predominantly in the elderly. Thus, lymphomas account for 25 per cent of testicular tumours in males over the age of 50 and 2 per cent of testicular tumours in males less than 50 years (Pugh and Cameron, 1976). This chapter is concerned with the investigation and management of the patient with a primary testicular presentation.

Clinical presentation

Since primary presentation of malignant lymphomas in the testis is rare, most series include patients investigated and treated over a span of several decades and detailed staging information is, therefore, scanty. Table 18.1 summarizes data from a selected series of publications and shows the main clinical features of importance.

1. Although a few younger patients are encountered in all series, testicular lymphoma is predominantly a disease of old age, occurring at a median age of 60 to 70 years.

Table 18.1 Clinical features of lymphomas presenting in the testis

References	No. of patients	Age (years)		Presentation with painless swelling	Length of history	Bilateral tumours	History of maldescent
		Range	Median				
Gowing (1976)	128	1½–90+	60–80	47/62	weeks–months	28/128 (20%)	1/128
Talerman (1977)	32	21–82	30/32 > 50	23/32	days–3 years most < 6/12	5/32 (16%)	0/32
Sussman et al. (1977)	37	4–85	63	30/37	2 weeks–2 years mean 5 months	14/37 (38%)	1/37
Paladugu et al. (1980)	27	8–78	64	21/27	10 days–10 years 11/27 < 3 months	3/27 (11%)	0/27
Duncan et al. (1980)	24	23–82	62	21/24	median 2 months	2/24 (8%)	0/23

2. Painless enlargement of the testis is the most common presenting feature, occurring in more than two-thirds of patients.

3. The length of history is usually, but not invariably, short. Most men have a history of swelling of less than six months.

4. The incidence of bilateral testicular involvement is variable (8 to 38 per cent) but higher than that encountered in germ-cell tumours. In a minority of patients, bilateral tumours are diagnosed at presentation, but in most cases there is an interval of months or years between the appearance of the first and second tumour, although most second tumours appear within one year of the first (Fig. 18.1). The rapid demise of the majority of testicular lymphoma patients leaves little time for the manifestation of a contralateral tumour and improved therapy could modify the frequency of bilateralism.

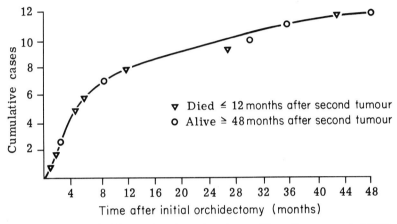

Fig. 18.1 Bilateral incidence of testicular lymphoma. (From Duncan *et al.*, 1980.)

5. A history of testicular maldescent is extremely uncommon, occurring in only 2 out of 247 patients, as shown in Table 18.1. This is in contrast to the association of maldescent with germ-cell tumour development.

6. The presence of systemic symptoms should be noted, since this appears to be an adverse prognostic sign (Paladugu *et al.*, 1980).

Staging

Staging in most reported series has been inadequate by current criteria, since many patients presented before the advent of lymphography and before marrow sampling was performed routinely. Following histological diagnosis, the patient should be examined carefully for evidence of disease in the contralateral testis, abnormal nodes in the groins, abdomen or supradiaphragmatic areas. Examination of the lymphoid tissue in Waldeyer's ring is mandatory. Evidence of hepatomegaly and splenomegaly should be sought. In considering more intensive staging procedures it is necessary to bear in mind that the majority of patients will be elderly. Unless contraindicated by age or infirmity, lymphangiography should be carried out. A full blood count, including differential white count and examination of the buffy coat for abnormal cells, should be performed. Bone marrow aspirate and trephine biopsy should be carried out routinely in view of the propensity of these aggressive neoplasms to involve the marrow. In view of the high incidence of pulmonary involvement at autopsy in patients with testicular lymphomas (Paladugu *et al.*, 1980), chest radiography including tomography is advocated. In patients with clinical evidence suggestive of liver involvement, a percutaneous needle biopsy may be indicated. Involvement of the marrow is not uncommonly associated, particularly with the histological subtype encountered in testicular lymphomas with meningeal involvement and, in marrow-positive patients, lumbar puncture and CSF cytology should be considered. Serum immunoglobulin abnormalities including the presence of paraproteins should be excluded. Other investigations, for example of the gastrointestinal tract and skeletal system, are carried out if clinically indicated.

Although this provides a broad guide to patient evaluation, flexibility is essential in view of the older age of presentation. In younger patients, staging laparotomy may be indicated if there is no clinical evidence of extratesticular disease; however, it is impossible to be dogmatic about the value of this procedure in non-Hodgkin lymphoma. It is of interest that of 4 patients whose disease was apparently confined to the testis in the series reported by Paladugu, 3 subsequently relapsed.

Stage distribution at presentation

In the Royal Marsden series of 24 patients, 18 were clinical Stage I or II and 6 Stage III or IV (Duncan *et al.*, 1980). Detailed staging data are scanty. One patient with clinical Stage I disease was staged by laparotomy, which was negative. Lymphography in 8 clinical Stage II patients showed involvement in 7 with the typical lymphoma appearance of lacy, enlarged lymph nodes. Paladugu *et al.* (1980) have described laparotomy findings in 7 histiocytic lymphomas of the testis, the spleen was positive in 2 of 6 patients sampled, the liver was involved in 4 patients, para-aortic nodes in 5 and marrow in 4. Because of the long-term survival of a minority of patients, it appears to be worthwhile to stage patients as precisely as possible, and careful clinical staging in many patients will disclose evidence of dissemination, thus rendering laparotomy inessential.

Pathological features

Table 18.2 summarizes the collected data from five series. It is seen that the tumour-bearing testis is frequently large and involvement of epididymis and spermatic cord are common. Furthermore, invasion of veins within the tumour is a frequently observed feature. It is seen also that a nodular architecture is exceptional and for all practical purposes the histology is diffuse in pattern. The criteria used for histological classification have tended to vary from series to series, but in two series (Sussman *et al.*, 1977; Paladugu *et al.*, 1980) diffuse histiocytic lymphoma is the predominant cell type. It is of interest that infiltration by macrophages producing the so-called 'starry-sky' appearance was

Table 18.2 Pathological features of testicular lymphoma

| References | No. of patients | Size of tumours (cm) | Tumour involvement | | | Architecture | | Histology* | | | 'Starry sky' appearance |
			Epididymis	Spermatic cord	Intratumour vascular	Nodular	Diffuse	DH	PDLD	Other	
Gowing (1976)	128	up to 16 × 9	Frequent	Frequent	Very frequent	0	128	—	41%	59% large cell undifferentiated lymphoma	NS
Talerman (1977)	32	7–15	21/27	18/26	NS	1	31	No detailed breakdown			NS
Sussman et al. (1977)	37	2.5–15.5	14/35	11/37	(67%)	0	37	34/37	—	(3 lymphocytic)	12/37
Paladugu et al. (1980)	27	1.5–11.0	10/27	5/27	11/27	0	27	20	2	Burkitt 1 Lymphoblastic 1 Plasmacytoma 1	14/27
Duncan et al. (1980)	24	—	—	—	—	0	24	9	15		NS

* According to the classification of Rappaport (1966). NS, not stated.

not uncommon. This feature has been associated with rapid proliferating lymphomas and a poor prognosis.

During the past few years it has become clear that the majority of non-Hodgkin lymphomas are derived from follicular centre cells and are B lymphocyte in origin (Lukes and Collins, 1974). As shown in Table 18.3, 31 out of 35 testicular non-Hodgkin lymphomas fall into the follicular centre cell category, the majority of which, in the series reported by Paladugu *et al.* (1980), are of large, non-cleaved type. This subtype is associated with a worse prognosis and a poorer response to chemotherapy than large, cleaved follicular centre cell lymphoma, although both are classified as histiocytic in the Rappaport classification (Strauchen *et al.*, 1978).

Table 18.3 Testicular lymphoma by Lukes and Collins' classification (Lukes and Collins, 1974)

Lukes and Collins' classification	Royal Marsden series	Paladugu et al. (1980)
Follicular centre cell		
small cleaved	0	2
large cleaved	4	1
small, non-cleaved non-Burkitt	3	—
small, non-cleaved Burkitt	0	1
large non-cleaved	1	19
Convoluted lymphocyte		1
B—immunoblastic sarcoma		3

Pattern of dissemination

In the Royal Marsden series (Duncan *et al.*, 1980), 3 clinical Stage I and II patients developed bone involvement and, 2 developed extradural lymphoma. Overall, 5 out of 24 patients subsequently manifested lymphoma of Waldeyer's ring, and 7 developed positive cerebrospinal fluid cytology. Although the retroperitoneal nodes appear to be involved with high frequency in a testicular lymphoma, the pattern of spread differs markedly from that of germ-cell tumours, and is in keeping with the spread pattern of aggressive, diffuse non-Hodgkin lymphoma as a whole.

Management

Hitherto, the treatment of these tumours has yielded very poor results. As is the case for non-Hodgkin lymphomas in general, despite their responsiveness to chemotherapy, progress in terms of curability has been slow to come. Because of their high propensity to disseminate, patients with testicular lymphoma should receive chemotherapy. It is the policy at the Royal Marsden Hospital to use a combination of cyclosphosphamide, adriamycin, vincristine and prednisone (CHOP) if the age and general condition of the patient permit. In diffuse histiocytic lymphoma, patients who enter complete remission with these agents alone or in combination with methotrexate or bleomycin show a superior survival to those who do not and long-term disease-free survivals are achieved (for general review see Canellos, 1980). As noted above, there is some evidence suggesting that the large, cleaved follicular centre cell lymphomas show the best survival characteristics and, if lymphomas of the testis are predominantly large non-cleaved, the outlook may not necessarily be improved by intensive chemotherapy.

In patients with Stage I or II disease, post-chemotherapy irradiation to the para-aortic, pelvic and inguinal nodes is advocated. Whether or not irradiation of the contralateral testis in the early stage patients is of value is unknown, but it has been recent policy in the Royal Marsden series to advise this in view of the high bilateral incidence.

Prognosis

As shown in Table 18.4, the prognosis for patients with testicular lymphoma is extremely poor, with the majority of patients dying of disseminated disease

Table 18.4 Survival of patients with testicular lymphoma

References	Total no. of patients	Outcome
Gowing (1976)	128	62% died within 2 years; 15/124 survived >5 years
Talerman (1977)	32	72% died 6–12 months
Sussman et al. (1977)	37	65% died with disseminated disease; 88% of deaths in first 2 years
Paladugu et al. (1980)	27	74% died 2–64 months

within the first two years after presentation. Of a series reported from the Royal Marsden Hospital and South West Thames Cancer Registry, only 6 out of 53 (11 per cent) patients were long-term, disease-free survivors. In a recent literature review by Paladugu et al. (1980), of 242 patients only 26 (10.7 per cent) had survived more than five years. Factors influencing outcome include stage (including systemic symptoms), size of the testicular mass at presentation, and involvement of epididymis and spermatic cord. Histology is more difficult to assess in the report from Paladugu et al. (1980). Patients with poorly differentiated lymphocytic lymphomas survived longer than those with diffuse histiocytic lymphomas, whereas, in the Royal Marsden series no difference between these two histologies was observed (Duncan et al., 1980). In the latter series there was a significant difference between Stage I and II patients and Stage III and IV patients in terms of lymphoma-free survival and overall survival (Fig. 18.2). No difference was observed between the disease-free survival of 10 Stage I and 8 Stage II patients.

Sertoli-cell tumours

Two distinct cell populations are present within the seminiferous tubules of the testis, germ cells and Sertoli cells. Sertoli cells are closely applied to the various cells of the germ-cell series which appear to be enmeshed by their cytoplasm, which is seen on electron microscopy as ramifying extensions separating germinal cells from each other. The cellular processes interdigitate

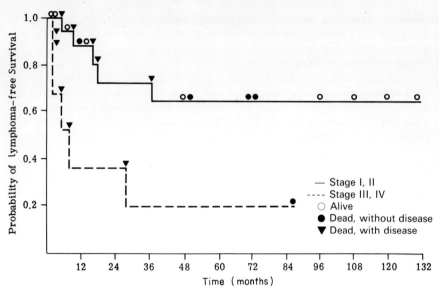

Fig. 18.2 Survival of testicular lymphoma by stage (Royal Marsden Hospital). (Data from Duncan *et al.*, 1980.)

with processes from other Sertoli cells. The function of Sertoli cells is unknown; they appear to be phagocytic, and supportive or nutritive functions have been ascribed to them. Tumours from the Sertoli-cell population are rare, accounting for 1.2 per cent of the Testicular Tumour Panel series. They are slow growing and may occur from childhood to old age, although predominantly before the age of 40 years. The tumours tend to be clearly demarcated and readily shelled out from the surrounding testis. The consistency is white or creamy yellow and cystic change is common. Of the 32 patients presenting to the Testicular Tumour Panel, 3 presented with gynaecomastia and 1 of these patients had high urinary gonadotrophin levels (Symington and Cameron, 1976). Increased urinary levels of androgens, oestrogens and pregnanediol have been recorded in Sertoli-cell tumours, but most patients have been investigated inadequately. Gynaecomastia has been reported to resolve after removal of the primary tumour. Shiffman (1967) reported a total of 15 cases of gynaecomastia of a total of 57 men with Sertoli-cell tumours.

Course of disease and prognosis

Sertoli-cell tumours were regarded initially as uniformly benign, but it is now clear that malignant variants can occur. In a literature review, Morin and Loening (1975) described 67 patients, 7 of whom developed metastases (10.4 per cent). Examples of malignant behaviour have occurred in all age groups. In patients with metastatic disease it is of interest that no elevation of urinary gonadotrophin or oestrogen levels has been recorded. In most cases metastases occurred in the draining lymph nodes. In an example of metastasizing Sertoli-cell tumour reported by Morin and Loening, there was involvement of the rete

testis, epididymis and spermatic cord as well as lymphatic and vascular permeation. The patient was treated with actinomycin-D, cyclophosphamide and
vincristine, but eventually died. At autopsy there was extensive Sertoli-cell
tumour in the lungs but none in the abdomen.

Of the series of 32 patients recorded by the British Testicular Tumour Panel
(Symington and Cameron, 1976), 6 patients are considered to have died from
metastatic tumour, 5 within eighteen months of orchidectomy and 1 at eighteen
years. A further patient developed metastases in the retroperitoneal nodes and
was reported well after node dissection at eight years. The incidence of malignancy in this series is thus 7 out of 32 (22 per cent), although it should be
noted that only in 2 cases were metastases confirmed histologically. Of these
7 patients, involvement of the rete, epididymis or lower cord had occurred in
4 and lymphatic and/or vascular invasion in all 7. Sites of metastases were
retroperitoneal and mediastinal nodes, liver, lung, brain and bone.

Conclusion and proposed management

The incidence of malignancy of 22 per cent in the series quoted above is higher
than that generally reported. Mostofi (1973) has reported an incidence of
approximately 10 per cent. Malignant potential appears to be associated with
involvement of the rete testis, epididymis and cord and with lymphatic and
vascular invasion. Clearly, orchidectomy is the initial treatment of choice
followed by careful pathological staging of the primary tumour. The humoral
status of the patient should be investigated, although there is no evidence that
oestrogen or gonadotrophin elevation correlates with prognosis or is useful as
a monitor of disease. If the pathological features described above are present,
it is wise to stage the patient carefully, as described in Chapter 7. The rarity
of these tumours precludes any meaningful statement with respect to the
efficacy or otherwise of node dissection, radiotherapy or chemotherapy.

Interstitial (Leydig)-cell tumours

Leydig cells constitute an endocrine organ which, under the influence of
gonadotrophin, produces androgenic hormones. Leydig-cell hyperplasia may
occur in association with atrophy of the seminiferous epithelium or failure of
development. Thus, it occurs in the cryptorchid, in testicular feminization and
in testes which have atrophied as a result of age, injury, ischaemia or irradiation. Interstitial-cell tumours are usually benign and may or may not be
associated with endocrine activity. They account for less than 2 per cent of
testicular tumours—43 out of 2739 cases seen by the British Testicular Tumour
Panel (Symington and Cameron, 1976)—and most occur in men between the
ages of 20 and 60, although childhood cases are reported.

The patient presents with, or is noted to have, a testicular mass in most
cases, although gynaecomastia may be a presenting feature in adults. Precocious puberty due to androgen production may be a feature in children. A
raised output of 17-ketosteroids has been documented in adults and children.
Differences in hormone profile may occur. Thus, Urban et al. (1978) reported
2 boys with Leydig-cell tumour in whom the hormone profiles were different,
suggesting differences in steroid biosynthesis by the tumours. It is important

in children with sexual precocity to distinguish between a Leydig-cell tumour and congenital virilizing adrenal hyperplasia by performing a dexamethasone suppression test.

In adults, Leydig-cell tumours may be associated with feminization due to oestrogen production by the tumour, although in most adults there is no humoral association. Gynaecomastia, impotence and loss of libido may occur and are associated with oestogen synthesis. Return to normal tends to occur after removing the tumour, although high oestrogen levels may persist (Herwig and Vinson, 1978).

Clinical course and prognosis

Deaths in 4 out of 43 patients (9.3 per cent) were reported by the British Testicular Tumour Panel (Symington and Cameron, 1976). Metastases occurred to retroperitoneal and mediastinal nodes, bone and lung. The tumours in these patients tended to be large, to have satellite nodules and in 3 cases a higher mitotic index and vascular invasion. Thus, although generally regarded as benign tumours, approximately 10 per cent behave in a more aggressive manner. Metastasizing tumours have only been encountered in adults. In adults, serum oestradiol levels may provide a useful monitor and correlate with tumour activity (Shimp et al., 1977).

Management

Orchidectomy is the initial treatment of choice, with careful pathological evaluation of the primary tumour for evidence of those features associated with metastastic potential described above. If these features are identified, clinical staging, as described in Chapter 7, should be performed. The efficacy of current chemotherapy, or indeed of radiotherapy, has not been evaluated because of the rarity of these tumours.

Mesothelioma of the tunica vaginalis

These rare tumours usually present with a hydrocele which may be blood stained. The tunica vaginalis is diffusely studded with papillary growths. The spread pattern is undocumented. One of 4 patients reported by the Testicular Tumour Panel (Gowing, 1976) developed local recurrence and a further patient, reported by Jaffe et al. (1978), developed local recurrence and involvement of para-aortic nodes, subsequently going on to develop pulmonary metastases. There was a transient response to adriamycin. It is of interest that this case showed electron microscopic evidence of mesothelial origin (long microvilli, cell junctions and basal laminae material). In a literature review, Jaffe et al. (1978) reported 8 patients, 6 of whom developed recurrent disease. Five patients subsequently died of their tumours. Treatment should include wide excision of the testis and scrotum. It appears that these tumours are refractory to drugs and radiation and behave like mesotheliomas at other sites.

Tumours associated with testicular feminization

The testicular feminization syndrome comprises a genetic male with the external appearances of a female and with undescended testis, absence of uterus or tubes and absent or scanty pubic and axillary hair (Morris, 1953). The syndrome is familial with inheritance by either an X-linked recessive or male-limited autosomal dominant gene (Symington and Cameron, 1976). The chromosome constitution is usually 46XY, although occasionally mosaics (XO/XY/XX or XY, XYY, XXY) occur. In addition to Sertoli-cell nodules, these patients are at risk of developing germ-cell tumours, particularly seminomas. An incidence of 22 per cent was reported by Morris and Mahesh (1963), but this is probably a reflection of case selection. Recently we have seen a patient with testicular feminization and seminoma. Because of the risk of tumour development, the patient was advised to have an abdominal exploration and a small seminoma was identified in an atrophic intra-abdominal testis. The patient was female in habitus. The usual clinical staging procedures for seminoma (see Chapter 10) were negative and follow up only was advised in view of the high probability of cure in a small, well-defined seminoma following surgery alone.

Tumours of dysgenetic gonads

So-called gonadoblastomas consisting of a tumour divided by fibrous septa in which two closely associated cell types can be identified (small deeply staining and large cell with vacuolated cytoplasm) occur in association with intersex states. Four examples are quoted by Symington and Cameron (1976) and in 3, small seminomas were associated with the lesion described as a gonadoblastoma. Seminoma metastases have been recorded (Schellhas *et al.*, 1971).

References

Canellos, G. (1980). *Cancer* **42** (Suppl. 2), 932.
Duncan, P. R., Checa, F., Gowing, N. F. C., McElwain, T. J. and Peckham, M. J. (1980). *Cancer* **45**, 1578.
Gowing, N. F. C. (1976). In *Pathology of the Testis*, p. 317. Ed. by R. C. B. Pugh. Blackwell Scientific, Oxford.
Herwig, K. R. and Vinson, R. K. (1978). *Urology* **11**, 283.
Jaffe, J., Roth, J. A. and Carter, H. (1978). *Urology* **11**, 647.
Lukes, R. J. and Collins, R. D. (1974). *Cancer* **34**, 1488.
Morin, L. J. and Loening, S. (1975). *Journal of Urology* **114**, 476.
Morris, J. McL. (1953). *American Journal of Obstetrics and Gynecology* **65**, 1192.
Morris, J. McL. and Mahesh, V. B. (1963). *American Journal of Obstetrics and Gynecology* **87**, 731.
Mostofi, F. K. (1973). *Cancer* **32**, 1186.
Paladugu, R. R., Bearman, R. M. and Rappaport, H. (1980). *Cancer* **45**, 561.
Pugh, R. C. B. and Cameron, K. M. (1976). In *Pathology of the Testis*, p. 199. Ed. by R. C. B. Pugh. Blackwell Scientific, London.
Rappaport, H. (1966). Tumors of the haematopoietic system. In *Atlas of Tumor Pathology*. Sect. 3. Fascicle 8. Armed Forces Institute of Pathology, Washington DC.
Schellhas, H. F., Trujillo, J. M., Rutledge, F. N. and Cork, A. (1971). *American Journal of Obstetrics and Gynecology* **109**, 1197.
Shiffman, M. A. (1967). *Journal of Urology* **98**, 493.

Shimp, W. S., Schultz, A. L., Hastings, J. R. and Anderson W. R. (1977). *American Journal of Clinical Pathology* **67**, 562.

Strauchen, J. A., Young, R. C. and DeVita, V. T. (1978). *New England Journal of Medicine* **299**, 1382.

Sussman, E. B., Hajdu, S. I., Lieberman, P. H. and Whitmore, W. S. (1977). *Journal of Urology* **118**, 1004.

Symington, T. and Cameron, K. (1976). Endocrine and genetic lesions. In *Pathology of the Testis*, p. 265. Ed. by R. C. B. Pugh. Blackwell Scientific, London.

Talerman, A. (1977). *Journal of Urology* **118**, 783.

Urban, M. D., Lee, P. A., Plotnick, L. P. and Migeon, C. J. (1978). *American Journal of Diseases of Childhood* **132**, 494.

Index